FRONTIERS IN BREAST CANCER RESEARCH

FRONTIERS IN BREAST CANCER RESEARCH

LOUIS P. FORTUGNO
Editor

Nova Biomedical Books
New York

Library of Congress Cataloging-in-Publication Data

Frontiers in breast cancer research / Louis P. Fortugno (editor).
p.; cm.
Includes bibliographical references and index.
ISBN-13: 978-1-60021-671-8 (hardcover)
ISBN-10: 1-60021-671-4 (hardcover)
1.Breast-- Cancer--Research. I. Fortugno, Louis P.
[DNLM: 1. Breast Neoplasms. 2. Research. WP 870 F935 2007]
RC280.B8F76 2007
616.99'449--dc22

2007012187

Published by Nova Science Publishers, Inc. ✣ New York

Contents

Preface

Breast cancer is a malignant tumor that has developed from cells of the breast. A malignant tumor is a group of cancer cells that may invade surrounding tissues or spread (metastasize) to distant areas of the body. The disease occurs almost entirely in women, but men can get it as well. The main types of breast cancer are ductal carcinoma in situ, invasive ductal carcinoma, lobular carcinoma in situ, invasive lobular carcinoma, medullary carcinoma, and Paget's disease of the nipple . About 1 of 8 women will get it in her lifetime. This new book presents the latest research in this field.

Chapter I - Transporters play a vital role in regulating movement of material into and out of the brain. In the brain capillaries, where tight junctions between endothelial cells limit paracellular flow, all material must pass across both the abluminal and luminal surfaces of the endothelium to enter the brain. In the choroidplexuses, where the capillaries are leaky, regulation of transport occurs at the apical and basolateral surfaces of the choroidal epithelium. Transporters strategically located at these cell surfaces scrutinise all material in the circulation and are well placed to efflux xenobiotics. Unlike the transporters that facilitate the transfer of nutrients into and waste material out of the brain, transporters that prevent entry of material to the brain must be capable of moving substances against a concentration gradient and of recognizing a wide range of different substrates. Such 'multidrug' transporters are members of the ATP binding cassette (ABC) family of proteins and use energy derived from ATP hydrolysis to power the movement of material across membranes. These include the transporters described in other chapters, i.e., P-glycoprotein (P-gp) and Multidrug Resistance-associated Proteins (MRPs). This chapter will examine Breast Cancer Resistance Protein (BCRP), a recently identified member of the ABC family of proteins (Allen and Schinkel, 2002a; Doyle and Ross, 2003). It will review what is currently known about BCRP in a rapidly moving field, make comparisons with P-gp and the MRPs, and discuss the implications of BCRP's characteristics in terms of the extent to which it might fulfil the roles required of an efflux transporter at the interfaces between blood BCRP was recognised initially in several drug resistant tumour cell lines and subsequently identified in certain tumour tissues where its presence has been putatively associated with poor clinical response to chemotherapy. However it is found in many normal, i.e., non-malignant, cells at a number of different sites in the body including in endothelial cells lining the brain capillaries. Clues to the possible physiological role of BCRP at the blood-brain barrier may be derived from the many studies that are now being conducted which examine its mechanisms of action and its substrate and inhibitor profiles in different cell systems or which analyse its influence on the distribution of drugs in whole animals.

Chapter II - The hyperandrogenic theory in the pathogenesis of breast cancer was conceived and developed in Milan at the Istituto Nazionale Tumori during the late 1960s and early 1970s, on based on endocrine, histological and clinical data. Patients with breast cancer were found to be frequently associated with high blood androgen levels, atypical endometrial hyperplasia, an index of chronic anovulation, and with ovarian interstitial cells hyperplasia, a finding suggesting that the ovary was the source of androgen excess. Increased amount of androgens and endometrial hyperplasia were also observed in women with hyperplastic alterations of breast epithelium, a condition predisposing to mammary cancer.

Case-control studies in the 1980s gave further substantial support to the theory, and in more recent years, prospective studies have confirmed beyond any doubt that increased testosterone levels are associated with increased risk of breast cancer. The relation with breast cancer was also reported for high levels of estrogens and low levels of sex hormone binding globulin (SHBG), in postmenopausal women, and low levels of progesterone in premenopausal women. Increased risk of breast cancer was also found to be linked with other metabolic and hormonal parameters, such as high levels of insulin, IGF-I, fasting glucose, abdominal obesity. Insulin is known to stimulate androgens synthesis in the ovary and to inhibit SHBG formation in the liver.

Two recent dietary intervention trials, aimed to keep low the insulin levels in the blood, have shown that an appropriate diet significantly reduced the circulating levels of sex hormones, mainly testosterone, both in healthy postmenopausal women (DIANA-1) and in breast cancer patients, who were relapse-free at recruitment (DIANA-2). These findings prove that a high testosterone level, with the associated endocrine-dismetabolic syndrome, is a factor of risk potentially curable with diet and discloses the way for large-scale dietary intervention trials of primary prevention of breast cancer.

In previous papers, the authors have suggested that women with breast cancer and high values of testosterone in urine were at increased risk of recurrence. More recently, data from the DIANA2 study, after 5 years of follow-up of the cohort, showed a significantly higher progression rate in patients with high serum testosterone levels compared to patients with low levels of the hormone. High value of testosterone seems, therefore, a powerful factor of risk of progressive disease, which can be corrected by diet and, if necessary, by pharmacological treatments.

Chapter III - Of all epigenetic modifications, hypermethylation is commonly considered as a critical causal event in silencing important classes of genes in cancer. In breast cancer, a series of tumor suppressor or related genes are frequently hypermethylated and which is associated with silencing of these genes. The authors now understand that DNA methylation mechanisms might include a number of DNA methyltransferases, proteins that direct DNA methyltransferases to specific promoters, chromatin modifying enzymes as well as demethylases. There are also data to suggest that pharmacological down regulation of some members of the DNA methylation machinery could inhibit cancer in vitro, in vivo and in clinical trials. The use of the methylation status of certain genes as a marker of cancer or cancerous conditions provides an additional weapon in early detection and prognosis of breast cancers. The authors describe the techniques used to decipher the complement of methylation-inactivated genes, discuss the epigenetic regulation of certain critical tumor suppressor and growth regulatory genes implicated in breast cancer and its relevance to breast cancer development, progression and therapy.

Chapter IV - Breast cancer incidence rates are higher among white than African-American (AA) women in the USA, although mortality rates from breast cancer are higher among AA women. Many published studies have shown trends towards younger age at diagnosis, worse prognostic features and lower survival rates for AA and other ethnic minority women with breast cancer compared with white women. Other studies have reported on racial and ethnic differences in patterns of care for women with breast cancer, suggesting that unequal access to care may in part explain the noted disparity in survival. While debate continues as to the relative degree in which tumor biology vs. socioeconomic factors influence racial differences in survival, cultural and behavioral differences play at least some role, and can partially explain the noted disparity in breast cancer survival seen among different racial and ethnic groups. Approximately 5 to 10% of all breast cancer in this country is associated with known hereditary mutations in the *BRCA1* and *BRCA2* genes, meaning nearly 22,000 breast cancer cases diagnosed per year are due to mutations in these cancer susceptibility genes. Hereditary breast cancer is more common among women with early age at diagnosis and is also more common among certain ethnic groups. While AA women are more likely to develop breast cancer at a younger age than white women, cancer risk assessment and testing for hereditary breast cancer syndromes is underutilized among AA women compared to non-minority women. It is incumbent on health care professionals to help develop solutions to the inequities in access to medical care for women with breast cancer in order to decrease the gap in breast cancer outcomes seen in this country. One way to achieve this is to improve access to screening and cancer risk assessment for all eligible women, and to make state of the art cancer treatment available for all women affected with breast cancer.

Chapter V - The presence of numerical and structural chromosome aberrations is a common characteristic of tumor cells. Accumulation of these aberrations leads to dramatic changes within the genome. These changes have tumor type and stage specific pattern of segmental losses and gains, resulting in gene losses and gene copy number imbalances. Tumor development and progression is driven by sequential acquisition of specific gene alterations, and chromosome aberrations contribute to these processes. Genomic instability in tumors can be classified as chromosome instability (CIN) and microsatellite instability (MIN). MIN is in general less frequent in tumors than CIN, but is rather frequent in some tumors of the digestive tract. This is mainly due to germline mutations in mismatch repair genes associated with the HNPCC cancer syndrome, but can also be due to somatic mutations and epigenetic mechanism. While MIN is rare in breast tumors, CIN is demonstrated in the majority of breast tumors (about 70%) by aneuploidy, deletions, amplifications and rearrangements. Although the reasons for CIN in breast tumors are not well understood, explanations can partly be obtained from deficient control of genes controlling cell proliferation, apoptosis, DNA repair or chromosome segregation. Among these genes are TP53, MYC, AURKA, BRCA1 and BRCA2. TP53 is relatively well studied and is believed to be a guardian of genome integrity. Myc seems to affect tumor pathogenesis in several ways, including increased proliferation and immortalization of the cancer cells and induction of CIN. The STK15 gene encodes the aurora A kinase, which has been shown to bind to centrosomes and is important in controlling their number and the segregation of correct chromosomes to the daughter cells during mitosis. Genomic instability is high in some hereditary breast cancer, particularly in tumors of BRCA1 and BRCA2 mutation carriers, a finding which is in line with the role of the gene products in DNA repair. Some recent developments in drug therapy are based on molecular and genomic findings about breast cancer pathogenesis. Defects in checkpoint control generate CIN and are believed to facilitate tumorigenesis, but additional disabling of checkpoint signaling is a possible anticancer strategy.

Chapter VI - The incidence of male breast cancer is rising, but it is still an uncommon condition. There are a limited number of large studies in male breast cancer, and most of the treatments are extrapolated from female breast cancer. This review aims to summarize the pathological similarities and differences between male and female breast cancer, with a specific emphasis on the genetic aspects, and molecular markers.

Chapter VII - *Introduction:* HER-2/neu protein is overexpressed in 15-20% of invasive breast carcinomas and has been reported to be an independently adverse prognostic and predictive factor in patients with breast cancer. Recently, HER-2/neu overexpression has gained therapeutic implications, because the use of trastuzumab/Herceptin^{TM}, recombinant humanized monoclonal antibody directed against extracellular domain of HER-2/neu molecule, has been shown to result in clinical response in patients with breast cancer overexpressing HER-2/neu.

Aims: As a result of these developments, there has been increasing demand for pathologists to perform exact evaluation of HER-2/neu in breast cancer specimens.

Methods and Results: In the authors series of 449 cases of breast cancer the authors have examined HER-2/neu protein and gene by means of immunohistochemistry and fluorescence in situ hybridization, respectively. The results of HER-2/neu study were compared with hormonal status, cancer grade and proliferative activity as assessed using immunohistochemistry with MIB1 antibody. Of these 449 cases 18 randomly chosen samples were examined for HER2/neu gene status. All 7 cases of breast cancer with strong overexpression of HER-2/neu (score 3+) revealed an amplification of the gene. In contrast, among 11 cases of breast cancers with mild HER-2/neu overexpression (score 2+), the gene amplification was demonstrated in 5 cases (45%).

Conclusions: Good concordance was achieved between immunohistochmistry in negative and strongly positive cases (score 3+). Immunohistochemical assessment and fluorescence in situ hybridization (FISH) are complementary methods for detection of HER-2/neu status in breast cancer. While immunohistochemistry is excellent screening method, FISH should be used for confirmation of positive result of HER-2/neu status analysis before Herceptin treatment.

Chapter VIII - In order to know possible associations of fruit consumption and the risk of breast cancer (BC) in Montevideo, the authors carried out a case-control study in the period 1999-2001. A total number of 333 women were interviewed with a specific questionnaire, 111 of which were certified cases of BC and 222 were frequency-matched healthy women, with a recent normal mammography (Birads 1). The questionnaire included a detailed 120-

item food frequency section, as well as sociodemographic, reproductive, familial, medical and lifestyle variables. There was particular emphasis set on types of fruits. After controlling for age, age at menarche, menopausal status, duration of menses, energy, family history of BC, smoking, total vegetables, total meat, dairy, frequency of exercise and number of live births, a multivariate analysis found that high intakes of orange (OR=0.51), orange juice (OR=0.26), citrus fruits (OR=0.27) and total fruits (OR=0.44) were associated with significant reduced risk of BC. The inclusion of dietary ascorbic acid in the regression models made even stronger the decrease of risk for orange (OR= 0.22) and citrus fruits (OR=0.13), suggesting that this constituent of fruits might be co-responsible for the results.

Chapter IX - *Background:* In Egypt, a study on 3747 mastectomies, showed that patients usually had poor presentation in terms of unfavorable histology, high tumor burden, and lymph node metastasis. Because advanced breast cancer has the poorest survival rate and is the most resource intensive to treat, measures to reduce the stage at diagnosis are likely to have the greatest benefit in terms of survival and costs. Mammography is the sole acceptable method for breast cancer screening, but its efficacy is still disputable.

The authors' objective was to evaluate the potential role of mammography in the diagnosis and screening of breast cancer among a cohort of Egyptian women.

Methods: From July 2002 to December 2003 a total of 7220 mammograms were performed in a private diagnostic centre in Cairo, Egypt and computerized data were retrieved for analysis. Pathology was confirmed in 504 cases.

Results: Screening as baseline, routine or in high risk groups was the basis in 49.4% of mammographic examinations, and diagnosis and follow-up in 50.6%. Median age was 48 (13-88) years and premenopausal represented 51.6%. As a whole, mammography was sensitive in detecting breast cancers in 80.3% of cases. Sensitivity was higher among those above age of 50 year, in postmenopausal women and with diagnostic mammography. Rate of false negatives was 6.6 %. Screening mammography was valuable in early detection of 2 cases with T1 stage tumors.

Conclusions: Mammography as a diagnostic tool was found to be of fair quality but poor in screening of the breasts among the Egyptian cohort. So, efforts of early detection could begin through public education to increase the awareness of breast cancer health care. Clinical breast examination should be considered as integral component of routine breast care especially in women with limited access to mammography. When needed and if resources permit expand early detection efforts to include mammographic screening.

Chapter X - Fanconi anaemia (FA) is one of the inherited anemias that characterized by congenital abnormalities, progressive bone marrow failure and cancer susceptibility. It is a recessive disorder: if both parents carry a mutation in the same FA gene, each of their children has a 25 per cent chance of inheriting the defective gene from both parents. Consequently, the child will have FA. Until recently all cloned FA genes considered being orphans, having nothing in common with any other known genes. However, recent discovery that the breast cancer susceptibility gene *BRCA2* is identical to the Fanconi anemia (FA) gene *FANCD1* made possible to reconsider this orphan status. In turn, FANCD2 Fanconi protein recruitment to chromatin is dependent on activation of another breast cancer susceptibility gene BRCA1 which seems to play a role of a switcher of the FA/BRCA pathway regulating chromosomal stability. Although cancer cells with non-functional *BRCA1* or *BRCA2* genes show chromosome damage similar to that in Fanconi anemia cells, it was not clear whether genetic mutations that cause Fanconi can also cause breast cancer. Then what is the connection between Fanconi anemia and breast cancer? Since the discovery of the new FA genes, it is becoming evident that there is a strong, yet unresolved, link between FA and BRCA pathway. For instance, children who inherited two copies of non-functional BRCA2-interecting protein, PALB2 (FANCN) developed a Fanconi anemia phenotype. At the same time, women inheriting one damaged copy of PALB2 have double risk of developing breast cancer. Mutations in another Fanconi gene FANCJ (*BRIP1*) is a risk factor for the breast cancer comprising a class with two breast cancer susceptibility genes, *CHEK2* and *ATM*, which upon exposure to other environmental risk factors may predispose a woman to cancer. Although all newly discovered FA genes are relatively small contributors to the overall incidence of breast cancers, their cumulative response may be amplified for maintaining the stability of the entire human genome. Accordingly, understanding the connection between the Fanconi genes and BRCA1/2 seems to hold potential for future cancer research.

In: Frontiers in Breast Cancer Research
Editor: Louis P. Fortugno, pp. 1-37

ISBN: 978-1-60021-671-8

Chapter I

The Potential Role of Breast Cancer Resistance Protein in the Blood-Brain Barrier

Margery A. Barrand*
Department of Pharmacology, University of Cambridge,
Cambridge, UK.

Introduction

Transporters play a vital role in regulating movement of material into and out of the brain. In the brain capillaries, where tight junctions between endothelial cells limit paracellular flow, all material must pass across both the abluminal and luminal surfaces of the endothelium to enter the brain. In the choroidplexuses, where the capillaries are leaky, regulation of transport occurs at the apical and basolateral surfaces of the choroidal epithelium. Transporters strategically located at these cell surfaces scrutinise all material in the circulation and are well placed to efflux xenobiotics. Unlike the transporters that facilitate the transfer of nutrients into and waste material out of the brain, transporters that prevent entry of material to the brain must be capable of moving substances against a concentration gradient and of recognizing a wide range of different substrates. Such 'multidrug' transporters are members of the ATP binding cassette (ABC) family of proteins and use energy derived from ATP hydrolysis to power the movement of material across membranes. These include the transporters described in other chapters, i.e., P-glycoprotein (P-gp) and Multidrug Resistance-associated Proteins (MRPs). This chapter will examine Breast Cancer Resistance Protein (BCRP), a recently identified member of the ABC family of proteins (Allen and Schinkel, 2002a; Doyle and Ross, 2003). It will review what is currently known about BCRP in a rapidly moving field, make comparisons with P-gp and the MRPs, and discuss the implications of BCRP's characteristics in terms of the extent to which it might fulfil the roles required of an efflux transporter at the interfaces between bloodBCRP was recognised initially in several drug resistant tumour cell lines and subsequently identified in certain tumour tissues where its presence has been putatively associated with poor clinical response to chemotherapy. However it is found in many normal, i.e., non-malignant, cells at a number of different sites in the body including in endothelial cells lining the brain capillaries. Clues to the possible physiological role of BCRP at the blood-brain barrier may be derived from the many studies that are now being conducted which examine its mechanisms of action and its substrate and inhibitor profiles in different cell systems or which analyse its influence on the distribution of drugs in whole animals.

Identification of BCRP as a Multidrug Transporter

P-gp was the first ABC transporter to be associated with multidrug resistance (MDR) (around the mid 1970s) with the MRPs being later discoveries (MRP1 sequenced in 1992). It was not until 1998 that BCRP was revealed as another MDR-associated ABC transporter. At that time, it was becoming apparent that there were certain tumour cell lines that showed resistance to several drugs, mainly mitoxantrone, bisantrene, topotecan and doxorubicin, and yet did not overexpress P-gp or MRPs. Recognition of this atypical, non-P-gp, non-MRP resistance phenotype initiated a search for another multidrug transporter. This led ultimately to the discovery of BCRP, otherwise termed Mitoxantrone Resistance Protein (MXR) or ABC transporter in Placenta (ABCP). The different names for this protein derive from the fact that it was cloned from three different sources in independent laboratories at about the same time: from a multidrug resistant breast cancer cell line selected in doxorubicin (MCF7/AdrVp), hence BCRP (Doyle et al., 1998), from a colon cancer line selected in mitoxantrone (S1-M1-80), hence MXR (Miyake et al., 1999), and from human placenta, hence ABCP (Allikmets et al., 1998).

A large number of cell lines that overexpress BCRP have now been developed either by selection with anticancer agents or by transfection with BCRP constructs (see Table I). These have provided a useful source of material for examining the structural and functional aspects of the protein, its substrate and inhibitor profiles, and the mechanistic basis of its action.

Though most commonly referred to as Breast Cancer Resistance Protein by virtue of its initial discovery in a drug-selected breast cancer cell line, it is not clear that the protein is actually often overexpressed in breast cancers in vivo (Faneyte et al., 2002; Doyle and Ross, 2003). Indeed only weak BCRP expression has been found in breast tumours (Diestra et al., 2002). There are however many different human tumours in which BCRP expression has been clearly demonstrated (see later section). This has prompted some intense investigation to elucidate its mechanisms of action and to identify effective inhibitors.

* Correspondence concerning this article should be addressed to Margery A. Barrand, Department of Pharmacology, University of Cambridge, Tennis Court Road, Cambridge CB2 1QJ, UK. Tel. +44 1223 334031, Fax. +44 1223 334040, E-mail: mb10002@cam.ac.uk.

Table I. Some human drug resistant cell lines showing high expression of BCRP

Cell line	Cell type	Selecting drug	Conc	RR
MCF-7/MX	breast cancer	mitoxantrone	80 nM	1208
MCF-7/AdrVp[a]	breast cancer	doxorubicin verapamil	1 μg/ml 2.5 μg/ml	
MCF-7/AdVp3000[b]	breast cancer	doxorubicin verapamil	3 μg/ml 5 μg/ml	
MCF-7/FLV1000[c]	breast cancer	flavopiridol	1 μM	
8226 MR 20	myeloma	mitoxantrone	20 nM	37
S1-M1-3.2	colon carcinoma	mitoxantrone	3.2 μM	
S1-M1-80	colon carcinoma	mitoxantrone	80 μM	
EPG85-257RNOV	gastric cells	mitoxantrone		
EPF86-079RNOV	fibrosarcoma	mitoxantrone		
Igrov 1 MX3	ovarian cells	mitoxantrone	340 nM	11
Igrov T8	ovarian cells	topotecan	950 nM	11

These cell lines have been developed by selection with different anticancer agents and are derived from several different cell types.

RR : relative resistance is obtained by dividing the IC50 for the selecting agent in the resistant cell line by the IC50 value for that in the appropriate parental cell line. Most of the cell lines listed above are mentioned in Litman et al 2001 or Doyle and Ross 2003. The concentrations and RR values are taken from Scheffer et al 2000. Other references are a.Doyle et al 1998; b.Miyake et al 1999; and c.Robey et al 2001.

Molecular Aspects of BCRP

Structural Organisation of BCRP

BCRP contains the distinctive ATP-binding domains that are characteristic of ABC proteins; i.e., the highly conserved Walker A and Walker B sequences and the additional ABC 'signature' sequence. It is a member of the ABC subfamily, ABCG(http://www.humanabc.org/) and is named as ABCG2.

The topology of BCRP contrasts with that of P-gp, a member of the ABC subfamily ABCB, and with the MRPs, members of the ABCC subfamily. As with many of the ABC transporters, P-gp (ABCB1) is constructed as a tandem repeat of a basic unit containing two domains: an N-terminal transmembrane domain (TD) of 6 to 11 α-helices which provide substrate specificity and a C-terminal nucleotide-binding domain (NBD) located in the cytoplasm which binds and cleaves ATP in order to generate the energy for substrate transport. Binding and subsequent hydrolysis of ATP results in a conformational change that causes the substrate to be translocated across the membrane. Many of the members of the MRP family are similarly constructed, though some, including the MRP1 (ABCC1) have an additional N-terminal TD of unknown function. By contrast BCRP and other proteins of the ABCG subfamily contain only one NBD and one TD (see Figure 1) arranged in reverse direction. The functional units of these 'half transporters' are thought to be dimers.

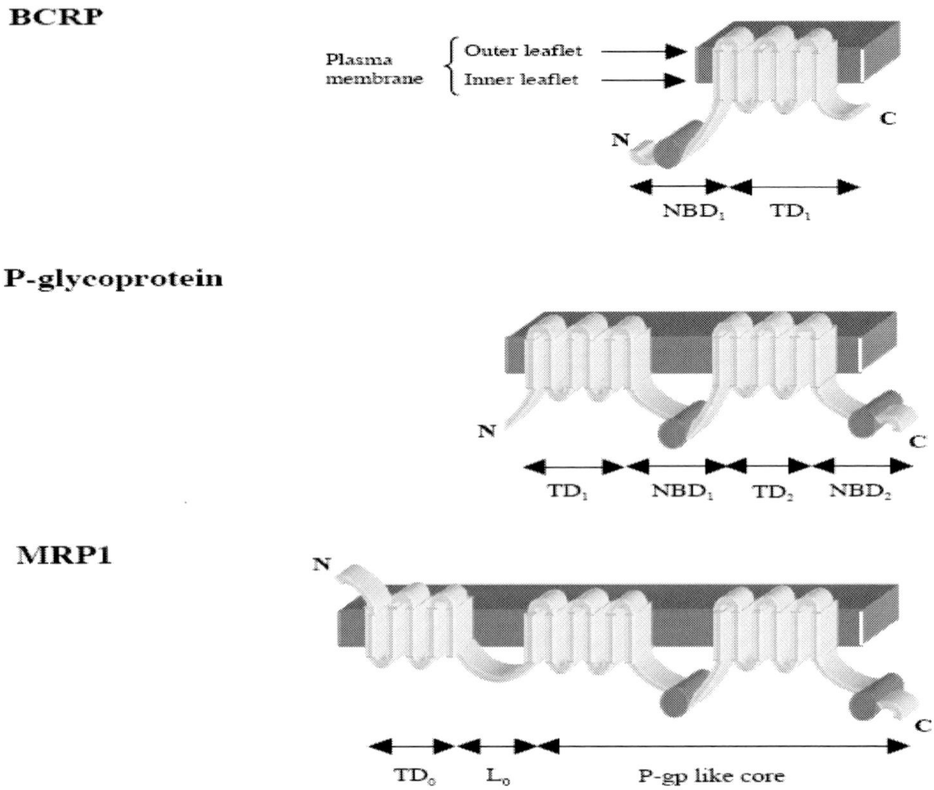

Figure 1. Topology of BCRP compared with that of other multidrug transporters, Pgp and MRP1. BCRP consists of one TD and an NBD orientated in reverse direction to that found in Pgp. P-glycoprotein itself is a 'full transporter' with a TD1-NBD1-TD2-NBD2 structure. Several of the MRP family members, including MRP1, have an additional N-terminal TD linked by a 'linker' region to a P-gp like core, while the other members have only the four-domain structure exemplified by P-gp. (TD-transmembrane domain; NBD- Nucleotide binding domain; 'N' and 'C' refer to the amino and carboxyl terminals of the transporter, respectively).

Relationship to other ABCG Family Members

The ABCG or White subfamily consists of eight proteins (see Table II), four of which have been well characterised (Schmitz et al., 2001). This family is so-called because of the close homology of its members with the Drosophila white gene protein. The protein products of the Drosophila white, brown and scarlet genes heterodimerise (white/brown and white/scarlet) to transport pigment precursors (guanine and tryptophan) in the Drosophila eye. The founding member of the ABCG subfamily, ABCG1, is essentially a human homologue of the Drosophila white gene. Various transcripts have been detected in different cells, probably due to alternative splicing events or use of different sites for initiation. The 12 amino acid linker region between the ATP-binding cassette and the transmembrane region is also subject to alternative splicing generating two major proteins. No such extensive variations have been reported with BCRP.

Table II. BCRP in relation to other member proteins of the ABCG (White) subfamily of transporters

Gene	Other names	Chromosomal location	Disease association	Tissue	Substrates
ABCG2	ABCP BCRP1 MXR	4q22	MDR	placenta breast liver	many chemo drugs
ABCG1	ABC8 White	21q22.3		ubiquitous	sterols lipids
ABCG3		8p12			
ABCG4	White 2	11q23			
ABCG5	White 3	2p21	β-sito-sterolemia	small intestine liver	sterols
ABCG6		7			
ABCG7		15			
ABCG8	White 4	2p21	β-sito-sterolemia	small intestine liver	sterols

Information taken from Schmitz et al 2001.

Ubiquitously expressed in tissues, ABCG1 appears to be involved in the regulation of cholesterol and phospholipid transport in macrophages, it itself being regulated in a sterol-sensitive manner. Two other ABCG transporters, ABCG5 and ABCG8, have been implicated in the efflux of dietary sterols from intestinal epithelial cells back into the gut lumen and from the liver to the bile duct. Abnormalities of these transporters have been linked to the human disease β-sitosterolemia which is characterised by altered handling of cholesterol and other sterols by the body including trapping within intestinal cells, lowered concentrations in the bile and strongly increased plasma levels (reviewed in Schmitz et al., 2001). There is conflicting evidence as to whether BCRP itself is involved in sterol transport and indeed whether it has a role to play in lipid movement (see later sections).

Evidence of Dimerisation

It has been shown that several of the mammalian ABCG half transporters, like their related proteins products of the Drosophila genes, dimerise with a partner protein (either with themselves to form a homodimer or with another protein to form a heterodimer) in order to be functional. BCRP may also act functionally as a dimer though there is some controversy on this point with suggestions of larger oligomers being formed (Xu et al., 2004). Currently, the bulk of the evidence points to BCRP being a homodimer, forming associations with itself but with no other proteins. Support for this idea has come from several studies including one in which separate BCRP constructs labelled either with Myc or with HA epitopes were co-transfected into cells (Kage et al., 2002). Immunoprecipitation with antibodies to one of the epitopes appeared to pull down constructs labelled with both epitopes as was apparent from subsequent western blot analysis. In the presence of reducing agents, BCRP migrated as a 70-kDa protein by SDS-PAGE but in the absence of reducing conditions it migrated as a 140-kDa protein presumed to be composed of BCRP molecules in the form of homodimers.

Indeed it was possible by probing with appropriate anti-Myc or anti-HA antibodies to determine the composition of these dimers.

In another study (Litman et al., 2002), chemical cross-linking methods were used to determine whether BCRP exists in the membrane in a greater than monomeric form. Chemical cross linking permanently links proteins that occur in close proximity to each other and so allows their subsequent analysis on SDS-PAGE. When used on BCRP, 3 bands with molecular masses of 180kDa or greater were identified on gels through which cell lysates of BCRP-overexpressing MCF-7 cells had been separated (Litman et al., 2002). Similar high molecular weight bands were also observed when cell lysates not subjected to cross-linking were run through SDS-PAGE under non-reducing conditions. Such high molecular weight bands are suggestive of oligomerisation occurring with BCRP either to itself or to another protein though it should be born in mind that non-specific protein complexes can be formed in the presence of chemical cross-linkers and under non-denaturating conditions.

Such studies demonstrate that BCRP, when highly expressed in cells, dimerises to itself but do not exclude the possibility that in other situations BCRP may have other partner proteins. However it is important to note in this context that BCRP has also been expressed and shown to be functional in heterologous expression systems ie oocytes, bacteria and insect cells where it is less likely that there are other partner ABC proteins with which it could bind. Even so, differences in functionality have been observed for the same construct when expressed in these different systems, an observation that has led to the suggestion that other partner proteins may nevertheless be involved (Yoshikawa et al., 2002). The importance of such associations of BCRP for its function has not been fully investigated.

Post-Translational Modification

As with many of the ABC transporters, BCRP can become post-translationally modified by addition of oligosaccharides at one or both of its potential N-linked glycosylation sites. This has been apparent from immunoblot analysis showing reduction in size of BCRP extracted from either membrane samples treated with N-glycosidase F which cleaves off the oligosaccharides or cells grown in the presence of tunicamycin to inhibit the N-glycosylation process (Litman et al., 2002). It has not been established whether glycosylation is important for BCRP function or possibly for routing or stability of the transporter within the cell, as has been shown for P-gp (Schinkel et al., 1993).

Promoter Organization and Regulation of Expression

Overexpression of proteins can be due to gene amplification, transcriptional upregulation, or post-translational events. The first of these mechanisms is quite common for both P-gp and MRP1 in highly resistant drug-selected cell lines but transcriptional activation is the usual mechanism in cell lines where only low level resistance develops. The ways in which BCRP expression is regulated in vivo are still far from understood but generally gene amplification is not the basis of the raised expression of MDR transporters found in clinical samples. An examination of the gene structure with particular reference to the promoter region has now been undertaken (Bailey-Dell et al., 2001).

It seems that the BCRP gene, which is located on chromosome 4q22, spans more than 66kb and consists of 16 exons varying in length from 60 to 532bp, i.e., equivalent to 20 to 74 codons; the introns range in size from 587bp to 18kbp. All splice junctions appear to conform to the GT/AG rule for splice donor and acceptor sites. The translation start site is in exon 2, the Walker A motif in exon 3, while exon 6 contains the nucleotide binding domain, ABC signature motif. The transmembrane regions of BCRP are coded in exons 10, 13, 14, 15 and 16 (see Figure 2).

The promoter organisation has features similar to those found in the promoters of both the MDR1 gene encoding human P-gp and the MRP1 gene. It is TATA-less with 5 putative Sp1 sites downstream from a putative CpG island and several AP1 sites. No sterol regulatory element was found in the BCRP promoter, unlike that of ABCG1 suggesting that BCRP is unlikely to act as a lipid transporter.

Analysis of promoter activity in the 5' upstream region of the BCRP gene was undertaken by inserting various portions of the promoter sequence attached to a reporter luciferase gene into four different human choriocarcinoma cell lines (Bailey-Dell et al., 2001). These particular lines were chosen since they naturally express BCRP, each to a different extent. In addition, such cells originate from the placenta, which shows high endogenous expression.

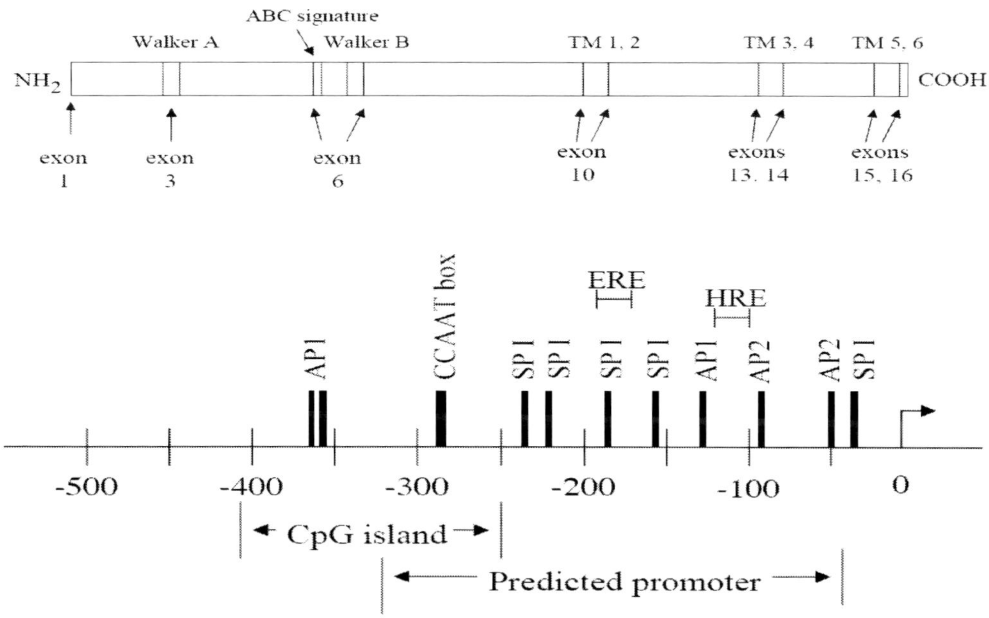

Figure 2. a) Diagram of human BCRP protein showing which exons encode the Walker A and Walker B motifs, the ABC signature and the transmembrane (TM) domains: b) 5' upstream region of the human BCRP gene showing putative promoter region, CpG island and potential transcription factor binding sites Also shown are the hypoxia-response element (HRE) sited at –116 to –112 and the putative estrogen response element (ERE) located at –187 to –173 in the promoter region (adapted from information taken from Bailey-Dell et al 2001, Ee et al 2004 and Krishnamurthy et al 2004).

These studies revealed the presence of both positive (between –1285 and –628 and between –312 and –115) and negative (between –628 and –312) regulatory elements but the identities of any trans-acting factors that may regulate expression was not established.

More recent analysis has identified hypoxia response elements at sites within the promoter region, the site binding most strongly to hypoxia-inducible factor (HIF-1) complexes being in region –116bp (see Figure 2). It was shown that hypoxia-induced transcriptional activation of the promoter led to upregulation of BCRP protein. This response was considered to be of survival value to cells exposed to hypoxia (Krishnamurthy et al., 2004). It was suggested that BCRP is able to expel various porphyrins in the heme pathway that would otherwise, under hypoxic conditions, accumulate and cause mitochondrial damage. Such an action might be of importance for endothelial cells lining brain microvessels, particularly following stroke (see later discussion).

Another study designed to explore factors that might regulate BCRP expression has revealed the presence of an estrogen response element (ERE), not identified in the earlier study (Bailey-Dell et al., 2001), in the 5' flanking region of the BCRP gene (Ee et al., 2004). To ascertain whether this putative ERE was functional, cells from two separate cancer cell lines, two lines derived from either breast or ovarian cancer, were exposed to physiological concentrations of estrogen (i.e., nM). Increased expression of BCRP was observed in the breast cancer cells that contained estrogen receptors and in the ovarian cells that had been stably transfected with the estrogen receptor (ERa) but not in untransfected ER-negative ovarian cells or in cells treated with antiestrogens. This raises the possibility that estrogens may directly stimulate production of BCRP in hormone-responsive tumours. To date, little correlation has been found between ER status, BCRP expression, and drug resistance in breast tumours (Kanzaki et al., 2001). Indeed there are few reports of overexpression of BCRP associated particularly with breast cancers. By contrast, BCRP is highly expressed in the placenta at the apical surface of the chorionic villus of the placenta, a site of production of estrogens. It is thought to play a crucial role here in protecting the fetus from toxic material in the maternal circulation. Thus induction of BCRP by estrogens that are produced locally and so reach high local concentrations would be important for ensuring adequate amounts of BCRP to protect the fetus.

BCRP Activity when Expressed in Heterologous Systems

The nature of BCRP's efflux actions has been examined in several heterologous expression systems including Lactococcus lactis (Janvilisri et al., 2003), insect cells (Ozvegy et al., 2001, 2002) and oocytes (Nakanishi et al., 2003), as well as in mammalian systems.

In each of these systems, BCRP functionality has been demonstrable. Expression of BCRP in the Gram-positive bacterium, Lactococcus lactis, was able to confer on the lactococcal cells a measure of resistance to certain agents known in mammalian cells to be transported by BCRP (e.g., Hoescht 33342). More direct evidence of functional BCRP efflux activity was obtained by monitoring the transport of Hoechst 33342 into inside-out membrane vesicles. In addition, in contrast to control inside-out membrane vesicles, BCRP-containing vesicles displayed a significant amount of orthovanadate-sensitive ATPase activity that was stimulated by daunomycin. Furthermore the BCRP-associated ATPase activity could be stimulated by sterols including cholesterol and estradiol as well as by steroids such as progesterone and testosterone and the estrogen antagonist, tamoxifen. It was suggested that the sterol stimulation could reflect a requirement by BCRP for sterols in its lipid environment (Janvilisri et al., 2003).

When expressed in Sf9 insect cells, BCRP shows membrane ATPase activity with a similar substrate stimulation specificity and inhibitor sensitivity to that of BCRP expressed in mammalian cells (Ozvegy et al., 2001). Interestingly, there was a relatively high level of basal ATPase activity in these ABCG2-expressing Sf9 membranes (i.e., in the absence of added substrate stimulation). This finding is in contrast to the low basal ATPase activity found if the MDR1 encoding P-gp is expressed in Sf9 cell membranes and suggests the presence of some endogenous substrate for BCRP, perhaps certain lipids or lipid derivatives.

Transfection of wild-type (R482) and a variant form (R482T) of BCRP into Xenopus oocytes has now been successfully accomplished (Nakanishi et al., 2003). In this system, the various BCRP forms were all well expressed at the cell surface and could be seen to be active as could be judged from the decreases in mitoxantrone accumulation. In agreement with what has been observed previously in mammalian systems, the R482T form, but not the R482 form, affected accumulation of daunorubicin. A mutation of a serine at codon 187 in the ABC signature motif led to complete absence of transport activity despite substantial expression of the protein at the oocyte cell surface. Significantly, this construct when co-transfected with either the R482 or R482T BCRP constructs acted as a dominant-negative inhibitor of BCRP function. These observations strongly support the idea that BCRP expressed in oocytes as in other expression system acts as a homodimer and does not interact with other proteins (as discussed earlier).

Substances That Interact with BCRP

BCRP's substrate and inhibitor profiles are currently the subject of extensive investigation. Examples of substances that have been shown to interact with or be transported by BCRP are shown in Table III. From the studies carried out so far, it is apparent that the MDR-associated ABC transporters identified at the blood-brain barrier or blood-CSF barrier differ somewhat in their mechanisms of action, substrate, and inhibitor profiles. BCRP has been said to confer an 'atypical' MDR (Ross et al., 1999) as compared with that conferred by the P-gp encoded by the human MDR1 gene. Nevertheless the MDR phenotype associated with BCRP does show some considerable similarities with that mediated by P-gp and some members of the MRP family. Thus there is a significant overlap in substrate profile between the various MDR-associated transporters. This is not an unexpected feature for a protective system. In the liver for example, there are a large number of closely similar enzymes involved in inactivation of xenobiotics, each with a broad range of substrates that overlap between the different enzymes.

Cell viability assays on both BCRP-overexpressing drug-selected and BCRP-transfected cell lines show that the transporter can confer resistance to several different types of anticancer agents including anthracyclines (doxorubicin, daunorubicin), anthracenediones (mitoxantrone), camptothecins (topotecan, irinotecan and its active metabolite, SN-38), and etoposide suggesting that these agents are effluxed by BCRP.

Table III. Substances that interact with BCRP

Anticancer drugs:	Dietary agents:	Fluorescent dyes:
mitoxantrone*	chlorophyll metabolites eg pheophorbide a[d]	Lysotracker Green
methotrexate*	polyphenols[e]	Rhodamine
doxorubicin*		Hoechst 33342
daunorubicin*	Endogenous lipophilic agents	
etoposide (VP-16)	steroids eg estradiol[f]	
topotecan[b]	estrone[g]	
SN-38[a]	diethylstilboestrol	
CPT-11	sulfated steroid conjugates[h]	
Other therapeutic drugs:		
prazosin	Estrogen anatagonists	
nucleoside reverse transcriptase inhibitors eg AZT and lamivudine[c]	tamoxifen[g]	

*depends on the amino acid at site 482.
A more comprehemsive list may be found in the review by Doyle and Ross 2003. Other references are:
[a]. Kawabata et al 2001.
[b]. Schellens et al 2000.
[c]. Wang et al 2003.
[d]. Jonker et al 2002.
[e]. Cooray et al 2004.
[f]. Janvilisri et al 2003.
[g]. Sugimoto et al 2003.
[h]. Suzuki et al 2003.

Furthermore, information about possible substrates has come from studies where the test substances have been shown to increase accumulation of proven substrates into whole cells or to block their ATP-dependent uptake into inside-out membrane vesicles prepared from BCRP-expressing cells. Studies of these sorts have identified a number of substances that interact with BCRP and so affect its efflux activity but such interactions do not prove that the substance itself is transported. More direct proof has to be obtained by monitoring the movement of the putative substrate in some way (e.g., via radio- or fluorescence labelling). The range of drugs to which BCRP confers resistance is slightly different from that found with P-gp and does not include typical P-gp substrates such as vinca alkaloids, paclitaxel, verapamil, or colchicine. However, the substrate profiles of the two transporters do overlap and some synthetic taxanes have recently been shown to be effective in preventing BCRP-mediated efflux activity (Minderman et al., 2004). Like P-gp, BCRP does not require GSH for the transport of electroneutral amphipathic drugs as is the case with MRP1.

Anticancer Agents

By contrast with P-gp, BCRP has been shown to transport the antifolate methotrexate, not only the unmodified drug but also the di- and tri-glutamylated derivatives (Volk and Schneider, 2003). This capability appears to be associated with the presence of the wild-type BCRP and is not seen in cell lines containing mutated forms of the transporter (Volk et al., 2002; Chen et al., 2003). Several members of the MRP family can also transport methotrexate with K_m values comparable to those of BCRP, but they are not able to transport polyglutamylated methotrexate. Thus BCRP is unique in this regard. The physiological significance of such BCRP-mediated methotrexate efflux is unclear since the K_m values are high and it is doubtful that intracellular levels of free methotrexate could ever reach levels of such magnitude in vivo. Indeed it has been estimated that the concentrations of methotrexate inside leukemic cells during treatment of pediatric leukaemia are 2-3 orders of magnitude below the K_m for BCRP as well as those for the MRPs. It is interesting to note that BCRP can also efflux folate. Indeed, in a recent report showing downregulation of BCRP during folate deficiency (Ifergan et al., 2004), it was suggested that BCRP might in fact play a role in regulating the folate status inside cells.

Another agent being tested as suitable for anticancer treatment because it causes cell cycle arrest and induces apoptosis is the chlorophenyl flavone, flavopiridol. This does not appear to be a substrate for P-gp and so might be regarded as potentially useful for avoiding resistance. However flavopiridol-resistance does occur and resistant cell lines have been developed. It seems that other transporters can bring about flavopiridol efflux including MRPs (Hooijberg et al., 1999) and BCRP (Robey et al., 2001).

Anti-HIV Agents

Resistance to drugs is a severe clinical problem not only with anticancer drugs but also with antiviral drugs. It has already been shown that over expression of P-gp or MRPs can reduce antiviral activity of AZT and HIV protease inhibitors (Washington et al., 1998). More recently it has been established that high levels of BCRP in CD4 +ve cells can bring about reduced anti-HIV-1 activity of nucleoside reverse transcriptase inhibitors such as AZT and lamivutrine (Wang et al., 2003). No studies have yet been undertaken to determine whether high in vivo expression of BCRP is indeed related to treatment failure and re-emergence of drug resistance in HIV-infected patients. In this context it is relevant to note that HIV infection can lead at the later stages of the disease to CNS disorders including encephalopathy and dementia. Although development of highly active antiretroviral therapy or HAART has decreased the incidence rates, most of the licensed anti-HIV drugs have a limited capacity to enter the brain. It is possible that expression of BCRP at the blood-brain barrier (see later section) may contribute to this poor access.

Dietary Components

Due to the perceived importance of BCRP in anticancer and in anti-HIV drug resistance, much attention has been given to identifying the therapeutic agents that may be transported by BCRP. However there are many dietary components that may also interact with and/or be transported by BCRP. Clues to the identities of some of these have come from studies on knock-out mice. Such studies have already shown the importance of the mouse equivalent, Bcrp1, for influencing the availability of dietary pheophorbide, a phototoxic porphyrin catabolite of chlorophyll (Jonker et al., 2002). Unlike the normal wild-type animals, mice lacking Bcrp1 developed hypersensitivity to pheophorbide fed in the diet and displayed extreme photosensitivity. It was subsequently established in overexpressing cell lines that both murine Bcrp1 and human BCRP can transport, and so influence the intracellular accumulation of, pheophorbiride. This raises questions about the possibility of other plant derived substances being substrates for the transporter.

Indeed it has been shown that certain plant polyphenols can interact with BCRP (Cooray et al., 2004). These are substances that may be taken into the circulation in substantial amounts from the diet. They can be classified into flavonoids, stilbenes (such as resveratrol), phenolic acids, and lignans. Flavonoids are particularly abundant in fruits and vegetables, providing much of the flavour and colour, and also in nuts, stems, flowers, wine and tea. Several hundred milligrams a day of flavonoids may be consumed as part of the western diet (Ross et al., 2002). Resveratrol, found in high concentrations in red wine, is another polyphenol with a structure similar to diethylstilbestrol, a known inhibitor of BCRP function (Sugimoto et al., 2003).

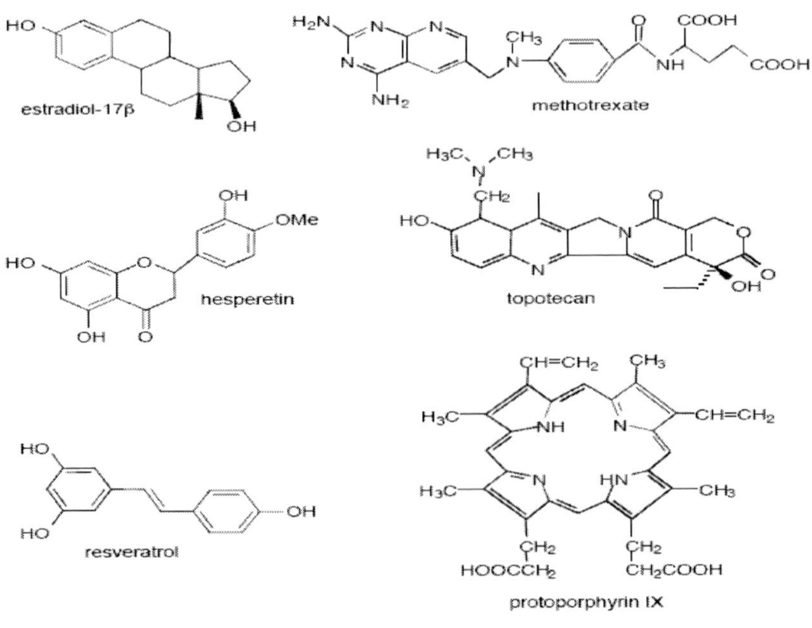

Figure 3. Chemical structures of some substances known to interact with BCRP.

Several studies have shown that flavonoids can modulate the activities of both P-gp (Zhang and Morris, 2003) and MRP1 (Bobrowska-Hagerstrand et al., 2003) affecting drug accumulation, cell viability following cytotoxic drug exposure, and the ATPase activity of P-gp. More recently, it has been reported that at least some polyphenols (see Figure 3) interact with BCRP (Cooray et al., 2004). These included the flavonoids quercetin, hesperetin, silymarin and daidzein, and the stilbene resveratrol. They were shown to interfere with BCRP-mediated efflux activity. Increases in accumulation (see Figure 4) of two separate BCRP substrates, mitoxantrone and bodipy-fl-prazosin, were observed in two different BCRP overexpressing cell types.

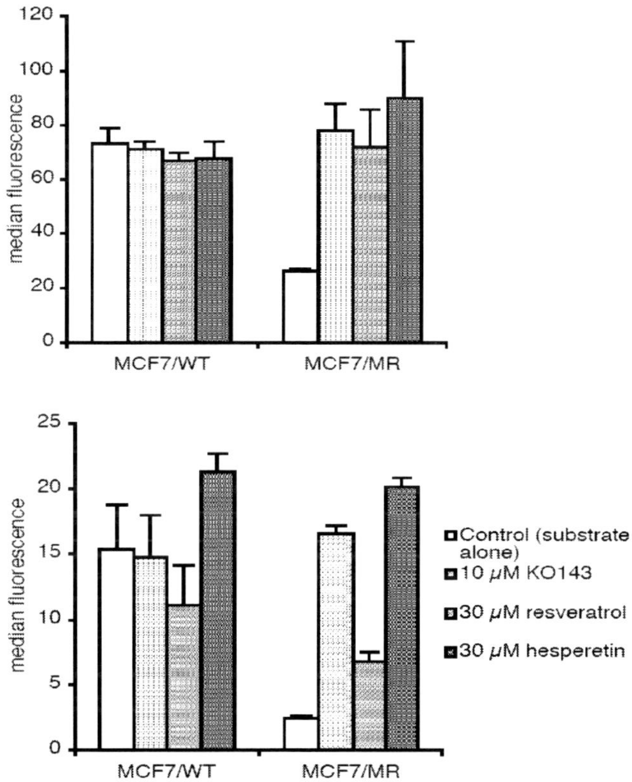

Figure 4. Effects of polyphenols or Ko143 on BCRP efflux activity in cells of a mitoxantrone-resistant BCRP-expressing cell line, MCF-7/MR, and the drug sensitive parental MCF-7/WT cell line. Values shown correspond to the median fluorescence of 5000 cells (mean±s.e.m, n=3) as measured by flow cytometry after exposure to a) 5 μM mitoxantrone or b) 250 nM bodipy-FL FL-prazosin. With each substrate, there is significantly less accumulation ie lower fluorescence in the BCRP-expressing MCF7/MR cells than in the MCF/WT cells under control conditions ie in the presence of the substrate alone. In the presence of the BCRP inhibitor KO143 or of the polyphenols, resveratrol and hesperetin, substrate accumulation ie level of fluorescence is increased in the BCRP-expressing MCF/MR cells to values comparable to those measured in the drug-sensitive MCF/WT cells. p values (repeated measures ANOVA, relative to control) were 0.19 (mitoxantrone) and 0.32 (bodipy-FL FL-prazosin) for the MCF7/WT cells and 0.0004 (mitoxantrone) and <0.0001 (bodipy-FL FL-prazosin) for the MCF7/MR cells. Dunnet's post hoc test showed all treatments differed from control (p < 0:05) for the drug resistant BCRP-expressing MCF/MR cells but not for the drug sensitive MCF/WT cells. (data taken from Cooray et al 2004).

They were also seen to stimulate BCRP-associated ATPase activity in inside-out vesicles prepared from BCRP-transformed L.lactis bacterial cells. Such interactions suggest that these polyphenols are substrates for BCRP. Given that the daily dietary intake of polyphenols could result in relatively high concentrations in the gut and circulation, these interactions could be of some significance for the in vivo activity of BCRP (see tissue location in later section).

Another dietary substance shown to be transported by the mouse Bcrp1 is the heterocyclic amine, 2-amino-1-methyl-6-phenylimidazo[4,5-b]pyridine (PhIP) (van Herwaarden et al., 2003). Heterocyclic amines are mutagenic and carcinogenic substances that are formed during the cooking of protein-containing foods; PhIP is one of the most abundant of these and is present in cooked meat and fish. Studies in Bcrp1 deficient and in Mdr1a/1b-deficient mice have shown that the absence of Bcrp1 but not of P-gp leads to profound effects on the distribution, availability and excretion of PhIP.These observations are of interest in demonstrating the importance of BCRP in providing protection against potential carcinogenic substances that may become ingested in the diet.

Endogenous Substances Including Lipophilic Agents

In addition to exogenous substances, there are certain endogenous agents that may be transported by BCRP. A number of estrogens and their derivatives are thought to interact with BCRP (Imai et al., 2002b). This has been shown for BCRP expressed in a bacterial expression system (Janvilisri et al., 2003) as well as in transfected mammalian cells (Sugimoto et al., 2003; Suzuki et al., 2003) where increased drug accumulation and restoration of drug sensitivities to, e.g., mitoxantrone and SN-38, have been observed in the presence of various estrogen agonists and antagonists. It has been suggested that, in the case of estrone and estradiol, these effects may be due to the actions of their conjugates rather than the unmodified steroids (Imai et al., 2003). However it is extremely difficult to obtain direct evidence of transport of very lipophilic substances using uptake into inside-out membranes because of the very high back diffusion of the material from the vesicles. It is nevertheless clear that BCRP is able to transport estrogen conjugates which could well have some bearing on its physiological roles in the body (see later section). In addition, some interesting interactions of heme with BCRP-mediated transport of estrone-sulphate have been observed (Krishnamurthy et al., 2004). This has led to the suggestion that BCRP may be involved in expelling such molecules and so help to regulate levels of porphyrins within cells.

Given the observed interactions of hormonal steroids with BCRP, there has been some interest in seeing whether BCRP may be able to transport sterols such as cholesterol and the plant derived sitosterols. Other members of the ABCG family to which BCRP belongs (i.e., ABCG5 and ABCG8) are thought to transport sterols and abnormalities in the genes encoding these transporters are associated with impaired sterol efflux from the intestines and liver. However, Albrecht et al. (2002) were unable to demonstrate any interactions of cholesterol or sitosterol with P-gp, MRP1, or BCRP present in cells of the mesenteric lymph nodes from mdr1a/1b knock-out mice.

There are several members of the ABC superfamily of proteins that do appear to transport lipids and lipid analogues (Borst and Oude Elferink, 2002). These include the P-gp (ABCB4) encoded by the MDR3 gene which can expel phosphatidylcholine from cells. Even the P-gp (ABCB1) encoded by the MDR1 gene is able to transfer various lipid analogues and certain endogenous lipids (e.g., platelet-activating factor, phosphatidylserine, glucosylceramide) from the inner to the outer leaflet of the plasma membrane. A role for MRP1 (ABCC1), a member of the ABCC family, in the outward translocation of phospholipids has also been demonstrated and within the ABCA family, ABCA1 has been shown to be involved in transport of phosphatidylserine in several cell types. In addition to these full transporters, several of the half transporters in the ABCG subfamily to which BCRP belongs have also been implicated in lipid transfer (Schmitz et al., 2001). ABCG1 is thought to be involved in regulation of cholesterol and phospholipid transport and ABCG5/ABCG8, associated together as heterodimers, may act as a choline flippase facilitating exposure of membrane-bound cholesterol to bile salts. It has recently been suggested that BCRP (ABCG2) itself may be involved in transport of endogenous phospholipids. Evidence for this has come from studies comparing levels of phosphatidylserine on the outer leaflet in BCRP high, low, and non-expressing cells and also following transbilayer movement of fluorescent phospholipid analogues (Woehlecke et al., 2003a). It may thus be able to bring about changes in the asymmetry of lipids in the cell membrane. Such redistribution could significantly impact on cell surface properties and cell-cell interactions.

Agents Used to Inhibit BCRP Activity

Several compounds have been investigated for their ability to block BCRP efflux activity. The compound GF 120918 (see Figure 5) is a known modulator of P-gp but also blocks BCRP-mediated drug efflux. Fumitremorgin C is an inhibitor of efflux more specific for BCRP (Rabindran et al., 2000). This is a natural product of fungal origin which also influences cell cycle arrest. Unfortunately it has tremor-inducing activity which precludes its use in vivo (van Loevezijn et al., 2001). Thus, newer less toxic analogues are being sought. Some of the most promising to emerge from further development are Ko132, Ko134 and Ko143 (Allen et al., 2002c), the last of these proving to be an excellent agent for studies where selective inhibition of BCRP is required. Another natural product of the same class of substances (i.e., diketopiperazines) is trypostatin A, another blocker of cell cycle progression. This has been shown at non-toxic concentrations to reverse resistance against mitoxantrone in various BCRP-expressing cell lines (Woehlecke et al., 2003b). In addition, the coumermycin derivative novobiocin, which blocks prokaryotic gyrases, has also been revealed as an effective competitive blocker of BCRP-mediated efflux (Shiozawa et al., 2004), reversing resistance to topotecan, SN-38, and mitoxantrone at micromolar doses in BCRP-expressing cell lines and competitively inhibiting topotecan transport into BCRP-expressing membrane vesicles at nanomolar levels.

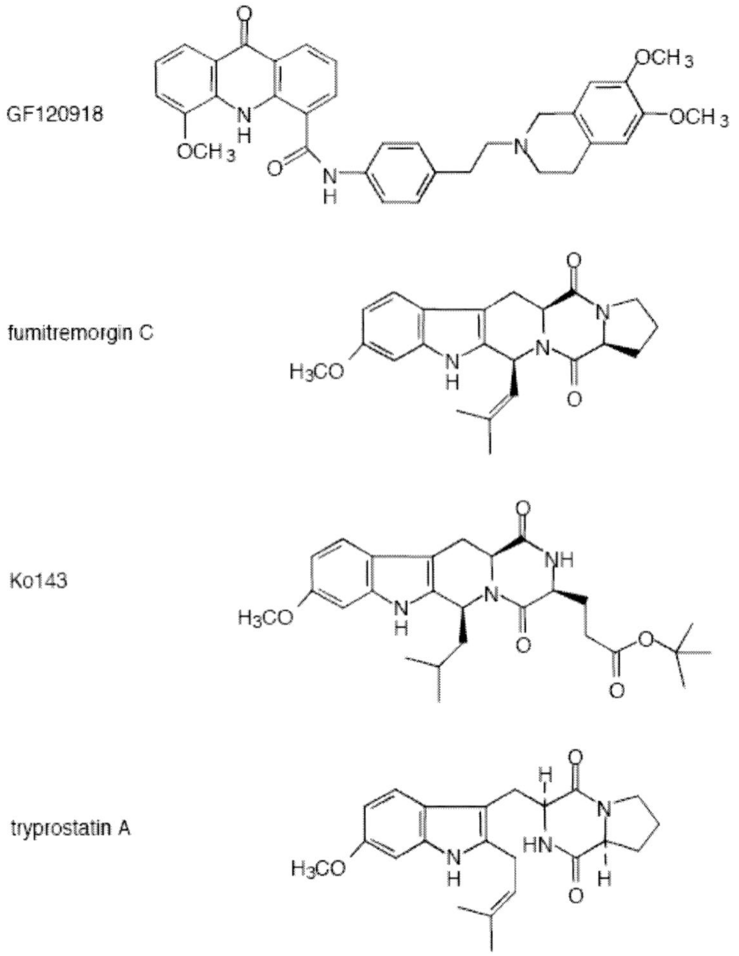

Figure 5. Structures of some agents used as inhibitors of BCRP.

Single Nucleotide Differences in the ABCG2 Gene and How these Impact on Substrate Profile

From the functionality studies described above, it became apparent that the substrate profile of BCRP was not always the same in each overexpressing cell line studied but differed in particular cell lines. It was later shown that such differences were due to single nucleotide polymorphisms in the BCRP expressed in the different cell lines or tissue from which BCRP was originally cloned. Hence the form cloned from human placenta, originally termed ABCP (Allikmets et al., 1998) has an arginine at position 482. This is a site close to the 3rd transmembrane domain (TMD) that appears critical for determining substrate specificity of BCRP. By contrast the form cloned from the doxorubicin-selected breast cancer cells (Doyle et al., 1998) has a glycine at this position whilst the BCRP cloned from a mitoxantrone-selected colon cancer line possesses a threonine at this site (Miyake et al., 1999). What is now considered to be the wild-type of BCRP (i.e., the form with an arginine at position 482) is unable to transport rhodamine 123 or LysoTracker Green and shows low resistance to anthracyclines but high resistance to mitoxantrone and topotecan. Variants containing a glycine or threonine in this position show a different substrate preference. Replacement of Arg482 by Gly or Thr provides a broader spectrum BCRP which shows higher levels of mitoxantrone resistance. Such variants are able to transport rhodamine 123 and LysoTracker Green and to show higher resistance to doxorubicin. On the other hand, they are unable to transport methotrexate (Chen et al., 2003). Mutations at amino acid 482 of the mouse Bcrp1 have also been observed in mouse fibroblast lines selected for resistance to doxorubicin (Allen et al., 2002b). These amino acid substitutions are distinct from those seen in human cell lines (i.e., replacement of arginine 482 by methionine or serine in the mouse), but they have similar consequences including greater resistance to anthracyclines, relatively lower resistance to topotecan, and greatly enhanced efflux of rhodamine 123. Indeed the amino acid at position 482 is regarded as a 'hot spot' for possible mutations. In this context, it is interesting to note the observations of Robey et al. (2003) in their comparative study of the substrate profiles of these 482 mutants. They noted that the inhibitor novobiocin was less effective in blocking the activity of the mutant forms than the wild-type BCRP thus raising the discomforting idea that, were there to be such mutations present at this position in BCRP expressed in human cancers, this might jeopardise the clinical effectiveness of such agents used to overcome BCRP-mediated resistance.

Miwa et al. (2003) have investigated further the effects of amino acid substitutions in the transmembrane domains by creating a number of different BCRP mutants with different substitutions not only at R482 on TMD 3 but also at E446 on TMD 2, at N557 on TMD 5, and at H630 on TMD 6. When transfected into mouse fibroblast cells most, though not all, constructs were expressed at the plasma membrane and conferred varying levels of resistance to SN-38, mitoxantrone, and methotrexate; this implied that each of these TMDs in BCRP may play an important role in drug recognition.

Table IV. Some cell lines in which single nucleotide differences in the ABCG2 gene have been identified

Cell line	Cell type	Selecting drug/s	Amino acidposition 482
MCF-7/MX[a]	human breast cancer	mitoxantrone	R
MCF-7/AdVp3000[a]	human breast cancer	doxorubicin verapamil	T
MCF-7/FLV1000[a]	human breast cancer	flavopiridol	R
S1-M1-80[a]	human coloncarcinoma	mitoxantrone	G
MT-4/DOX$_{500}$[b]	human T cell	doxorubicin	M
88.6/D800-A[c]	murine fibroblast	doxorubicin	M
88.6/D800-B[c]	murine fibroblast	doxorubicin	S
KOT52/D320[c]		doxorubicin	R/M 40/60%

Further information on the characteristics of these lines can be obtained from a Honjo et al 2001; b Miwa et al 2003; and c Allen et al 2002b.

They divided the transfectants into four groups; those showing higher resistance to SN-38 than to mitoxantrone (these included forms in which the substituted amino acids contained relatively large side chains), those showing higher resistance to mitoxantrone than to SN-38 (these included forms in which the positively charged amino acid present in the wild type was replaced by a negatively charge moiety), those in which resistance to SN-38 and to mitoxantrone were similar, and those conferring little resistance. Despite these differences, both fumitremorgin C and estrone showed equivalent effects on the reversal of resistance conferred by these constructs suggesting that the mutant BCRP proteins all retain similar binding properties for these particular inhibitors. The authors raised the interesting point that most of the mutations observed resulted in increased resistance to the challenging drugs used. They therefore asked why it should be that the apparently less efficient form of BCRP is the one present in normal tissues. This they suggested may point to the existence of important, as yet unidentified, physiological substrates that are transported more efficiently by the wild-type form of BCRP.

It was clear from these drug-selected cell lines that variations in amino acid sequence, particularly in the TMDs, can have a bearing on substrate specificity of BCRP. Thus, BCRP expression has been investigated in a number of different cell lines not subjected to drug selection (Imai et al., 2002a). In a panel of 59 cancer cell lines, high expression was found in two colon cancer, two lung cancer, one ovarian, and one leukaemia line. The whole coding sequence was determined in 11 of the lines including some showing high expression and some with low expression. Three variant BCRP cDNAs were identified including a deletion and a C to A change at base position 421 (C421A) leading to an amino acid substitution from lysine to glutamine at amino acid position 141 (Q141K). Cells transfected with this C421A variant were significantly more sensitive to anticancer agents and allowed higher intracellular accumulation of topotecan. Further analysis revealed similar transcript levels but lower protein levels. It was suggested that the change from lysine to glutamine would result in a different electronic charge that could alter tertiary structure sufficiently to lead to greater susceptibility to degradation. Despite this suggested lower stability of the mutated protein, one of the lung cancer lines that contained this substitution still showed high BCRP expression so additional factors must influence expression levels.

The possibility that similar single nucleotide polymorphisms leading to functional differences might be found in the general population prompted a search for such mutations amongst different ethnic populations including Japanese (Iida et al., 2002; Imai et al., 2002a) and Swedish (Backstrom et al., 2003). In another study, Honjo et al. (2002) sequenced 90 ethnically diverse DNAs obtained from the Single Nucleotide Polymorphism Discovery resource and representing the spectrum of human genotypes. Though a number of polymorphisms were discovered in these studies, many in untranslated regions, no polymorphisms at amino acid 482 corresponding to the arginine to glycine or arginine to threonine changes seen in the drug-selected cell lines were found. In contrast, the Q141K substitution was detected and with a higher frequency in the Japanese (Imai et al., 2002a) than in the Swedish (Backstrom et al., 2003) populations. The results of Zamber et al. (2003) suggest that, despite there being an almost 80-fold variation in the level of BCRP expression in the intestines of different individuals, there was no obvious correlation between expression level and any particular allelic change. Thus the clinical relevance of these and other polymorphisms in BCRP is not yet clear but certainly warrants further investigation since genetic variants of some ABC transporters have been linked to certain disease states (Oude-Elferink and Groen, 2002) and variants of others including P-gp may affect drug pharmacokinetics (see discussions in Schwab et al., 2003 and Sparreboom et al., 2003).

Subcellular Location of BCRP

BCRP seems to be predominantly localized to the plasma membrane (see Figure 6) of both drug selected and transfected cell lines (Rocchi et al., 2000; Scheffer et al., 2000). This has been established using mouse monoclonal antibodies, BXP-21 and BXP-34. Most recently, polyclonal antibodies have been generated against various cytoplasmic regions of the protein including those in the vicinity of the Walker A sequence and of the C signature region. These antibodies have been used in either confocal or electron microscopical analysis to confirm a plasma membrane localization of BCRP in various BCRP-overexpressing cell lines (Litman et al., 2002). Such localization sets BCRP apart from other half-transporters that are sited mainly in intracellular membranes such as the mitochondrion (ABCB7), the peroxisome (ALD subfamily), and the endoplasmic reticulum (Tap1/Tap2). A plasma membrane location for BCRP is consistent with a putative role in the efflux of substrates from the cell.

In polarized cell lines, such as BCRP-transfected MDCK-II Madine Darby Canine Kidney cells, BCRP becomes localized primarily to the plasma membrane on the apical aspect of the cells, thus being situated so as to cause the movement of material from basal to apical side.

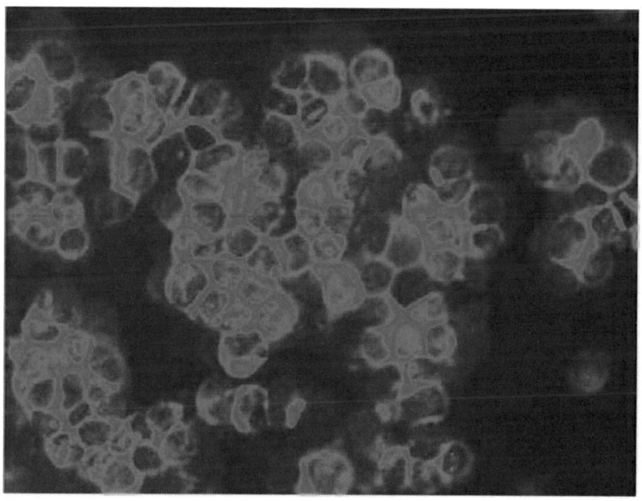

Figure 6. Immunofluorescent staining for BCRP in mitoxantrone-resistant breast cancer cells. Cytospins of cells from the MCF-7/MR cell line were fixed in methanol and exposed firstly to anti-BCRP antibody, BXP-21 followed by fluorescent linked anti-mouse secondary antibody to detect the location of BCRP. Fluorescent staining is localised mainly to the plasma membrane (courtesy of H.C.Cooray, unpublished).

However, a role for the transporter in intracellular trafficking of molecules cannot be ruled out as some immunohistological studies have reported perinuclear staining of BCRP in several topotecan and mitoxantrone resistant cell lines (Rajagopal and Simon, 2003). There are also reports of intracellular staining for mouse Bcrp1; this was detected in smooth muscle cells derived from the lung and in certain cell types from the distal air spaces (Summer et al., 2003).

Distribution and Putative Roles of BCRP in Normal Tissues and in Tumours

The subcellular locations of BCRP are of particular relevance to the possible role or roles of BCRP in normal tissues including the blood-brain barrier. The protein is found in many tissues, particularly at barrier sites where it appears to be localised to the apical surfaces of the epithelial cells (Maliepaard et al., 2001), as outlined in Table V.

Table V. Tissue distribution and cellular location of BCRP

Tissue location	Possible function
Placenta - syncytiotrophoblast[a]	Protection of fetus excretion of substrates into maternal circulation
Apical membranes of small intestine and colon epithelium[a]	Reduced uptake/excretion of substrates
Proximal tubular epithelium of kidney[a]	Excretion?
Canalicular membrane of liver[a]	Excretion of substrates by the liver
Apical membrane of ductal epithelial cells of the breast[a]	Unknown
'Side' population of stem cells[b, c]	Unknown
Endothelium of blood capillaries and veins[a]	Unknown

[a]Maliepaard et al 2001
[s]Kim et al 2002
[c]Scharenberg et al 2002
Further information on tissue distribution can be obtained in the review by Doyle and Ross 2003.

This distribution of BCRP shows similarities to that of the multidrug transporter, P-gp which is also expressed in various epithelia, particularly in organs associated with drug absorption and disposition including the hepatocyte canalicular membrane, renal proximal tubules, and the intestinal mucosa. P-gp is known to provide a first line of defence against the entry of many types of xenobiotics into the body (Schinkel, 1999). BCRP's distribution however contrasts with that of the MRPs many of which are widely distributed throughout the body in tissues including the choroid plexus, oral mucosa, small intestine, testis, and respiratory tract.

BCRP in the Placenta

Highest BCRP expression in human tissues is found in the placenta on the syncytiotrophoblast facing the maternal circulation. This suggests a role for the protein in either elimination of substrates from the fetus or preventing entry of material from the maternal circulation. Such ability has been demonstrated for the mouse Bcrp1; in both wild-type and P-gp knockout mice, inhibition of Bcrp1 by GF120918 (a common inhibitor of human and mouse P-gp and BCRP) resulted in around a 3-fold increase in the fetal uptake of intravenously administered topotecan, a BCRP substrate (Jonker et al., 2000).

BCRP in Small Intestine, Liver and Kidney

BCRP is also expressed at more modest levels in the colon, small intestine, liver and ovary where it may prevent entry or mediate elimination of unwanted material from these tissues. In the same study on P-gp knockout mice by Jonker et al. (2000), it was shown that co-administration of GF120918 with orally administered topotecan resulted in approximately 6-fold increases in area under the curve for topotecan, suggesting that Bcrp1 is a major determinant of topotecan oral bioavailability. Similar increases in oral availability of topotecan were seen in a subsequent study in which Bcrp1-knockout animals were investigated (Jonker et al., 2002).

It is not always appropriate to extrapolate from events occurring in mice to the human situation, particularly since it seems relative levels of BCRP may differ in human and in mouse tissues; for example in contrast to human tissues, there is higher expression of Bcrp1 in kidney and more modest expression in placenta in the mouse (Jonker et al., 2000). Nevertheless it is interesting to note the similarity in results to those found in mice in a recent clinical study in which GF120918 was co-administered with topotecan (Kruijtzer et al., 2002). Here it was shown that the oral bioavailability of topotecan more than doubled (from 40% to 97%) when the drug was co-administered with the inhibitor. The plasma concentration time curves indicated that there was an increased peak plasma level compatible with increased absorption. Thus, as in mice, blockade of BCRP in humans can lead to increased systemic exposure to oral topotecan. This emphasises the functional significance of BCRP expression in the intestine.

Such effects will however depend on the nature of the drug under investigation and are not observed when etoposide availability is monitored (Allen et al., 2003). Etoposide is a good substrate for P-gp and absence of this transporter alone (i.e., in mdr1a/1b knockout mice) results in much higher etoposide plasma levels compared to those found in the wild-type animals with no further increases being seen if Bcrp1 activity is inhibited by GF120918.

The relative importance of these two transporters for handling various substances in the body can vary and, in the case of the dietary carcinogen, PhIP, it is Bcrp1 rather than P-gp that has the most pronounced effect on the pharmacokinetics of this substance (van Herwaarden et al., 2003). It seems from Bcrp1 knock-out studies that Bcrp1 is responsible for hepatobiliary and direct intestinal excretion of PhIP, such that fecal elimination represents the major exit route, but in the absence of Bcrp1 this is changed to urinary elimination.

BCRP in Stem Cells

Both BCRP and P-gp are consistently expressed in stem cells. It is becoming increasingly apparent that, even in adult animals, there are stem cells present within various tissues including bone marrow (Zhou et al., 2001), skeletal muscle (Zhou et al., 2001; Tamaki et al., 2002), brain (Reynolds and Weiss, 1992; Johansson et al., 1999), and lung (Summer et al., 2003). These cells exhibit a high degree of plasticity (Bunting 2002) and can differentiate into different cell types; in the case of neural precursor cells they can differentiate into neurones and different types of glial cells. Those found in the bone marrow can give rise not only to all cells of haematological lineage but also skeletal and cardiac muscle and endothelial cells. Identification of stem cells has been aided by the discovery that these cells exclude the fluoresecent dye, rhodamine 123, (Zijlmans et al., 1995), a capability that has been attributed to the presence of P-gp activity. Another fluorescent dye, Hoechst 33342, has been useful in revealing the existence of a smaller stem cell fraction, the so-called 'side population'; these cells represent a mere 0.05% of cells in the bone marrow and are detectable since they exclude the dye. In this case it is BCRP that is thought to be the transporter responsible. It is known that BCRP can efflux Hoechst 33342 and that it is highly expressed in haematopoietic stem cells (Kim et al., 2002; Scharenberg et al., 2002). Furthermore, in mice lacking the Bcrp1 gene, this efflux is absent (Zhou et al., 2002).

Many of the observations on stem cells have come from studies on skeletal muscle or bone marrow in the mouse where Bcrp1, the murine equivalent of human BCRP, is expressed. There are however reports of progenitor cells with similar Hoechst efflux characteristics that have been isolated from human pancreatic islets of Langerhans (Lechner et al., 2002). These cells stain positively for the intermediate filament protein, nestin which is a marker of neural stems but also show high expression of both BCRP and MDR1 P-gp. Stem cells expressing BCRP have also been identified within the liver of rats (Shimano et al., 2003). When hepatocytes are prevented from proliferating in response to liver damage, a population of cells called 'hepatic oval cells' emerge that have the capability to differentiate into hepatocytes or cholangiocytes. These cells have characteristics similar to those of stem cells from other sources, i.e. exclusion of Hoechst 33342, and this capacity is associated with expression of rat BCRP.

The roles of the two transporters in stem cell function may be different. Overexpression of P-gp in bone marrow cells leads to an expansion of the side population, their prolonged survival in culture, and an enhanced repopulating activity after transplantation into mice (Bunting 2002). P-gp thus seems to be implicated in stem cell expansion. Bcrp by contrast appears associated with quiescent stem cells. Its expression is sharply down-regulated upon haematological maturation and is not detected in mature blood cells. Furthermore overexpression of Bcrp significantly blocks hematopoietic development (Zhou et al., 2001). It has been suggested (Bunting, 2002) that BCRP expression may play a role in early stem cell self-renewal by partially blocking differentiation whilst P-gp expression serves to promote differentiation and expansion. However, definitive roles for these transporters in stem cells are unclear. Bcrp1-null mice still retain normal steady-state haematopoiesis and stem cell number.

Mice have now been generated that lack both P-gp and Bcrp. Analysis of these animals has revealed that these transporters do not appear to be required for normal development of hematopoietic cells (Zhou et al., 2003). It has been suggested however that they may provide additive protection to stem cells against toxicity of xenobiotics despite their relatively modest levels of expression in the wild-type animals (Zhou et al., 2003). In this context, it is interesting to note the influence on stem cells of the Akt pathway which is an important regulator of cell survival. Akt-deficient mice display a reduction in side population fraction as defined by the ability of the cells to efflux Hoechst 33342. Furthermore blockade of the Akt pathway in vitro in bone marrow cells almost completely abrogates detection of side population stem cells. It seems that acute inhibition of the Akt pathway affects the localisation of Bcrp1 within these stem cells causing it to become translocated from plasma membrane to intracellular compartment (Mogi et al., 2003) and hence impairing its ability to efflux Hoechst 33342. This link between the Akt pathway and Bcrp1 location raises the question as to whether or not Bcrp1-mediated efflux activity might be required for stem cell survival.

This question has more recently been addressed by Krishnamurthy et al. (2004). These authors observed that Bcrp1-deficient mice accumulate more porphyrins in their hematopoietic cells as compared to their wild-type counterparts. They note that progenitor cells in these animals appear particularly sensitive to low oxygen tension but their survival under these conditions can be improved by blocking heme synthesis. They suggest that Bcrp1 in wild-type animals assists in protection from hypoxic damage by expelling potentially damaging porphyrin molecules and so minimising their accumulation within the cells.

BCRP in Tumours

BCRP appears to be widely present in untreated human solid tumours of many types (Diestra et al., 2002) though it has been observed more frequently in adenomas of the digestive tract, endometrium, lung, and in melanoma. Whether it provides a clinically relevant mechanism of drug resistance is unclear. Studies relating BCRP expression with response rate have shown a trend towards poorer survival in breast cancer patients with higher BCRP mRNA detectable in sections of frozen biopsy material but this did not reach statistical significance (Burger et al., 2003). The role of BCRP in acute lymphoblastic leukaemia has also been explored (Plasschaert et al., 2003). The study showed that the BCRP protein is expressed at a higher level and has more impact on drug accumulation in cells of B-lineage than of T-lineage. The BCRP substrates anthracycline, mitoxantrone, and methotrexate are used frequently to treat patients with acute lymphoblastic leukaemia. Thus the presence of BCRP could potentially impact on clinical response in these patients. In a separate study, a correlation was reported between BCRP mRNA expression and in vitro resistance to Ara-C in leukemic cells isolated from patients with pediatric acute lymphoblastic leukaemia but the significance of this finding is unclear since Ara-C is not apparently a substrate for BCRP (Stam et al., 2003).

BCRP in Vascular Endothelia

Other sites where BCRP is consistently observed are the endothelia lining the vasculature supplying many tissues. In this, it differs from P-gp which is present only on vessels supplying the brain, testis and skin. Nevertheless, the presence of multidrug transporters on vascular endothelial cells at special barrier sites such as the blood-brain and blood-testis barriers is of particular importance since here the vessels possess tight junctions which place severe restrictions on the free paracellular diffusion of substances seen in peripheral endothelia. Clearly, the presence of multidrug efflux transporters at these sites contributes to the creation of 'pharmacological sanctuaries' within the body. This permits these organs and tissues to function in relative isolation from the rest of the body. Indeed in P-gp knock-out mice, the integrity of the blood-brain barrier is shown to be significantly compromised with much higher brain penetration of P-gp substrates such as vinblastine and ivermectin being possible. However there is as yet no evidence from knock-out mouse studies that BCRP plays a similar role at the blood brain barrier.

Interestingly BCRP is said to occur on venules and capillaries (Maliepaard et al., 2001) but not in arterioles. This means that BCRP is distributed in the regions of the vasculature where most of the exchange of materials between blood and tissues occurs. On endothelial cells of vasculature supplying tumours (e.g., testicular germ cell tumours, endometrial, ovarian and colon carcinomas, and brain tumours) antibody staining for BCRP has been described as moderate to strong, stronger indeed than on the vascular endothelium in the surrounding normal regions (Diestra et al., 2002). This raises the interesting possibility that BCRP expression is perhaps upregulated in the endothelium of blood vessels during neoplastic vasculogenesis. This may relate to endothelial cell proliferation or possibly reflect the differing requirement of blood vessels supplying highly metabolising tumour tissue. Relevant to this is the observation of Zhang et al. (2003) that BCRP mRNA levels are significantly higher in the blood vessels of gliomas than of normal brain samples (see later).

BCRP in Brain Tissue

BCRP has been detected in brain tissue. There appears to be only very modest expression of Bcrp1 in mouse brain (Jonker et al., 2000) but expression of BCRP in human material may well be more substantial. Recent studies have explored the distribution of BCRP in human brain samples. In both normal and tumour brain sections (meningiomas and gliomas), the expression of BCRP has been characterized using RT-PCR, western blotting, and immunohistochemistry (Cooray et al., 2002). BCRP was detectable in brain tissue by western blot analysis and seemed to be expressed in higher amounts in the gliomas than in the normal or in the meningioma samples. Immunohistochemistry revealed that the staining of BCRP was restricted mainly to the brain vasculature (see Figure 7). The exceptions to this were found in samples of meningiomas where parenchymal staining was also evident.

Expression of BCRP in blood vessels supplying brain tumours has also been reported by Diestra et al., 2002) using immunohistochemical staining methods.

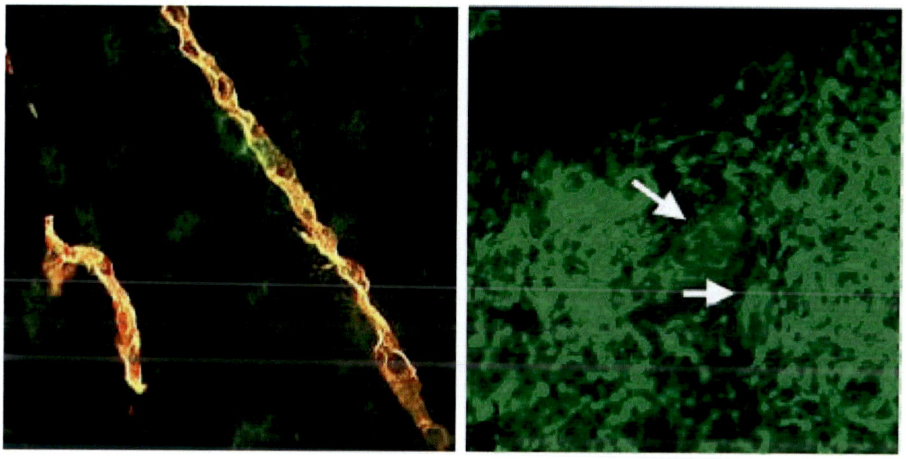

Figure 7. Immunofluorescent staining for BCRP in frozen sections of human brain samples using anti-BCRP antibody, BXP-21. BCRP staining a) in a normal human brain sample is restricted primarily to the vasculature but b) in a meningioma sample additional extensive parenchymal staining can be observed around the vessels indicated by the arrows.

Localisation of BCRP in the Specialised Endothelium of the Human Blood-Brain Barrier

Within the brain tissue, BCRP is primarily expressed on brain vasculature. Using confocal microscopy it has been possible to gain some understanding of the subcellular distribution of BCRP within the brain microvessels. Utilizing the fact that the brain endothelial glucose transporter GLUT-1 is normally located on both sides of brain endothelial cells (both luminal and abluminal membranes), dual-staining with antibodies for GLUT-1 and for BCRP revealed the main sites of BCRP expression in microvessels of both normal and tumour brain. The distribution of BCRP staining was seen to be inner to that of GLUT-1 in all microvessels viewed, which tends to suggest that BCRP is localized towards the luminal membrane of human brain endothelial cells in the in vivo blood-brain barrier (Cooray et al., 2002). An illustration of this point is shown in Figure 8.

Levels of BCRP mRNA in brain microvessels have also been analysed. This was accomplished using the highly intricate method of laser capture microdissection to lift blood vessels from frozen sections of brain, extract the RNA and analyse it for gene expression (Zhang et al., 2003). An earlier study (Bennett et al., 2001) undertaken in rat brain tissue showed this technique to be suitable for harvesting brain microvessels (see Figure 9) and for analysing them for the various gene transcripts they contain. The later study (Zhang et al., 2003) was able to report clearly the presence of BCRP mRNA in RNA extracted from microvessels lifted from human brain tissue sections and using a semi quantitative approach to reveal clear differences in expression in vessels from normal and from glioma brain samples. The method is not however without its difficulties. These are mainly concerned with RNA degradation and the requirement for a large number of vessels to be harvested to able to detect transcripts other than the highly expressing housekeeping genes.

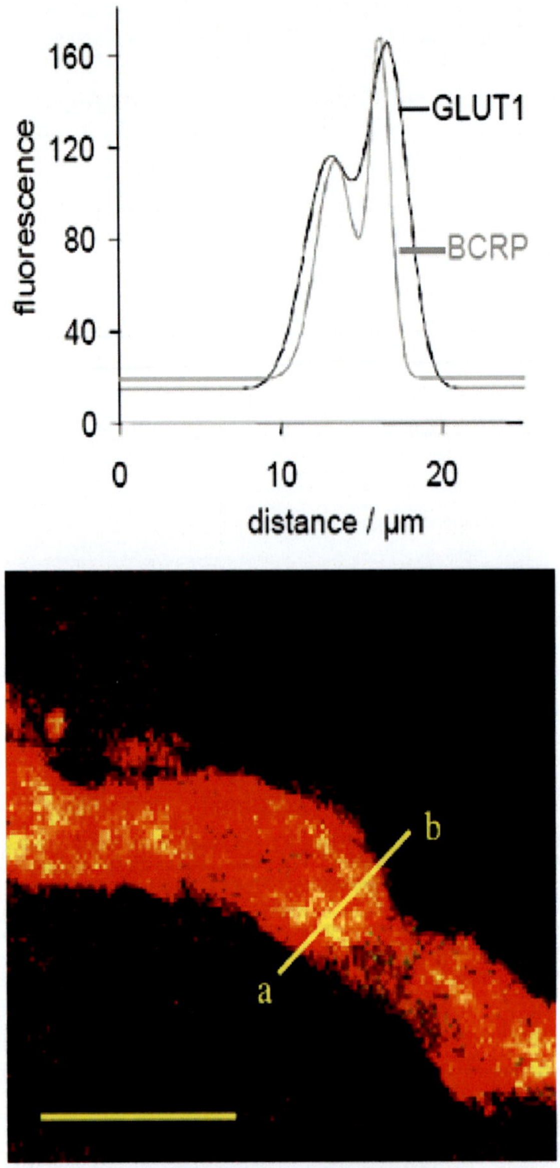

Figure 8. Cross sectional profile of human brain microvessel stained for BCRP and for GLUT-1 showing the variation in intensity of fluorescence immunostaining across the vessel as measured under the confocal microscope. In the original, GLUT1 is stained red and BCRP is stained green with sites of superimposition being in yellow. Scale bar = 20μm. The red and green fluorescence intensity profiles were determined along the path AB as shown in a). Each of these was then fitted using a baseline and two Gaussian peaks. The resulting fitted curves are shown in b) with GLUT staining represented by the black curve and BCRP by the grey curve. The fluorescence intensity for BCRP staining has been scaled so as to be comparable with that for GLUT1 so that the relative separation of the peaks can be seen by eye. The BCRP fluorescence peaks are seen to be closer together than those for GLUT1 suggesting that BCRP is located more towards the lumen of the vessel than is GLUT1. In 8 similar segments analysed, the difference in the separation of the peaks was 0.46±0.16 μm (mean±s.e.m., $p<0.02$) (Cooray, Hladky and Barrand, unpublished results).

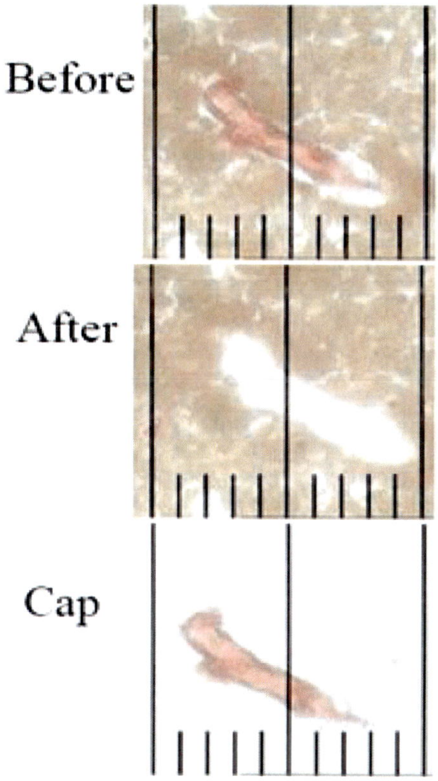

Figure 9. Laser capture of a microvessel from a frozen and dehydrated section of rat brain. The microvessel has been visualised by staining for alkaline phosphatase activity and the three images show in sequence the vessel in situ before being lifted from the section, the section after the microvessel has been removed and the microvessel now retained on the plastic cap. Note the precise microdissection of the vessel that is possible with this method. (courtesy of Dr G.C.Bennett, unpublished).

It is also more difficult to apply to human brain material where there may be a lag before samples can be frozen and so RNA degradation presents a particular problem. Furthermore interpretation of the levels of expression may be confounded by the necessity to ligate blood vessels supplying the region to be removed during surgery. This may mean that the microvessels to be analysed may have suffered severe anoxia before removal and thus show changes in mRNA expression as a result. Despite these caveats, the method has great potential for comparing expression in vessels from different regions and in vessels from damaged versus undamaged areas.

Detection of BCRP in the Brain Tissue of Other Species

It is not only in human and mouse tissues in which a BCRP-like transporter has been identified. Recently, a homologue of BCRP has been described in porcine brain endothelial cells by Eisenblatter et al. (2003). This protein, named as Brain Multidrug-resistance Protein

(BMDP), shows 86% amino acid identity with human BCRP and is predicted to have the typical architecture of a 'reverse' half-transporter. BMDP was shown, using immunohistochemistry, to be localized to the cell membrane of cultured porcine brain endothelial cells. A blood vessel location in vivo for the message was inferred from RNA isolation experiments in which the mRNA of BMDP appeared to be concentrated in the brain microvessels, levels of transcript being higher in isolated capillaries than in homogenised brain tissue.

High levels of BMDP transcript were also detectable in cultured porcine brain endothelial cells. These appeared approximately 30-times higher than P-gp expression, suggesting that at least in the porcine endothelium, BMDP plays a more prominent role than P-gp. This was corroborated via functional studies using the radiolabeled substrate ^{3}H-daunorubicin performed on cultured PBCEC grown as monolayers. While GF120918, a common inhibitor of P-gp and BCRP, abrogated almost completely the transport of daunorubicin from the basolateral to the apical side of the porcine brain endothelial cell monolayer, a number of specific Pgp inhibitors gave only moderate inhibition. This strongly suggests that the contribution by BMDP to transport of substrates across the porcine blood-brain barrier may be greater than with P-gp. These studies are the first to report functional BCRP (or rather, a porcine homologue) in cells derived from the blood-brain barrier.

The Possible Roles of BCRP at the Blood-Brain Barrier

Based on its expression at the luminal membrane of endothelial cells, it would seem that BCRP is well situated to efflux material from the endothelial layer. This may indicate a protective function for BCRP at the blood-brain barrier in limiting entry of substrates into the brain. It is already well documented that P-gp, similarly located at the luminal aspect of the brain capillary endothelium, performs such a 'gatekeeper' role at the blood brain barrier, pumping out a variety of xenobiotics; these compounds would otherwise gain access to the brain via the transcellular pathway due to their lipophilicity (Schinkel, 1999). The additional protection BCRP may bring to bear is as yet not well defined. The number of drugs known to be excluded from the brain by P-gp is large, ranging from non-sedating antihistamines, anti-epileptics, and beta-blockers to anti-HIV reverse transcriptase inhibitors. BCRP has a more limited range but does have some additional substrates not handled by P-gp.

Early studies using Bcrp1-knockout mouse or inhibitors of BCRP in mice already deficient in P-gp (i.e., mdr1a/mdr1b knock-outs) failed to show any changes in distribution of substances in the brain. Despite its effects on availability and hepatobiliary excretion, inhibition of Bcrp1 in P-gp-deficient mice (Jonker et al., 2000) did not result in enhanced accumulation in the brain of either topotecan or mitoxantrone, both good substrates for Bcrp1. Nor indeed was there any significant increase observed in brain penetration of another Bcrp1 substrate, the heterocyclic amine, PhIP in Bcrp1 knockout mice (van Herwaarden et al., 2003). However in a more recent study in which an in situ method of brain perfusion was used to measure drug uptake into the brain (Cisternino et al., 2004) clear increases in the brain transport coefficients of mitoxantrone were seen in both P-gp-deficient and wild-type mice when the activity of the mouse Bcrp1 was inhibited by GF120918. This appears to be the first evidence that impairment of BCRP activity at the blood-brain barrier has an effect on the transfer of substances into or out of the brain. Whether BCRP on human brain blood vessels likewise limits entry of drugs to the brain has not been directly demonstrated but may well be the case. Nevertheless it should be born in mind that there may be species differences. Indeed it has already been noted that the relative BCRP levels between tissues are different in human and in mouse.

Another role for BCRP on the luminal surface of the endothelium lining the brain microvessels may be in the secretion of endogenous substances into the blood, particularly substances relevant to endothelial cell function or those related to endothelial cell survival. There are a large number of possible candidates if one considers the extensive range of different types of substances that are already known to interact with BCRP (see above) from steroids, large natural product anticancer agents, chlorophyll metabolites and polyphenols to relatively small charged species such as the folate analogue, methotrexate. Indeed BCRP is known to be able to efflux endogenous folate which may suggest a role for the transporter in regulating intracellular folate status (Ifergan et al., 2004). Other endogenous substances that BCRP may assist in regulating are porphyrins. Of note in this context are the ideas of Krishnamurthy et al. (2004) that BCRP is able to protect cells from hypoxic damage by removing porphyrins that would otherwise accumulate to the detriment of the cell. These ideas were suggested with regard to the possible role of BCRP in hematopoietic stem cells (see above). They could however be applicable to other cell types not so extensively engaged in heme synthesis (i.e., the endothelial cells lining blood vessels that are likely to face interruption in blood flow and resultant hypoxia). Survival of endothelial cells would be necessary to prevent vessel damage but be particularly important in brain microvessels for maintaining blood-brain barrier integrity.

Conclusion

BCRP has only relatively recently been identified and many questions still remain regarding its in vivo functionality. Unlike any of the other multidrug transporters including P-gp and the MRPs, BCRP is expressed on endothelia of veins and capillaries in every tissue so far examined and this suggests the possibility that it effluxes a substrate which may have toxicity to many tissues but is incapable of passing between endothelial cells, or is a non-diffusible product of endothelial cell metabolism. Thus within the brain, expression of BCRP on the brain blood vessels may be of significance in limiting entry of certain substances to the brain but equally may point to a role in efflux of material either from the brain or more locally from the endothelial cells themselves. However, there is as yet though no direct evidence for this. The vast body of research available on P-gp and members of the MRP family has pointed to specific in vivo roles for these transporters. For BCRP, the situation is less clear, at least at certain sites in the body, and most certainly its role at the blood-brain barrier has still to be unravelled.

Acknowledgements

MAB wishes to express her gratitude to her colleagues, Dr SB Hladky and Mr HC Cooray for their help in the preparation of this chapter.

References

Albrecht C, Elliott JI, Sardini A, Litman T, Stieger B, Meier PJ and Higgins CF (2002). Functional analysis of candidate ABC transporter proteins for sitosterol transport. *Biochim. Biophys. Acta, 1567(1-2):* 133-142.

Allen JD and Schinkel AH (2002). Multidrug resistance and pharmacological protection mediated by the breast cancer resistance protein (BCRP/ABCG2). *Mol. Cancer Ther., 1(6):* 427-434.

Allen JD, Jackson SC and Schinkel AH (2002). A mutation hot spot in the Bcrp1 (Abcg2) multidrug transporter in mouse cell lines selected for Doxorubicin resistance. *Cancer Res., 62(8):* 2294-2299.

Allen JD, Van Dort SC, Buitelaar M, van Tellingen O and Schinkel AH (2003). Mouse breast cancer resistance protein (Bcrp1/Abcg2) mediates etoposide resistance and transport, but etoposide oral availability is limited primarily by P-glycoprotein. *Cancer Res., 63(6):* 1339-1344.

Allen JD, van Loevezijn A, Lakhai JM, van der Valk M, van Tellingen O, Reid G, Schellens JH, Koomen GJ and Schinkel AH (2002). Potent and specific inhibition of the breast cancer resistance protein multidrug transporter in vitro and in mouse intestine by a novel analogue of fumitremorgin C. *Mol. Cancer Ther., 1(6):* 417-425.

Allikmets R, Schriml LM, Hutchinson A, Romano-Spica V and Dean M (1998) A human placenta-specific ATP-binding cassette gene (ABCP) on chromosome 4q22 that is involved in multidrug resistance. *Cancer Res., 58(23):* 5337-5339.

Backstrom G, Taipalensuu J, Melhus H, Brandstrom H, Svensson AC, Artursson P and Kindmark A (2003). Genetic variation in the ATP-binding cassette transporter gene ABCG2 (BCRP) in a Swedish population. *Eur J Pharm Sci, 18(5):* 359-364.

Bailey-Dell KJ, Hassel B, Doyle LA and Ross DD (2001). Promoter characterization and genomic organization of the human breast cancer resistance protein (ATP-binding cassette transporter G2) gene. *Biochim. Biophys. Acta, 1520(3):* 234-241.

Bennett GC, Felix RA, Chew JE, Richardson PJ and Barrand MA (2001). Use of laser capture microdissection to analyse gene expression at the blood-brain barrier (BBB. *Endothelium, 8(4):* 309.

Bobrowska-Hagerstrand M, Wrobel A, Mrowczynska L, Soderstrom T, Shirataki Y, Motohashi N, Molnar J, Michalak K and Hagerstrand H (2003). Flavonoids as inhibitors of MRP1-like efflux activity in human erythrocytes. A structure-activity relationship study. *Oncol. Res., 13(11):* 463-469.

Borst P and Oude Elferink R (2002) Mammalian ABC transporters in health and disease. *Annu. Rev. Biochem., 71:* 537-592.

Bunting KD (2002). ABC transporters as phenotypic markers and functional regulators of stem cells. *Stem Cells, 20(1):* 11-20.

Burger H, Foekens JA, Look MP, Meijer-van Gelder ME, Klijn JG, Wiemer EA, Stoter G and Nooter K (2003). RNA expression of breast cancer resistance protein, lung resistance-related protein, multidrug resistance-associated proteins 1 and 2, and multidrug resistance gene 1 in breast cancer: correlation with chemotherapeutic response. *Clin. Cancer Res., 9(2):* 827-836.

Chen ZS, Robey RW, Belinsky MG, Shchaveleva I, Ren XQ, Sugimoto Y, Ross DD, Bates SE and Kruh GD (2003). Transport of methotrexate, methotrexate polyglutamates, and 17beta-estradiol 17-(beta-D-glucuronide) by ABCG2: effects of acquired mutations at R482 on methotrexate transport. *Cancer Res., 63(14):* 4048-4054.

Cisternino S, Mercier C, Bourasset F, Roux F and Scherrmann J-M (2004) Expression, up-regulation, and transport activity of the multidrug-resistance protein Abcg2 at the mouse blood-brain barrier. *Cancer Res., 64:* 3296-3301.

Cooray HC, Blackmore CG, Maskell L and Barrand MA (2002). Localisation of breast cancer resistance protein in microvessel endothelium of human brain. *NeuroReport, 13(6):* 2059-2063.

Cooray HC, Janvilisri T, van Veen HW, Hladky SB and Barrand MA (2004). Interaction of the breast cancer resistance protein with plant polyphenols. *Biochem Biophys. Res. Comm., 317(1):* 269-275.

Diestra JE, Scheffer GL, Catala I, Maliepaard M, Schellens JH, Scheper RJ, Germa-Lluch JR and Izquierdo MA (2002). Frequent expression of the multi-drug resistance-associated protein BCRP/MXR/ABCP/ABCG2 in human tumours detected by the BXP-21 monoclonal antibody in paraffin-embedded material. *J. Pathol., 198(2):* 213-219.

Doyle LA and Ross DD (2003). Multidrug resistance mediated by the breast cancer resistance protein BCRP (ABCG2). *Oncogene, 22(47):* 7340-7358.

Doyle LA, Yang W, Abruzzo LV, Krogmann T, Gao Y, Rishi AK and Ross DD (1998). A multidrug resistance transporter from human MCF-7 breast cancer cells. *Proc. Natl. Acad. Sci USA, 95(26):* 15665-15670.

Ee PL, Kamalakaran S, Tonetti D, He X, Ross DD and Beck WT (2004). Identification of a novel estrogen response element in the breast cancer resistance protein (ABCG2) gene. *Cancer Res., 64(4):* 1247-1251.

Eisenblatter T, Huwel S and Galla HJ (2003). Characterisation of the brain multidrug resistance protein (BMDP/ABCG2/BCRP) expressed at the blood-brain barrier. *Brain Res, 971(2):* 221-231.

Faneyte IF, Kristel PM, Maliepaard M, Scheffer GL, Scheper RJ, Schellens JH and van de Vijver MJ (2002). Expression of the breast cancer resistance protein in breast cancer. *Clin Cancer Res, 8(4):* 1068-1074.

Honjo Y, Morisaki K, Huff LM, Robey RW, Hung J, Dean M and Bates SE (2002). Single-nucleotide polymorphism (SNP) analysis in the ABC half-transporter ABCG2 (MXR/BCRP/ABCP1). *Cancer Biol Ther., 1(6):* 696-702.

Hooijberg JH, Broxterman HJ, Scheffer GL, Vrasdonk C, Heijn M, de Jong MC, Scheper RJ, Lankelma J and Pinedo HM (1999). Potent interaction of flavopiridol with MRP1. *Br. J. Cancer, 81(2):* 269-276.

Ifergan I, Shafran A, Jansen G, Hooijberg JH, Scheffer GL and Assaraf YG (2004). Folate deprivation results in the loss of breast cancer resistance protein (BCRP/ABCG2) expression: a role for BCRP in cellular folate homeostasis. *J. Biol. Chem., 279(24):*25527-25534.

Iida A, Saito S, Sekine A, Mishima C, Kitamura Y, Kondo K, Harigae S, Osawa S and Nakamura Y (2002). Catalog of 605 single-nucleotide polymorphisms (SNPs) among 13 genes encoding human ATP-binding cassette transporters: ABCA4, ABCA7, ABCA8, ABCD1, ABCD3, ABCD4, ABCE1, ABCF1, ABCG1, ABCG2, ABCG4, ABCG5, and ABCG8. *J. Hum. Genet., 47(6):* 285-310.

Imai Y, Asada S, Tsukahara S, Ishikawa E, Tsuruo T and Sugimoto Y (2003). Breast cancer resistance protein exports sulfated estrogens but not free estrogens. *Mol. Pharmacol., 64(3):* 610-618.

Imai Y, Nakane M, Kage K, Tsukahara S, Ishikawa E, Tsuruo T, Miki Y and Sugimoto Y (2002a). C421A polymorphism in the human breast cancer resistance protein gene is associated with low expression of Q141K protein and low-level drug resistance. *Mol Cancer Ther., 1(8):* 611-616.

Imai Y, Tsukahara S, Ishikawa E, Tsuruo T and Sugimoto Y (2002b). Estrone and 17beta-estradiol reverse breast cancer resistance protein-mediated multidrug resistance. *Jpn. J. Cancer Res, 93(3):* 231-235.

Janvilisri T, Venter H, Shahi S, Reuter G, Balakrishnan L and van Veen HW (2003). Sterol transport by the human breast cancer resistance protein (ABCG2) expressed in Lactococcus lactis. *J. Biol. Chem., 278(23):* 20645-20651.

Johansson CB, Momma S, Clarke DL, Risling M, Lendahl U and Frisen J (1999). Identification of a neural stem cell in the adult mammalian central nervous system. *Cell, 96:* 25-34.

Jonker JW, Buitelaar M, Wagenaar E, Van Der Valk MA, Scheffer GL, Scheper RJ, Plosch T, Kuipers F, Elferink RP, Rosing H, Beijnen JH and Schinkel AH (2002). The breast cancer resistance protein protects against a major chlorophyll-derived dietary phototoxin and protoporphyria. *Proc. Natl. Acad. Sci. USA, 99(24):* 15649-15654.

Jonker JW, Smit JW, Brinkhuis RF, Maliepaard M, Beijnen JH, Schellens JH and Schinkel AH (2000). Role of breast cancer resistance protein in the bioavailability and fetal penetration of topotecan. *J. Natl. Cancer Inst., 92(20):* 1651-1656.

Kage K, Tsukahara S, Sugiyama T, Asada S, Ishikawa E, Tsuruo T and Sugimoto Y (2002). Dominant-negative inhibition of breast cancer resistance protein as drug efflux pump through the inhibition of S-S dependent homodimerization. *Int. J. Cancer, 97(5):* 626-630.

Kanzaki A, Toi M, Nakayama K, Bando H, Mutoh M, Uchida T, Fukumoto M and Takebayashi Y (2001). Expression of multidrug resistance-related transporters in human breast carcinoma. *Jpn. J. Cancer Res., 92(4):* 452-458.

Kawabata S, Oka M, Shiozawa K, Tsukamoto K, Nakatomi K, Soda H, Fukuda M, Ikegami Y, Sugahara K, Yamada Y, Kamihira S, Doyle LA, Ross DD and Kohno S (2001). Breast cancer resistance protein directly confers SN-38 resistance of lung cancer cells. *Biochem. Biophys. Res. Commun., 280(5):* 1216-1223.

Kim M, Turnquist H, Jackson J, Sgagias M, Yan Y, Gong M, Dean M, Sharp JG and Cowan K (2002). The multidrug resistance transporter ABCG2 (breast cancer resistance protein 1) effluxes Hoechst 33342 and is overexpressed in hematopoietic stem cells. *Clin. Cancer Res., 8(1):* 22-28.

Krishnamurthy P, Ross DD, Nakanishi T, Bailey-Dell K, Zhou S, Mercer KE, Sarkadi B, Sorrentino BP and Schuetz JD (2004). The stem cell marker Bcrp/ABCG2 enhances hypoxic survival through interactions with heme. *J. Biol. Chem., 279(23):*24218-24225.

Kruijtzer CM, Beijnen JH, Rosing H, ten Bokkel Huinink WW, Schot M, Jewell RC, Paul EM and Schellens JH (2002). Increased oral bioavailability of topotecan in combination with the breast cancer resistance protein and P-glycoprotein inhibitor GF120918. *J. Clin. Oncol., 20(13):* 2943-2950.

Lechner A, Leech CA, Abraham EJ, Nolan AL and Habener JF (2002). Nestin-positive progenitor cells derived from adult human pancreatic islets of Langerhans contain side population (SP) cells defined by expression of the ABCG2 (BCRP1) ATP-binding cassette transporter. *Biochem. Biophys Res. Commun., 293(2):* 670-674.

Litman T, Druley TE, Stein WD and Bates SE (2001). From MDR to MXR: new understanding of multidrug resistance systems, their properties and clinical significance. *Cell Mol. Life Sci., 58(7):* 931-959.

Litman T, Jensen U, Hansen A, Covitz KM, Zhan Z, Fetsch P, Abati A, Hansen PR, Horn T, Skovsgaard T and Bates SE (2002). Use of peptide antibodies to probe for the mitoxantrone resistance-associated protein MXR/BCRP/ABCP/ABCG2. *Biochim. Biophys. Acta, 1565(1):* 6-16.

Maliepaard M, Scheffer GL, Faneyte IF, van Gastelen MA, Pijnenborg AC, Schinkel AH, van De Vijver MJ, Scheper RJ and Schellens JH (2001). Subcellular localization and distribution of the breast cancer resistance protein transporter in normal human tissues. *Cancer Res., 61(8):* 3458-3464.

Minderman H, Brooks TA, O'Loughlin KL, Ojima I, Bernacki RJ and Baer MR (2004) Broad-spectrum modulation of ATP-binding cassette transport proteins by the taxane derivatives ortataxel (IDN-5109, BAY 59-8862) and tRA96023. *Cancer Chemother. Pharmacol., 53:* 363-369.

Miwa M, Tsukahara S, Ishikawa E, Asada S, Imai Y and Sugimoto Y (2003). Single amino acid substitutions in the transmembrane domains of breast cancer resistance protein (BCRP) alter cross resistance patterns in transfectants. *Int J Cancer, 107(5):* 757-763.

Miyake K, Mickley L, Litman T, Zhan Z, Robey R, Cristensen B, Brangi M, Greenberger L, Dean M, Fojo T and Bates SE (1999). Molecular cloning of cDNAs which are highly overexpressed in mitoxantrone-resistant cells: demonstration of homology to ABC transport genes. *Cancer Res., 59(1):* 8-13.

Mogi M, Yang J, Lambert JF, Colvin GA, Shiojima I, Skurk C, Summer R, Fine A, Quesenberry PJ and Walsh K (2003). Akt signaling regulates side population cell phenotype via Bcrp1 translocation. *J. Biol. Chem., 278(40):* 39068-39075.

Nakanishi T, Doyle LA, Hassel B, Wei Y, Bauer KS, Wu S, Pumplin DW, Fang HB and Ross DD (2003). Functional characterization of human breast cancer resistance protein (BCRP, ABCG2) expressed in the oocytes of Xenopus laevis. *Mol. Pharmacol., 64(6):* 1452-1462.

Oude Elferink R and Groen AK (2002). Genetic defects in hepatobiliary transport. *Biochim. Biophys. Acta, 1586:* 129-145.

Ozvegy C, Litman T, Szakacs G, Nagy Z, Bates S, Varadi A and Sarkadi B (2001). Functional characterization of the human multidrug transporter, ABCG2, expressed in insect cells. *Biochem. Biophys Res. Commun., 285(1):* 111-117.

Ozvegy C, Varadi A and Sarkadi B (2002). Characterization of drug transport, ATP hydrolysis, and nucleotide trapping by the human ABCG2 multidrug transporter. Modulation of substrate specificity by a point mutation. *J. Biol. Chem., 277(50):* 47980-47990.

Plasschaert SL, van der Kolk DM, de Bont ES, Kamps WA, Morisaki K, Bates SE, Scheffer GL, Scheper RJ, Vellenga E and de Vries EG (2003). The role of breast cancer resistance protein in acute lymphoblastic leukemia. *Clin. Cancer Res., 9(14):* 5171-5177.

Rabindran SK, Ross DD, Doyle LA, Yang W and Greenberger LM (2000). Fumitremorgin C reverses multidrug resistance in cells transfected with the breast cancer resistance protein. *Cancer Res., 60(1):* 47-50.

Rajagopal A and Simon SM (2003) Subcellular localization and activity of multidrug resistance proteins. *Molec Biol. Cell, 14:* 3389-3399.

Reynolds BA and Weiss S (1992) Generation of neurons and astrocytes from isolated cells of the adult mammalian central nervous system. *Science, 255:* 1707-1710.

Robey RW, Honjo Y, Morisaki K, Nadjem TA, Runge S, Risbood M, Poruchynsky MS and Bates SE (2003). Mutations at amino-acid 482 in the ABCG2 gene affect substrate and antagonist specificity. *Br. J. Cancer, 89(10):* 1971-1978.

Robey RW, Medina-Perez WY, Nishiyama K, Lahusen T, Miyake K, Litman T, Senderowicz AM, Ross DD and Bates SE (2001). Overexpression of the ATP-binding cassette half-transporter, ABCG2 (Mxr/BCrp/ABCP1), in flavopiridol-resistant human breast cancer cells. *Clin. Cancer Res., 7(1):* 145-152.

Rocchi E, Khodjakov A, Volk EL, Yang CH, Litman T, Bates SE and Schneider E (2000). The product of the ABC half-transporter gene ABCG2 (BCRP/MXR/ABCP) is expressed in the plasma membrane. *Biochem. Biophys Res. Commun., 271(1):* 42-46.

Ross DD, Yang W, Abruzzo LV, Dalton WS, Schneider E, Lage H, Dietel M, Greenberger L, Cole SP and Doyle LA (1999). Atypical multidrug resistance: breast cancer resistance protein messenger RNA expression in mitoxantrone-selected cell lines. *J. Natl. Cancer Inst., 91(5):* 429-433.

Ross JA and Kasum CM (2002). Dietary flavonoids: bioavailability, metabolic effects, and safety. *Annu. Rev. Nutr., 22:* 19-34.

Scharenberg CW, Harkey MA and Torok-Storb B (2002). The ABCG2 transporter is an efficient Hoechst 33342 efflux pump and is preferentially expressed by immature human hematopoietic progenitors. *Blood, 99(2):* 507-512.

Scheffer GL, Maliepaard M, Pijnenborg AC, van Gastelen MA, de Jong MC, Schroeijers AB, van der Kolk DM, Allen JD, Ross DD, van der Valk P, Dalton WS, Schellens JH and Scheper RJ (2000). Breast cancer resistance protein is localized at the plasma membrane in mitoxantrone- and topotecan-resistant cell lines. *Cancer Res., 60(10):* 2589-2593.

Schellens JH, Maliepaard M, Scheper RJ, Scheffer GL, Jonker JW, Smit JW, Beijnen JH and Schinkel AH (2000). Transport of topoisomerase I inhibitors by the breast cancer resistance protein. Potential clinical implications. *Ann. NY Acad. Sci., 922:* 188-194.

Schinkel AH (1999). P-Glycoprotein, a gatekeeper in the blood-brain barrier. *Adv Drug Deliv Rev, 36(2-3):* 179-194.

Schinkel AH, Kemp S, Dolle M, Rudenko G and Wagenaar E (1993). N-glycosylation and deletion mutants of the human MDR1 P-glycoprotein. *J. Biol. Chem. 268(10):* 7474-81.

Schmitz G, Langmann T and Heimerl S (2001) Role of ABCG1 and other ABCG family members in lipid metabolism. *J. Lipid Res., 42:* 1513-1520.

Schwab M, Eichelbaum M and Fromm MF (2003). Genetic polymorphisms of the human MDR1 drug transporter. *Annu. Rev. Pharmacol Toxicol., 43:* 285-307.

Shimano K, Satake M, Okaya A, Kitanaka J, Kitanaka N, Takemura M, Sakagami M, Terada N and Tsujimura T (2003). Hepatic oval cells have the side population phenotype defined by expression of ATP-binding cassette transporter ABCG2/BCRP1. *Am. J. Pathol., 163(1):* 3-9.

Shiozawa K, Oka M, Soda H, Yoshikawa M, Ikegami Y, Tsurutani J, Nakatomi K, Nakamura Y, Doi S, Kitazaki T, Mizuta Y, Murase K, Yoshida H, Ross DD and Kohno S (2004). Reversal of breast cancer resistance protein (BCRP/ABCG2)-mediated drug resistance by novobiocin, a coumermycin antibiotic. *Int. J. Cancer, 108(1):* 146-151.

Small D (2003). Role of ABC transporters in secretion of cholesterol from liver into bile. *Proc. Natl. Acad. Sci. USA, 100:* 4-6.

Sparreboom A, Danesi R, Ando Y, Chan J and Figg WD (2003). Pharmacogenomics of ABC transporters and its role in cancer chemotherapy. *Drug Resist. Updat, 6(2):* 71-84.

Stam RW, van den Heuvel-Eibrink MM, den Boer ML, Ebus MEG, Janka-Schaub GE, Allen JD and Pieters R (2003). Multidrug resistance genes in infant acute lymphoblastic leukemia: Ara-C is not a substrate for the breast cancer resistance protein. *Leukemia, 18(1):*78-83.

Sugimoto Y, Tsukahara S, Imai Y, Ueda K and Tsuruo T (2003). Reversal of breast cancer resistance protein-mediated drug resistance by estrogen antagonists and agonists. *Mol. Cancer Ther., 2(1):* 105-112.

Summer R, Kotton DN, Sun X, Ma B, Fitzsimmons K and Fine A (2003). Side population cells and Bcrp1 expression in lung. *Am. J. Physiol. Lung Cell Mol. Physiol., 285(1):* L97-104.

Suzuki M, Suzuki H, Sugimoto Y and Sugiyama Y (2003). ABCG2 transports sulfated conjugates of steroids and xenobiotics. *J. Biol. Chem., 278(25):* 22644-22649.

Tamaki T, Akatsuka A, Ando K, Nakamura Y, Matsuzawa H, Hotta T, Roy RR and Edgerton VR (2002). Identification of myogenic-endothelial progenitor cells in the interstitial spaces of skeletal muscle. *J. Cell Biol., 157(4):* 571-577.

van Herwaarden AE, Jonker JW, Wagenaar E, Brinkhuis RF, Schellens JH, Beijnen JH and Schinkel AH (2003). The breast cancer resistance protein (Bcrp1/Abcg2) restricts exposure to the dietary carcinogen 2-amino-1-methyl-6-phenylimidazo[4,5-b]pyridine. *Cancer Res., 63(19):* 6447-6452.

van Loevezijn A, Allen JD, Schinkel AH and Koomen GJ (2001). Inhibition of BCRP-mediated drug efflux by fumitremorgin-type indolyl diketopiperazines. *Bioorg. Med. Chem. Lett., 11(1):* 29-32.

Volk EL and Schneider E (2003). Wild-type breast cancer resistance protein (BCRP/ABCG2) is a methotrexate polyglutamate transporter. *Cancer Res., 63(17):* 5538-5543.

Volk EL, Farley KM, Wu Y, Li F, Robey RW and Schneider E (2002). Overexpression of wild-type breast cancer resistance protein mediates methotrexate resistance. *Cancer Res., 62(17):* 5035-5040.

Wang X, Furukawa T, Nitanda T, Okamoto M, Sugimoto Y, Akiyama S and Baba M (2003). Breast cancer resistance protein (BCRP/ABCG2) induces cellular resistance to HIV-1 nucleoside reverse transcriptase inhibitors. *Mol. Pharmacol., 63(1):* 65-72.

Washington CB, Duran GE, Man MC, Sikic BI and Blaschke TF (1998). Interaction of anti-HIV protease inhibitors with the multidrug transporter P-glycoprotein (P-gp) in human cultures cells. *J. Acquir. Immune Defic. Syndr. Hum. Retrovirol., 19:* 203-209.

Woehlecke H, Osada H, Herrmann A and Lage H (2003). Reversal of breast cancer resistance protein-mediated drug resistance by tryprostatin A. *Int. J. Cancer, 107(5):* 721-728.

Woehlecke H, Pohl A, Alder-Baerens N, Lage H and Herrmann A (2003). Enhanced exposure of phosphatidylserine in human gastric carcinoma cells overexpressing the half-size ABC transporter BCRP (ABCG2). *Biochem J., 376(Pt 2):* 489-495.

Xu J, Liu Y, Yang Y, Bates S and Zhang JT (2004). Characterization of oligomeric human half ABC transporter ABCG2/BCRP/MXR/ABCP in plasma membranes. *J. Biol. Chem., 279(19):*19781-19789.

Yoshikawa M, Kasamatsu S, Yasunaga M, Wang G, Ikegami Y, Yoshida H, Tarui S, Yabuuchi H and Ishikawa T (2002). Does ABCG2 need a heterodimer partner? Expression and functional evaluation of ABCG2 (Arg 482). *Drug Metab. Pharmacokin., 17(2):* 130-135.

Zamber CP, Lamba JK, Yasuda K, Farnum J, Thummel K, Schuetz JD and Schuetz EG (2003). Natural allelic variants of breast cancer resistance protein (BCRP) and their relationship to BCRP expression in human intestine. *Pharmacogenetics, 13(1):* 19-28.

Zhang S and Morris ME (2003). Effects of the flavonoids biochanin A, morin, phloretin, and silymarin on P-glycoprotein-mediated transport. *J. Pharmacol. Exp. Ther., 304(3):* 1258-1267.

Zhang W, Mojsilovic-Petrovic J, Andrade MF, Zhang H, Ball M and Stanimirovic DB (2003). The expression and functional characterization of ABCG2 in brain endothelial cells and vessels. *Faseb J., 17(14):* 2085-2087.

Zhou S, Morris JJ, Barnes Y, Lan L, Schuetz JD and Sorrentino BP (2002). Bcrp1 gene expression is required for normal numbers of side population stem cells in mice, and confers relative protection to mitoxantrone in hematopoietic cells in vivo. *Proc. Natl. Acad. Sci. USA, 99(19):* 12339-12344.

Zhou S, Schuetz JD, Bunting KD, Colapietro AM, Sampath J, Morris JJ, Lagutina I, Grosveld GC, Osawa M, Nakauchi H and Sorrentino BP (2001). The ABC transporter Bcrp1/ABCG2 is expressed in a wide variety of stem cells and is a molecular determinant of the side-population phenotype. *Nat. Med., 7(9):* 1028-1034.

Zhou S, Zong Y, Lu T and Sorrentino BP (2003). Hematopoietic cells from mice that are deficient in both Bcrp1/Abcg2 and Mdr1a/1b develop normally but are sensitized to mitoxantrone. *Biotechniques 35(6):* 1248-52.

Zijlmans JM, Visser JW, Laterveer L, Kleiverda K, Heemskerk DP, Kluin PM, Willemze R and Fibbe WE (1998). The early phase of engraftment after murine blood cell transplantation is mediated by hematopoietic stem cells. *Proc. Natl. Acad. Sci. USA 95(2):* 725-9.

In: Frontiers in Breast Cancer Research
Editor: Louis P. Fortugno, pp. 39-70

ISBN: 978-1-60021-671-8

Chapter II

Androgens and Breast Cancer. The Hyperandrogenic Theory of Breast Cancer: Past, Present and Future

Giorgio Secreto, Elisabetta Venturelli, Patrizia Pasanisi and Franco Berrino
Dept. of Preventive and predictive medicine,
National Cancer Institute, Milan, Italy

Abstract

The hyperandrogenic theory in the pathogenesis of breast cancer was conceived and developed in Milan at the Istituto Nazionale Tumori during the late 1960s and early 1970s, on based on endocrine, histological and clinical data. Patients with breast cancer were found to be frequently associated with high blood androgen levels, atypical endometrial hyperplasia, an index of chronic anovulation, and with ovarian interstitial cells hyperplasia, a finding suggesting that the ovary was the source of androgen excess. Increased amount of androgens and endometrial hyperplasia were also observed in women with hyperplastic alterations of breast epithelium, a condition predisposing to mammary cancer.

Case-control studies in the 1980s gave further substantial support to the theory, and in more recent years, prospective studies have confirmed beyond any doubt that increased testosterone levels are associated with increased risk of breast cancer. The relation with breast cancer was also reported for high levels of estrogens and low levels of sex hormone binding globulin (SHBG), in postmenopausal women, and low levels of progesterone in premenopausal women. Increased risk of breast cancer was also found to be linked with other metabolic and hormonal parameters, such as high levels of insulin, IGF-I, fasting glucose, abdominal obesity. Insulin is known to stimulate androgens synthesis in the ovary and to inhibit SHBG formation in the liver.

Two recent dietary intervention trials, aimed to keep low the insulin levels in the blood, have shown that an appropriate diet significantly reduced the circulating levels of sex hormones, mainly testosterone, both in healthy postmenopausal women (DIANA-1) and in breast cancer patients, who were relapse-free at recruitment (DIANA-2). These findings prove that a high testosterone level, with the associated endocrine-dismetabolic syndrome, is a factor of risk potentially curable with diet and discloses the way for large-scale dietary intervention trials of primary prevention of breast cancer.

In previous papers, we have suggested that women with breast cancer and high values of testosterone in urine were at increased risk of recurrence. More recently, data from the DIANA2 study, after 5 years of follow-up of the cohort, showed a significantly higher progression rate in patients with high serum testosterone levels compared to patients with low levels of the hormone. High value of testosterone seems, therefore, a powerful factor of risk of progressive disease, which can be corrected by diet and, if necessary, by pharmacological treatments.

Introduction

Mammary changes during a woman's life (puberty, reproductive age, menopause) and during each menstrual cycle require balanced stimulation of epithelial, stromal and adipose cells of the breast by several proteic and steroid hormones [1]. A still more subtle regulation is obtained by local production of polypeptide growth factors which can mediate and modulate the steroid action trough autocrine and paracrine mechanisms. Growth factors, steroids and proteic hormones operate in harmonious equilibrium to regulate the normal growth and differentiation of breast cells. The critical role of female sex steroids, estradiol and progesterone, in the development of the mammary gland is well known. The effect of prolactin, insulin, glucocorticoids, thyroid and pituitary hormones is recognised, while a possible role for androgens, other than to be the substrate for the local synthesis of estrogens, has been poorly investigated. This is rather surprising in light of two facts: first, the mammary gland is a cutaneous organ with the same embryological origin of the sweating apocrine glands [2, 3], and the apocrine epithelium is under the government of androgens. Like the skin, the breast is the site of intensive androgen metabolism, and is able to convert testosterone in its more active metabolite, dihydrotestosterone (DHT), which is not aromatizable to estrogen [2]. Isles of apocrine metaplasia are frequently associated with hyperplasia and cancer of the breast [4, 5]. Second, the first onset of breast development in girls occurs about 2 years before the appearance of the menarche, and only with the menarche the cyclic ovarian estrogens production begins. The years preceding menarche are characterised by a sharp increase in adrenal androgens, with the associated appearance of the first pubic and axillaries hairs, and the first enlargement of the breast [6]. At this age adrenal androgens play an important role in inducing hypothalamic changes leading to menarche.

The present review reports the published evidence, largely from our laboratory, that androgen excess is a major endocrine abnormality which characterizes women with breast cancer. We also suggest that androgen excess is indicative of a complex hormonal unbalance that involves estrogen and other hormones and that favours the development of breast cancer and its diffusion.

The Hyperestrogenic Hypotheses

Endogenous estrogens are thought to play a leading role in mammary carcinogenesis, although contrasting evidence of increased estrogenic activity has been reported in women with breast cancer, whether absolute excess of estrogen, excess relative to progesterone or balance between different estrogen fractions [7]. In the past years, several hyperestrogenic hypotheses have been proposed: the hypothesis of the estriol, of the estrone, of the luteal inadequacy, of the estrogen window, of the free-estradiol, of the 16-hydroxylation versus 2-hydroxylation of estradiol, of the total estrogen *plus* progesterone excess just to remember some of the most important [7, 8]. All these hypotheses present some weaknesses and all have been criticised. Several of them have been discarded by the same proponent authors. It should be noted, however, that results from large prospective studies published in the past ten years showed increased risk of breast cancer associated with high serum levels of estrogens. Subsequently in this chapter, we will present extensive data from these studies.

The free estradiol hypothesis is worthy to be mentioned in this context. The hypothesis was proposed in 1981 by Siiteri et al. [9], who found increased levels of free estradiol in breast cancer patients. Sex steroids circulate in the blood stream bound to proteins, aspecifically to albumin and specifically to sex hormone-binding globulin (SHBG). The free fraction of a hormone is the fraction biologically active, and the authors suggested that increased levels of free estradiol could have been responsible for tumour promotion even in the presence of normal concentrations of total estradiol. Results of this study [9] were confirmed by some groups of researchers but not by others, and Siiteri et al. themselves repeated the study in 1986 [10], but were unable to confirm their previous findings and, perhaps prematurely, discarded the hypothesis. It should be noted that estrogen stimulates and androgen inhibits SHBG production [11]. Because testosterone has much higher binding affinity for SHBG than estradiol, it is conceivable that an increased amount of free estradiol is frequently present in hyperandrogenemic women. Thus, the free estradiol hypothesis may be in good agreement with the hyperandrogenic theory.

The luteal inadequacy [12] and the estrogen window hypotheses [13] assumed that the excess of estrogens was not absolute, but relative to low levels of progesterone, in anovulatory and low ovulatory menstrual cycles. However, Grattarola R. in 1964 [14] found that chronic anovulation was frequently present in hyperandrogenic women with breast cancer, and, in more recent years, prospective studies showed that low progesterone levels in the luteal phase were associated with increased risk of breast cancer in premenopausal women [15,16].

The Hyperandrogenic Theory

In apparent contrast to the dominant hyperestrogenic hypotheses, since the late 1960s a possible role for androgens in the pathogenesis of breast cancer was originally claimed from our laboratory based on endocrine, histological and clinical data. According to the theory, androgen excess is the endocrine abnormality that characterizes patients with breast cancer and accounts for a complex hormonal disorder that involves estrogens as well as other hormones and metabolic factors.

The Core of the Theory

The hyperandrogenic theory originated from a study by Grattarola R. [14], who performed endometrial biopsies in the second half of the menstrual cycle in premenopausal patients with breast cancer and in premenopausal normal controls (table 1).

Table 1. Histological characteristic of premenstrual endometrium in breast cancer patients and in healthy controls (Modified from: Grattarola R. *Cancer,* 1964 17, 1119)

Endometrial picture	Patients		Controls	
	N.*	%	N.*	%
Progestational (ovulatory)	15	17.2	45	67.8
Proliferative (anovulatory)	34	39.1	12	28.8
Glandular hyperplasia	9	10.3	2	3.4
Atypical hyperplasia	29	33.3	0	0.0

*N. = number of subjects.

At histological examination, the author observed that glandular hyperplasia or atypical adenomatous hyperplasia, a pattern which affords unquestionable proof of nonovulatory menstrual cycle, was present in 43% of breast cancer patients; another 39% displayed a simple proliferative endometrium, presumptive of a nonovulatory cycle, whereas progestational endometrium, presumptive of an ovulatory cycle, was found only in 17% of patients versus 68% of controls.

The frequent association of endometrial hyperplasia and breast cancer suggested that a common endocrine abnormality should be involved in the pathogenesis of both diseases. Initially, according to a widely accepted opinion, Grattarola hypothesized that continuous ovarian estrogen stimulation, unopposed by progesterone in chronic anovulatory menstrual cycles, had to be considered the hormonal abnormality underlining endometrial hyperplasia and breast cancer, but soon after, new evidence suggested that some other factor should occur to drive the proliferative process started by estrogens towards atypical endometrial hyperplasia and breast cancer. This factor was identified with increased androgen production in a series of papers that we will briefly summarize:

(1) In anovulatory menstrual cycles, atypical endometrial hyperplasia occurred only in the presence of increased androgen excretion values, while anovulatory cycles without increased androgen excretion showed a simple proliferative pattern of the endometrium [17, 18].
(2) Urinary androgen excretion levels were found significantly higher in patients with breast cancer, in patients with atypical endometrial hyperplasia and in patients with endometrial adenocarcinoma than in normal subjects [17-21] (table 2).

(3) Endometrial atypia was to a high degree misdiagnosed as adenocarcinoma in an androgenized woman with polycystic ovarian disease [22] and in another woman with androgen secreting adrenal adenoma [23]. After partial bilateral ovarian resection and monolateral adrenalectomy, respectively, the androgenic activity normalized and the endometrium reverted to a normal progestative pattern.
(4) Increased urinary testosterone levels were associated with well differentiated endometrial adenocarcinoma, whereas in undifferentiated endometrial carcinomas testosterone levels were normal [24].
(5) Patients who showed disease progression 5-15 years after diagnosis of breast cancer had urinary testosterone concentrations significantly higher than patients who did not develop metastases in the same period of time [21].

On these findings, the situation: atypical endometrial hyperplasia *plus* increased androgenic activity was considered representative of hormone dependent breast cancer. Patients with these characteristics were offered oophorectomy, and the histological examination of the removed ovaries, showed, in every case, islets of enlarged hyperplastic interstitial cells [19, 25]. This finding fitted in with previous reports that ovarian interstitial hyperplasia was frequently present in breast cancer patients [26] and that the incidence of positive responses to oophorectomy was higher in patients whose ovaries presented interstitial cells hyperplasia [27].

Table 2. Urinary testosterone excretion values in 3 groups of premenopausal and of postmenopausal subjects: normal controls; patients with endometrial disease; patients with breast cancer (Modified from: Grattarola, R. *Am. J. Obstet. Gynecol.*, 1973 116, 423 and from: Grattarola, R; et al. *Am J Obstet Gynecol*, 1974 121, 169)

PREMENOPAUSAL			POSTMENOPAUSAL		
Subjects	N*	Testosterone μg/24 h (mean±S.E.)	Subjects	N*	Testosterone μg/24 h (mean±S.E.)
Normal controls			Normal controls		
Progestational endometrium	7	5.5±1.3	*Hypotrophic endometrium*	12	7.6±1.46
Endometrial disease			Endometrial disease		
atypical endometrium	11	53.2±11.4	*Endometrial adenocarcinoma*	8	20.1±2.50
Breast cancer			Breast cancer		
Progestational endometrium	9	16.1± 2.1	*hypotrophic endometrium*	8	10.9±3.2
atypical endometrium	10	68.1±13.0	*atypical endometrium*	9	32.1±2.97

*N. = number of subjects.

The interstitial cells of the ovary are physiologically concerned with the synthesis of androgens [28]: their hyperplastic pattern gives anatomical support to the biochemical evidence of increased androgen production in these patients and proves the ovarian origin of the androgen excess, as confirmed by the significant reduction of testosterone excretion values after oophorectomy [19,25]. Before the menopause, ovarian interstitial cells hyperplasia is characteristic of polycystic ovaries, a frequent endocrine abnormality of premenopausal women not always clinically detectable. Such an ovary may be responsible for sterility or sub fertility, a known factor of risk for breast cancer, while pregnancy at early age may correct the functional irregularity, playing a protective role. After the menopause, ovarian follicles disappear while the interstitial compartment of the ovary persists and preserves its steroidogenic activity. If polycystic ovarian disease, even at a mild degree of severity, occurred during the fertile life, at menopause the continuous stimulation of the ovaries by large amounts of gonadotropins may lead to interstitial cells hyperplasia. The later the menopause, the larger the amount of interstitial tissue at its onset. Late menopause is a known factor of risk for breast cancer. Oophorectomy can, therefore, be proposed to hyperandrogenic patients irrespectively of their menopausal status.

Patients with high testosterone excretion values submitted to oophorectomy were subsequently followed up with repeated measurement of urinary androgens. We observed that testosterone levels, which had decreased to normal after surgery, started again to rise some months later, suggesting that adrenal glands were also involved. We offered low-dose short-time dexamethasone (DXM) therapy to these patients and obtained reversion to normal of urinary testosterone values [25], confirming the adrenal origin of androgen increase after oophorectomy.

Further Support to the Theory

The reported studies constitute the "core" of the hyperandrogenic theory, which identifies in the ovarian interstitial cells hyperplasia the source of a hormonal unbalance characterized by increased androgen production (Figure 1).

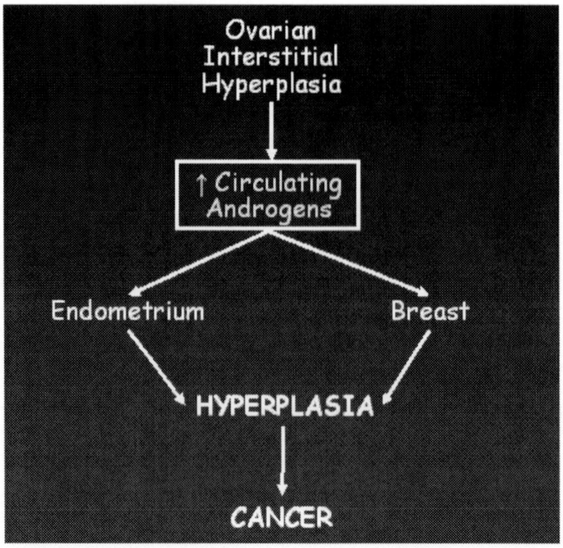

Figure 1. Synopsis of hyperandrogenic theory.

Starting from these premises, we published in the 1980s a series of case–control studies which confirmed and extended the original findings of Grattarola. Some of these studies will be reported in the next section on benign breast disease. Increased levels of circulating testosterone, but not of estradiol, luteinizing hormone, and prolactin, were found in postmenopausal women with breast cancer [29]. In a series of case –control studies [30-32] we found a positive association between risk of breast cancer and androgen concentrations in blood (testosterone, DHT, dehydroepiandrosterone-sulphate (DHEA-S), androstenedione) and in urine (5α-androstan, 3α,17α, diol (androstandiol) and testosterone), both in premenopausal and in postmenopausal women. In premenopausal women, a great increase in risk of subsequent breast cancer was found for low levels of progesterone in one study [30], but we were unable to confirm this finding in a subsequent work on a larger number of subjects [31]. However, the association between low progesterone levels and increased risk of breast cancer has been established in recently published data from prospective studies (see the "Prospective Studies" section).

Relationship between Polycystic Ovary Syndrome (PCOS) and Breast Cancer

According to the theory, polycystic ovaries are responsible for chronic anovulation and increased androgen production in breast cancer patients. We would therefore expect a strong association between PCOS or PCO-like syndromes and increased risk of breast cancer, but the few studies on the argument gave contradictory results, and, in the whole, do not support the expected association [33-38].

In women with PCO, increased risk was suggested only for postmenopausal breast cancer [35], but not for premenopausal cancer [38]. A possible explanation of this finding is that treatment of PCOS was not taken into account in these studies. PCOS and PCO-like syndromes are typical of women at young age, and we believe that when the disease is diagnosed, patients are submitted to treatment with the aim to lower hyperandrogenemia and to induce ovulation. Therapy is usually protracted for many years and it is suspended around the menopausal age. Treatment could be therefore effective in lowering the risk in premenopausal women, during therapy, but, as already mentioned, the ovary is still susceptible to synthesize androgens after the menopause and increased androgen production can occur under stimulation by gonadotropins if treatments performed at a young age had not been able to cure the disease. We think that persistence of polycystic ovaries might be a factor of increased risk for postmenopausal breast cancer, as suggested by Coulam et al [35], although not confirmed by Anderson et al [34]. It should be noted, however, that a great difference exists in the two studies. Coulam et al [35] reported on 1270 patients with documented chronic anovulation syndrome, whereas Anderson et al [34] enrolled women on the basis of a self-administered questionnaire. The prevalence of PCOS in the cohort of Anderson et al was only 1.35%, a rate much lower than expected in a normal population that casts some doubt on the sensitivity of the method used for recruitment.

Androgens in Benign Breast Disease

Mammary epithelial hyperplasia is a recognized factor of risk for breast cancer [39] and is often associated with cancer in the same or in the contralateral breast [40]. Benign and malignant disease of the breast share several factors of risk [41], suggesting a common hormonal cause in the pathogenesis of both diseases. The same hormonal status observed in breast cancer patients, namely anovulatory menstrual cycles, endometrial hyperplasia and increased androgenic activity was also found in patients with benign breast disease [42]. In this study, the urinary excretion values of testosterone and androstandiol were measured in a group of patients with simple moderate hyperplasia of breast epithelium, in a group with marked atypical hyperplasia and in a control group. Considering together the 2 groups of patients, women with breast fibrocystic disease showed significantly higher concentration of both androgens compared with controls (table 3). However, patients with only moderate epithelial hyperplasia had levels of androstandiol significantly higher than normal, whereas patients with atypical hyperplasia presented supranormal levels of testosterone. The author surmised that high levels of androstandiol in patients with moderate epithelial proliferation were suggestive of increased metabolism and conversion of the strong androgen DHT into the weaker androstandiol, resulting in decreased androgenic activity and, as a consequence, in reduced androgenic stimulation in the breast. It is well known that the mammary gland is capable of converting testosterone into its still more active metabolite, DHT, which, in turn, metabolizes to androstandiol, a weak androgen, thereby losing androgenic "aggressiveness". For better comprehension, we report the metabolic pathway of androgens in figure 2.

A role for androgens to drive benign breast disease towards malignancy has been suggested by results of a clinical study, in which the incidence of breast cancer was found 4.5 times higher than expected in women with breast fibrocystic disease treated with androgenic drugs [43].

In a further study [44], we measured urinary testosterone and androstandiol levels in 4 groups of subjects: patients with breast cancer, patients with breast epithelial hyperplasia, women with a family history of breast cancer, and normal controls. We detected a significantly higher amount of testosterone in cancer patients and of androstandiol in hyperplasia patients, compared with the controls. Considering together the two androgens, we found increased levels of testosterone or androstandiol in more than 60% of the cancer group and in about 40% in the hyperplasia group, but only in the 4.7% of familiarity group, a frequency similar to that of controls (3.5%). We concluded that increased androgen excretion is a hormonal abnormality common to benign and malignant breast disease (table 4).

In a subsequent study [45], the blood levels of testosterone, progesterone and SHBG were determined in the second half of the menstrual cycle of patients with breast cancer, of women with breast epithelial hyperplasia, and of normal controls.

In subjects with malignant and with benign breast disease, testosterone values were significantly higher and progesterone levels significantly lower than in controls while SHBG concentrations did not differ among groups (table 5). These data confirmed that in patients with hyperplasia and cancer of the breast, hyperandrogenemia was associated with anovulatory menstrual cycles or luteal inadequacy. Androgen excess together with normal

SHBG concentration also suggested that increased availability of free testosterone was present in these patients.

Table 3. Progestational endometrial pattern and urinary excretion levels of testosterone and androstandiol in normal healthy women and in women with breast epithelial hyperplasia (Modified from: Grattarola, R. *Cancer Res* 1978 38, 3051)

Group	N.*	Testosterone μg/24 mean±SE	Androstandiol μg/24 h mean±SE	Progestational endometrium N.* (%)
Normal	18	6.5±0.8	35.0±3.4	18 (100%)
Hyperplasia	26	17.4±2.3	68.5±8.2	9 (36.6%)

*N. = number of subjects.

Table 4. Urinary excretion values of testosterone and androstandiol and number of cases with increased androgenic activity (i.e. testosterone ≥13.0 μg/24 h or androstandiol ≥60.0 μg/24 h) in 4 groups of subjects: 1. normal controls, 2. women with a family history of breast cancer, 3. women with breast epithelial hyperplasia, 4. women with breast cancer (Modified from: Secreto, G; et. al. *Eur J Cancer Clin Oncol,* 1983 19, 5)

Group	N*	Testosterone μg/24 h (mean ± SD)	Androstandiol μg/24 h (mean ± SD)	Increased Androgen Activity N.*	%	P
Normal	22	6.25±3.48	32.55±20.00	1	4.5	
Familial	21	5.41±3.60	29.38±15.89	1	4.7	NS
Hyperplasia	39	6.97±4.44	47.25±31.0§§	15	38.5	<0.01
Breast cancer	18	11.30±6.78§	44.96±33.90	11	61.1	<0.001

*N. = number of subjects.

§ P<0.01, Breast cancer vs. other groups.

§§ P<0.05, Hyperplasia vs. Normal control.

Table 5. Circulating levels of testosterone, progesterone and SHBG in normal healthy women in patients with breast epithelial hyperplasia and patients with breast cancer (Modified from: Secreto, G; et al. *Cancer Res,* 1984 44, 841)

	Normal		Hyperplasia		Cancer	
	N*	Mean±SD	N	Mean±SD	N.	Mean±SD
Testosterone (ng/ml)	55	0.47±0.16	31	0.55±0.20°	23	0.62±0.22**
Progesterone (ng/ml)	55	17.6±8.11	31	13.90±8.60°	23	11.40±8.0**
SHBG (μg DHT/100ml)	42	2.04±0.48	23	2.33±0.61	14	2.13±0.78

*N. = number of subjects.

° significance Vs controls: p<0.05.

* significance Vs controls: p<0.005.

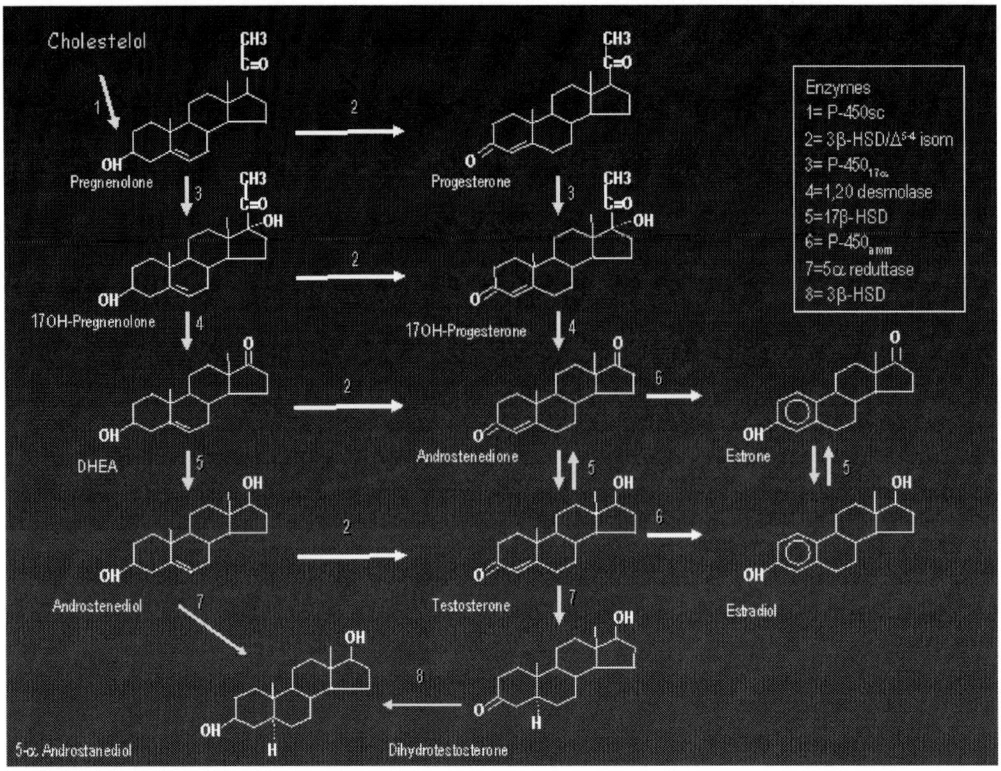

Enzymes:
1= P-450sc=20-22 desmolase
2= 3β-HSD/Δ5-4 isom= 3β-hydroxy steroid dehydrogenase/ /Δ5-4 isomerase
3= P-450 17α= 17α hydroxylase
4=1,20 desmolase
5=17β-HSD= 17 β-hydroxy steroid dehydrogenase
6= P-450arom = aromatase
7=5α reduttase
8=3β-hydroxy steroid dehydrogenase

Figure 2. Sex steroid metabolic pathway.

Androgen Levels as a Marker of Response to Therapeutic Oophorectomy

In an observational study, we divided patients with metastatic breast cancer into 3 groups according to androgen levels, normal or above normal, and to type of treatment, oophorectomy alone or oophorectomy plus DXM [25]. According to data of our laboratory, testosterone values higher than 13.0 μg/24 h or androstandiol values higher than 60.0 μg/24 h were considered above normal. Remission of metastases was more frequent and long-lasting in the group of patients with high testosterone values treated with oophorectomy and DXM. This finding was subsequently confirmed on a larger number of patients [46] (table 6) and led to a study, in which the ability to anticipate the clinical response to oophorectomy was contemporarily evaluated for the estrogen receptor (ER) content of the tumour (positive or negative) and for the amount of urinary androgens (normal or supranormal) (both the laboratories and the clinicians were blind) [47]. Results of this study, which have been later confirmed on a larger number of cases [48], showed that both ER and urinary androgens were able to predict the outcome to treatment with about the same ability (table 7).

Table 6. Objective remission of metastases after oophorectomy alone or oophorectomy plus dexamethasone in 133 patients with advanced breast cancer (Modified from: Secreto, G; et al *Endocrine-Related Cancer,* 1984 14, 55)

Groups	Treatment			Remission
		N.*	N.	%
1. Normal androgens	oophorectomy	61	16	26.2
2. High androgens**	oophorectomy	46	25	54.3
3. High androgens	oophorectomy +DXM	26	24	92.3

*N. = number of subjects.

** Testosterone ≥13.0 µg/24 h or androstandiol ≥60.0 µg/24 h.

Table 7. Evaluation of clinical response to oophorectomy in patients with advanced breast cancer according to the estrogen receptor content of metastases (ER+ present, ER- absent) and urinary androgen excretion levels normal (A-) or above normal (A+). (Modified from: Oriana, S; et al. *Breast Cancer Res. Treat*, 1982 2, 101)

Groups**	Patients		Remission		Progression
	N*.	N*.	%	N*.	%
A+	24	15	62.5	9	37.5
A-	29	8	27.6	21	72.4
ER+	38	20	52.6	18	47.4
ER-	24	5	20.8	19	79.2

*N. = number of subjects.

**A+ = testosterone ≥13.0 µg/24h or androstandiol ≥60.0 µg/24h); ER+ >5fmoles/mg protein.

Table 8. Relationship between clinical response to oophorectomy, ER content of metastases and urinary androgen excretion in 50 breast cancer patients with metastatic disease (Modified from: Oriana, S; et al. *Breast Cancer Res. Treat*, 1987 9, 201)

Group**	Remission		Months of remission		
	N.*	%	Mean	Median	Range
ER+A+	14/16	87.5	28.8	14.0	19-58
ER+A-	10/15	66.7	11.9	9.0	7-30
ER-A+	5/10	50.0	16.2	18.0	10-33
ER-A-	0/ 9				

*N. = number of subjects.

** A+ = testosterone levels ≥13.0 µg/24h or androstandiol levels≥60.0 µg/24h; ER+ >5fmoles/mg protein.

Interestingly, 90% of patients with ER positive and supranormal androgen levels showed remission of metastases, whereas none of the 9 patients with ER negative and normal androgen levels benefited from oophorectomy [49] (table 8).

Testosterone as a Marker of Recurrence in Operable Breast Cancer

We have already reported in a previous section (The core of the theory) that persistence of hyperandrogenemia is associated with cancer recurrence even many years after diagnosis of the primary tumour [21].

In a subsequent study, urinary testosterone excretion was measured in 80 women with early breast cancer after mastectomy and in 93 women with advanced disease before therapeutic oophorectomy [50]. Supranormal testosterone values (>13.0 μg/24 h) were detected in 18% and in 31% of patients with early and advanced cancer, respectively. The nearly twice frequency of high testosterone excretors in the advanced disease group let us to suggest that the risk of disease progression in patients with supravalues of testosterone is about twice the risk of normal excretors [50]. Remission of metastases after oophorectomy was observed in 59% of high testosterone excretors and in 32% of normal excretors. After oophorectomy, testosterone concentration decreased significantly only in the high excretors group, suggesting that the ovary was the source of increased androgen production. No change in testosterone levels was observed in normal excretors. We concluded that supranormal testosterone excretion in premenopausal breast cancer patients was associated with 2 paradoxical effects: increased risk of post-mastectomy recurrence and higher remission rate after oophorectomy [50].

In 1993 [51], we reported on 70 premenopausal and 43 postmenopausal women with operable breast cancer, followed up for 5 years after primary surgical treatment of the disease. Urinary testosterone levels were repeatedly measured in each patient, who was considered "high excretor" when testosterone values were in the upper tertile of the distribution for premenopausal and postmenopausal patients, in at least 2 out of the first 3 measurements (pre-surgery, post-surgery, at six months).

Incidence of relapse in node-negative patients was too small to carry out any statistical analysis. In premenopausal node-positive patients, the rate of recurrence as function of testosterone levels was 77% in high vs. 28% in normal excretors ($p < 0.006$). The picture in postmenopausal node-positive patients was similar, 54% vs. 11%, but the difference was not statistically significant. We concluded that urinary testosterone was a prognostic indicator of early breast cancer recurrence in node-positive patients (table 9).

Recently published data from a dietary intervention study [52] convincingly support the role of testosterone as a marker of prognosis in early breast cancer. One hundred and ten postmenopausal breast cancer patients without clinical evidence of recurrence participated in the study and offered samples of blood for hormone analysis at baseline and at the end of the one year dietary intervention. After 5.5 years of follow-up, 31 patients showed progressive disease, either distant metastases, or local recurrence, or contralateral breast cancer. Progressions occurred in a substantially higher number of patients in the upper tertile of testosterone values compared with patients in the lower tertile of the hormone (HR=7.2; 95%

CI=2.4-24.4). Interestingly, comparing basal and final testosterone determinations, disease progression occurred in 20 of the 39 patients whose testosterone values persisted above the median value of 0.4 ng/ml, but only in 2 of 13 patients (HR=0.15, 95% CI=0.03-0.71 %) with high testosterone levels at baseline, which decreased under the median at the end of the dietary intervention (table 10).

Table 9. Distribution of recurrences after 5 years of follow-up in node-positive (N+) and node-negative (N-) patients according to testosterone levels (Modified from: Ballerini, P; et al. *Breast Cancer Res. Treat,* 1993 26, 1)

	N^+ PATIENTS*			N^- PATIENTS*		
	All	A+**	A-	All	A+	A-
Premenopausal	11/34	5/7	6/27	5/36	2/10	3/26
Postmenopausal	15/25	8/9	7/16	5/18	1/7	4/11
Total	26/59	13/16	13/43	10/54	3/17	7/37

*Number of relapsed/total number of patients.

**A+ = premenopause: testosterone levels > 8.0 μg/24h postmenopause: testosterone levels > 4.9 μg/24h.

Table 10. Distribution of recurrences over 5.5 years of follow-up according to serum testosterone levels before and after one-year of androgen lowering diet (Modified from Berrino, F; et al. *Int. J. Cancer,* 2005 113, 499)

Baseline	1-year	Disease free	Any recurrence**	Total	Hazard ratio (95% C.I)
High*	High	19	20^{ab}	39	1 (reference)
High	Low	11	2^{a}	13	0.15 (0.03-0.71)
Low	High	2	1	3	1.01 (0.13-7.81)
Low	Low	46	6b	52	0.15 (0.06-0.39)

*High= above the median value of 0.4 ng/ml.

** local, distant, contralateral.

Further evidence of testosterone as a marker of cancer progression derives from the yet unpublished data [A, Micheli, et al, Plasma Testosterone and Prognosis of Postmenopausal Breast Cancer Patients, submitted] of the analysis of 194 postmenopausal breast cancer patients who participated in the control group of a previous study of our Institute set up to evaluate the effect of fenretinide on the occurrence of contralateral breast cancer [53].

Results of these reports, although convincing, are based on a relative small number of subjects and need to be confirmed. For this purpose, we have set up a study specifically designed with a statistical power suitable to conclusively assess the role of endogenous testosterone as a predictor of breast cancer progression. In addition, we will investigate the prognostic value of estrogens, measured only in postmenopausal subjects, and of other androgens.

Androgen Receptors

The role of ER and progesterone receptors (PgR), as independent prognostic parameters, to identify patients who will benefit from hormonal treatment is well recognised [54]. Conversely, little is known about the role of androgen receptors (AR) and their prognostic value in breast carcinoma. AR were found in 50-90% of infiltrating breast tumours [55-59] and have also been detected in the majority of *in situ* carcinomas [59, 60]. AR has been associated with longer survival in operable disease [56, 61, 62] and with favourable response to hormonal therapy (tamoxifen) in advanced disease [56].

A strong positive correlation has been reported among the presence of AR, ER, and PgR in breast tumours [57, 63-65], however AR were also found in a significant number of ER and PgR negative tumours [59]. A new class of breast tumours was recently identified by microarray analysis of gene expression and was termed "molecular apocrine tumours", for their apocrine features at histological examination [66]. These tumours are ER negative/AR positive, frequently show ERBB2 amplification and represent the 8-14% of breast cancers [66]. Another recently published paper describes a subset of ER negative/PgR negative tumours, which paradoxically express genes usually expressed in ER positive breast cancers. These tumours are AR positive and respond to androgens for their growth [67].

The association found between AR and HER2/ neu [59, 66] is of particular interest. HER2/ neu is a protein codified by the ERBB2 gene, which belongs to the epidermal growth factor (EGF) receptor family. EGF receptor after binding to its ligand stimulates cells proliferation and differentiation [68-71]. Overexpression of HER2/ neu was found in about 30% of metastatic breast cancer and is considered a negative prognostic factor [68].

Regulation by androgens of EGF production has been shown already many years ago in mouse submandibular salivary gland [72, 73]. Salivary glands are specialised apocrine glands of cutaneous origin, the same embryological origin of the breast [74, 75]. Apocrine epithelium is under the influence of androgens and it is an active site for conversion of weak androgen precursors into more active compounds [74, 76]. Apocrine metaplasia is frequently present in the breast of women with mammary cancer [5, 4 77], and, in analogy to what has been observed in animals, androgens are thought to induce EGF secretion in apocrine cells of the human breast [4,5, 77-80]. Stimulation of EGF by androgens in humans is further supported by the finding of very high concentrations of EGF in prostate fluid, seminal fluid and sweat [81].

In conclusion, contemporary presence of AR, ER and PgR in breast cancer suggests that sex steroids act in concert in the growth regulation of mammary tumors. Existence of AR positive ER negative tumours, the prognostic value of AR and the association of AR with HER2/ *neu* indicate that a subpopulation of androgen dependent breast cancer exists.

Intratumour Concentrations of Sex Steroids

The aptitude of breast tumours to produce hormones is well recognized, and it is assumed that local production can influence the endocrine environment of the breast itself, thus playing a role in cancer development. The intratumour concentration of estrogens has been extensively studied, and was found substantially higher compared with circulating levels [82-84]. Significantly higher concentrations in tumour than in blood have also been observed for weak androgens (5-androsten-3β, 17β-diol (androstenediol), dehydroepiandrosterone (DHEA) and androstenedione), which can provide a substrate for the conversion to estrogens [58, 82, 85, 86]. Little interest has been given to the study of strong androgens, and only few papers dealt with intratumour concentrations of testosterone [83, 87, 88] and of its not aromatizable metabolite, DHT [87, 88]. The intratissue amount of DHT was significantly higher than in blood, in both the studies that measured this hormone, with a tissue/plasma ratio of 3. A strong positive, highly statistically significant, correlation between testosterone and DHT ($r = 0.71$) has been reported in both these studies [87, 88]. The tissue/plasma ratio of testosterone was found to vary widely, from 0.05 to 5.0 in one report [83] and from 0.3 to 4.0 in another study [88], suggesting that testosterone levels in a subgroup of tumours are substantially higher than in the blood but in another subgroup are lower. In a subsequent paper [89], we compared tumour and circulating levels of testosterone, DHT and estradiol in 2 groups of postmenopausal patients divided according to their age, under or over 70 years, and we found that a testosterone tissue/plasma ratio lower than 1 was characteristic of the older patients. We also observed a significant decrease in the intratumour concentrations of DHT in the older group, suggesting reduced 5α-reductase activity in these tumours. No significant difference between groups was observed for estradiol levels. We concluded that the hormonal environment of the tumour differs between younger and older postmenopausal patients, and that the difference mainly involves the intratumour amounts of androgens.

The mechanisms of action of androgens in regulation of breast cells proliferation has been widely debated and it is still an argument of discussion. However three mechanisms are commonly accepted and are briefly summarized in figure 3. An extensive description has been reported in the review by Liao et al [90] (Figure 3).

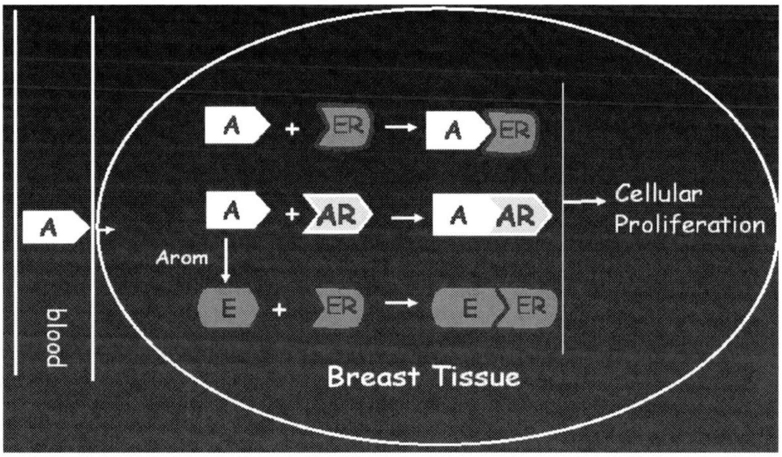

1. Interaction with specific receptors. 2.binding to estrogen receptor to elicit estrogenic effects on breast cells. 3. local aromatization of androgens into estrogens which, ultimately, would be the effectors of cell proliferation.

A= androgens; E= estrogens; arom= aromatase enzyme; AR= androgen receptor; ER= estrogen receptor.

Figure 3. Mechanisms of action of androgens in breast tissue.

Confirmation Studies

Besides our studies, most of the case-control studies in the literature reported testosterone levels higher than normal in breast cancer patients [see for review ref 91]. Testosterone levels were also found to be higher in healthy Caucasian women, a population at high risk for breast cancer, than in healthy Japanese [92] and Chinese [93, 94] women, populations at low risk for breast cancer. In the Chinese group the amount of testosterone was positively correlated with mortality for breast cancer [94].

Increased androgen levels in breast cancer patients seem therefore well documented. The question arises whether hyperandrogenemia is merely associated with breast cancer appearance or whether androgen excess precedes the clinical onset of the disease. Pre-existence of the endocrine abnormality would be of great importance to a select a group of healthy women at increased risk of cancer for a factor potentially curable such as hyperandrogenism. The association of increased androgen levels with ovarian interstitial cell hyperplasia [19, 20, 25], a characteristic that resembles polycystic ovaries, and the finding of increased androgen levels in women with hyperplasia of breast epithelium [42, 44, 45], a known factor of risk for breast cancer, indirectly suggest that the endocrine abnormality is present before the appearance of the tumour. However, unequivocal evidence could only derive by prospective studies.

In a publication of 1983, we reported our clinical observation of six breast cancer occurrences in women whose androgen levels were measured 17 to 69 earlier. Each of them showed excretion values of either testosterone or androstandiol or both higher than normal suggesting that androgen excess is a factor of risk which can be detected before the development of cancer [95]. This was a simple clinical observation, however we like to consider this paper as a sort of precursor of the large epidemiological prospective studies, which will be reported in the next section.

Prospective Studies

Starting from the second half of the 1990s, results from several prospective studies on the association between hormones and breast cancer in postmenopausal women [96] confirmed beyond any doubt that increased testosterone levels are associated with an increased risk of breast cancer. In addition to testosterone, the association with breast cancer was also reported for high levels of other androgens (androstenedione, DHEA, DHEA-S), for high levels of estrogens (estradiol, free-estradiolo, estrone, estrone sulphate) and for low levels of SHBG [96]. The observed association was independent of circulating estradiol These findings have been recently confirmed in the large cohort of the European Prospective Investigation into Cancer and Nutrition (EPIC) study [97] (table 11).

Consistent with the elevation in risk with increasing level of endogenous testosterone shown in these studies, women using testosterone as a part of postmenopausal hormone treatment have a significantly increased risk of invasive breast cancer [98]. These results are also consistent with studies showing that menopause hormonal treatment with synthetic 19-

nor-testosterone derived progestagens are associated with greater risk of breast cancer compared with those with natural (micronized) progesterone [99].

Only few studies investigated the relation between sex hormones and breast cancer in premenopausal women. No association with risk could be found for estrogens [100], possibly for the large intra-individual variation in hormone levels during the menstrual cycle. With regard to the androgens, a study conducted in our Institute (ORDET, Hormones and Diet) [15] showed increased risk of cancer associated with high levels of testosterone. Interestingly, a statistically significant risk was also found for low levels of progesterone. It should be noted that participants in ORDET provided blood samples between the 20th and 24th day after the start of their last menstrual flow, thus allowing to measure progesterone concentration, presumably, in the second half of the cycle. Finding of increased risk for testosterone levels and low progesterone levels, has been recently confirmed on a large number of subjects in the EPIC study [16] (table 12).

Table 11. Breast cancer risk according to circulating sex hormones and SHBG of postmenopausal women (677 cases and 1309 controls) within European Prospective Investigation into Cancer and Nutrition (EPIC) (Modified from Kaaks, A; et al. *Endocr Relat Cancer,* 2005 12, 1071)

	RR: 5° vs. 1°quintile		
	RR	95% CI	P trend
Free Testosterone	2.50	1.76-3.55	<0.0001
Testosterone	1.85	1.33-2.57	<0.0001
Androstenedione	1.94	1.40-2.69	<0.0001
DHEAS	1.69	1.23-2.33	0.0002
SHBG	0.61	0.44-0.84	0.004
Estrone	2.07	1.42-3.02	<0.0001
Estradiol	2.07	1.42-3.02	<0.0001
Free Estradiol	2.13	1.52-2.98	<0.0001

Further analyses of these prospective studies and other studies took into account several parameters which can be considered representative of the metabolic syndrome. In particular, increased risk of breast cancer [101,103] or breast cancer recurrences [102] was found for high levels of insulin, IGF-I, [104-108], fasting glucose [105], and for abdominal obesity [109, 110]. Hyperinsulinemia, consequent to insulin resistance, is known to stimulate androgens synthesis in the ovary and to inhibit SHBG formation in the liver [111], thus these findings could well be included to support the hyperandrogenic theory. Insulin itself has well recognised growth promoting effects [112, 113] and, in addition, it stimulates IGF-I proliferative activity in cells [114]. Growth hormone (GH) is the main regulator of IGF-I levels in the blood, although insulin and nutritional factors also have a role. In turn, the biological activity of IGF-I is modulated by the IGF-I binding proteins (IGFBPs) [115], two of which, IGFBP1 and IGFBP2 are synthesised in the liver under the control of insulin. The first prospective results on IGF-I and BC suggested that the association was present only in premenopausal women [105-107] but recently published studies [116,117], suggested that the relationship with age is more complex [116] showing an association with post-menopausal breast cancer [117].

Table 12. Breast cancer risk according to circulating sex hormones and SHBG of premenopausal women (370 cases and 726 controls) within European Prospective Investigation into Cancer and Nutrition (EPIC) (Modified from Kaaks, A; et al. *J Natl Cancer Inst,* 2005 97, 755)

	RR: 4° vs. 1°quartile			Cases younger than 50 years		
	RR	95% CI	P trend	OR	95% CI	P trend
Testosterone	1.73	1.16-2.57	0.01	2.22	(1.18-4.18)	0.02
Androstenedione	1.56	1.05-2.32	0.01	1.92	1.06-3.45	0.04
DHEAS	1.48	1.02-2.14	0.10	2.00	1.14-3.51	0.02
SHBG	0.95	0.65-1.40	0.72			
Estrone	1.16	0.72-1.85	0.46			
Estradiol	1.01	0.66-1.55	0.89			
Progesterone	0.61	0.38-0.98	0.06	0.52	0.28-0.95	0.4

Several studies suggested that the metabolic and anthropometric factors defining the metabolic syndrome [118] are associated with increased BC risk: hypertension [119, 120], low plasma HDL [121], high triglycerides [122-124] and high glucose [105]. Although the evidence of the link of the metabolic syndrome with breast cancer risk is not univocal, yet data from the literature give convincing support to the role of insulin resistance in the development of the disease. As a consequence, dietary intervention trials aimed to keep low the insulin levels in the blood might be useful to correct the endocrine abnormalities, namely hyperinsulinemia, hyperandrogenemia and increased IGF-I activity, thus protecting from the disease.

Dietary Intervention Trials. The DIANA (Diet and Androgens) Studies

A new dimension on the role of androgens in breast cancer was obtained by two recently performed randomized controlled studies of dietary intervention [125, 126]. The studies showed that a diet aimed to keep low the circulating insulin concentration was appropriate to reduce the circulating levels of sex hormones, mainly testosterone, both in healthy postmenopausal women [125] and in postmenopausal breast cancer patients, who were relapse-free at recruitment [126].

The dietary intervention has been described in detail [125], and can be summarized as follows:

(1) Increased consumption of low-glycemic-index food, and of monounsaturated and n-3 polyunsaturated fatty acids.
(2) Decreased consumption of refined carbohydrates and total and saturated fat.

(3) Augmented intake of phytoestrogens-rich foods, including soy products, legumes, flax and other seeds, and cruciferous vegetables.

The DIANA 1 Study

Three hundred and twelve healthy postmenopausal women agreed to take part in the study. The 104 subjects with circulating testosterone levels in the upper tertile of the distribution (>0.38 ng/ml) were randomized into an intervention and a control group (52 women each). Blood samples for hormonal and biochemical examinations were obtained at baseline and 4.5 months later, at the end of the study.

Main findings were a significant decrease in testosterone levels and a significant increase in SHBG concentrations in the intervention group. Estradiol levels also decreased but not significantly compared with the control group. A significant decrease was also observed for body weight, fasting glycaemia and for the total area under the insulin curve during oral glucose tolerance test [125]. A subsequent paper [127] reported a significant increase for serum levels of IGFBP1, IGFBP2 and GH binding protein and a significant decrease of C-peptide, whereas no change was observed in the serum levels of IGF-I (table 13)

Table 13. Effects of a 4,5 months of hypoglycemizing dietary intervention on biochemical and hormonal levels: the DIANA 1 study (Modified from Berrino. F; et al. . *Cancer Epidemiol Biomarkers Prev,* 2001 10, 25)

	% Change	P*		% Change	P*
SHBG	+25.2	0.0001	Glycaemia	-5.7	0.026
Testosterone	-18.3	0.004	Glycemic area	+4.8	0.85
Estradiol	-18.0	0.13	Growth hormone	+54.2	0.22
Free Testosterone	-28.6	<.0001	GHBP	+29.1	0.002
Free Estradiol	-23.4	0.05	IGF-1	-5.9	0.64
Insulin	-10.4	0.14	IGFBP-1	+12.2	0.015
Insulinemic area	-7.7	0.04	IGFBP-2	+30.4	0.0004
C-peptide	-19.1	0.03	IGFBP-3	-4.5	0.21

*P value of the statistical difference of mean change in the intervention group compared to control.

The DIANA 2 Study

The dietary intervention was applied to 114 postmenopausal women with breast cancer, who were disease free at recruitment [126]. Forty one of them were under tamoxifen adjuvant treatment. After an initial period of 3 months in which women were randomized into an intervention and a control group, all the patients followed the same diet up to the end of the study period (12 months), and showed a significant reduction in serum testosterone, fasting insulin, fasting glycaemia, cholesterol (total and LDL), triglycerides and body weight. Changes were less marked and not statistically significant in patients under tamoxifen treatment, while the effect in patients without tamoxifen was similar to that observed in women of the DIANA 1.

An interesting finding of the DIANA 2 study was the evidence of the role of testosterone as a marker of recurrence in women with early breast cancer, which we have already described in the previous section of "testosterone as a marker of recurrence in operable breast cancer" [52]. In addition, increased risk of cancer recurrence was also found for the presence of metabolic syndrome at baseline (RR=3.0, 95% CI 1.2-7.1). Combining the two parameters (metabolic syndrome and serum testosterone), the adjusted hazard ratio of recurrence among women with metabolic syndrome and testosterone levels higher than 0.40 ng/ml (median value) was 6.7 (95% CI 2.3-19.8) compared with that among women without metabolic syndrome and testosterone levels < or =0.40 ng/ml. The results suggest that the metabolic syndrome may be an important prognostic factor for breast cancer [128].

In conclusion, results of the DIANA studies indicate that a comprehensive change in diet is successful to improve the endogenous hormone metabolism which might eventually result in decreased risk of breast cancer in healthy women, and decreased risk of recurrence in patients with early disease.

Conclusion

Most of the known factors of risk for breast cancer, as familiarity, age at menarche, age at menopause, are not accountable for correction [129]. Other factors of risk, like anticipation of the first pregnancy at early age or increased number of children [129], are not socially sustainable. Only for nursing we can recommend a tenable preventive advice, but the benefit is certainly fairly small.

Finding of a powerful and potentially curable factor of risk is critical for planning both a primary prevention trial and clinical trials for optimization of standard treatments, or for testing new pharmacological approaches. Measurement of serum testosterone levels can be usefully employed for this purpose. Additional evaluation of other sex steroids and search for the presence of the metabolic syndrome may be helpful to identify subjects in the general population at increased risk of cancer and patients with early breast cancer at increased risk of relapse.

The Past

Taken together, results of case-control and prospective studies confirm that a complex hormonal disorder, involving both androgen and estrogen, favours the development of breast cancer and its progression. Usually androgen and estrogen are considered hormones with antagonistic actions, but it is true only in part. Hyperandrogenemia and hyperestrogenemia are often associated in the same patient and both concur to the full clinical outcome of endocrine disorders, as in the case of the PCO syndrome, a hyperandrogenic syndrome in which high estrogen levels are frequently present, or in the case of the upper body type (android) obesity in which testosterone and estradiol levels are both higher than in the lower body type (gynoid) obesity [130].

The reported examples suggest that hyperandrogenemia and hyperestrogenemia may be expressions of the same endocrine abnormality. We think, however, that hyperandrogenemia, associated with PCO-like abnormalities, can be easily detected at any time during a woman's life, whereas estrogen circulating levels are submitted to cyclical variations in menstruating women and are often under the sensitivity of the method in postmenopausal women. Together with hormonal unbalance, discovery of the metabolic syndrome may be useful to better categorize women at increased risk of breast cancer.

The Present

Therapeutic strategies for breast cancer take into account only the pathological features (grade, loco-regional nodes, pT) and the hormone receptor characteristic (ER, PgR, HER-2) of the tumour [54]. It should be stressed that hormone-dependence of the tumour is only a side, although of great importance, of a more general endocrine abnormality of women bearing cancer. Such an abnormality should be searched for and, possibly, corrected in each patient. In other words, together with the evaluation of the hormone-dependence of the tumour we should also characterize breast cancer patients, with particular reference to their endocrine and metabolic condition. We suggest that detection of hyperandrogenemia and of the metabolic syndrome is a useful tool to drive towards personalized treatments of women with breast cancer. Discovery of increased androgenic activity and of the metabolic syndrome is also suitable to select a group of otherwise healthy women at increased risk of breast cancer to submit to preventive interventions.

The Future

Cancer growth largely depends on the endocrine environment in which the tumour develops. We suggest that evaluation of androgenic activity lets us plan therapies with the double objective to treat breast cancer and, contemporarily, to correct the basic hormonal abnormality, thus reducing the probability of recurrences. We can also program an adequate endocrine follow-up, because androgen measurement can be repeated at any time we think necessary, contrary to the evaluation of the receptor content of the tumour. The same reasoning done for hyperandrogenemia can be applied to the metabolic syndrome, which is often associated with increased androgenic activity [131].

Obviously, hormonal and biological characterization of breast cancer patients adds information but do not substitute the pathological and endocrine features of the tumour to drive therapy.

Treatment of Advanced Disease

In hyperandrogenemic patients, medical (or surgical) oophorectomy is the first choice therapy and should be proposed independently from the menopausal status of the patient. Ovarian suppression will be associated with anti-estrogen or anti-aromatase drugs in women with ER positive tumours. Patients will be followed-up with repeated examination of circulating androgens, mainly testosterone, and short term-low-dose DXM treatment (1.5 mg of DXM a day for 30 days) will be administered every time testosterone levels increase over the cut off value, which we fixed at 0.4 ng/ml, in our laboratory. This corresponds to the median value in postmenopausal breast cancer patients and to the upper quartile in healthy postmenopausal women. In the presence of the metabolic syndrome, a suitable dietary intervention will be associated.

Adjuvant Therapies of Early Breast Cancer

Several randomized trials comparing medical oophorectomy (GnRH analogs) with classical CMF treatment [132-135] have shown similar results with both therapies in early breast cancer patients. It seems logical to suppose that better selection of patients to submit to endocrine treatments will lead to enhanced efficacy of the therapy, and to improved quality of life, without the adverse effects of chemotherapy. The same treatments proposed for the advanced disease can be also proposed in the early disease.

Primary Prevention of Breast Cancer

The opportunity to select a subgroup of otherwise healthy women at increased risk of breast cancer for metabolic and hormonal abnormalities, together with the ability to reverse to normal such abnormalities through a comprehensive change in diet (DIANA studies) [125-126] open the way to primary prevention. Dietetic approach is certainly physiological and virtually devoid from dangerous effects, however, it could be insufficient in some women. In the presence of hyperandrogenemia, diet should be associated with the usual hormonal treatments of increased androgen production: namely, induction of ovulation in women who wish pregnancy, and suppression of ovarian activity with antiandrogens and oral contraceptives in women who do not desire to become pregnant. It should be noted, however, that oral contraceptives, although reducing hyperandrogenemia, are ineffective on the other accompanying endocrine-metabolic anomalies such as insulin resistance [136]. The combination of antiandrogens with insulin sensitizers represents a new interesting approach to the treatment of hyperinsulinemic hyperandrogenism which seems to achieve the best control of the endocrine-metabolic abnormalities in women with PCOS [137, 138].

Whatever the treatment chosen, control of hyperandrogenemia and the associated metabolic syndrome seems the main objective to achieve for primary prevention of breast cancer. Large-scale intervention studies on diet and pharmacological treatments in women at increased risk of breast cancer are urgently needed to define the best approach to prevention.

In conclusion, we have reported in this review the evidence on the role of androgen excess on development and spread of breast cancer. The original findings of Grattarola, published already 40 years ago, were not deprived of their value during the years but, on the contrary, found substantial support in case-control studies and, more recently, obtained unequivocal confirmation in large prospective studies.

We think the time has arrived to turn to more personal treatments of breast cancer through a better selection of patients with endocrine abnormalities. We also suggest that detection of AR and HER2/ neu should be routinely performed to improve the hormonal characterization of the tumour.

The frequent association of hyperandrogenemia with the metabolic syndrome, and discovery that an appropriate change in diet is effective to revert to normal the endocrine and the metabolic disorder open a new prospective to the treatment and prevention of breast cancer.

References

[1] Broiling, F; Oak, T. Growth control and differentiation in mammary epithelial cells. *Envirom. Health Prospect.* 1989 80, 85-89.

[2] Miller, WR; Telford, J. Dixon, JM; Shivas, AA; Androgen metabolism and apocrine differentiation in human breast cancer. *Breast Cancer Res. Treat.* 1985 5, 67-73.

[3] Osborne, MP. Diseases of the Breast:. In: Harris J.R, Lippman M.E., Morrow M., Hellman S. (eds). *Breast development and anatomy.*Diseases of the Breast. Lippincot-Raven, Philadelphia, Pennsylvania, USA, 1996, pp. 1-14.

[4] Wellings, SR; Alpers, CE. Apocrine cystic metaplasia: subgross pathology and prevalence in cancer-associated versus random autopsy breasts. *Hum. Pathol.*, 1987 18, 381-6.

[5] Tavassoli, FA; Norris, HJ. A comparison of the results of long-term follow-up for atypical intraductal hyperplasia and intraductal hyperplasia of the breast. *Cancer*, 1990 65, 518-29.

[6] Stoll. BA; Secreto, G. New hormone-related markers of high risk to breast cancer. *Ann Oncol,* 1992 3, 435-438.

[7] Zumoff, B. Hormonal profiles in women with breast cancer. *Anticancer Res.,* 1988 8, 627-636.

[8] Key, TJ; Pike, MC. The role of oestrogens and progestagens in the epidemiology and prevention of breast cancer. *Eur. J. Cancer Clin. Oncol.*, 1988 24, 29-43. Review.

[9] Siiteri, PK; Hammond, GL; et al. Increased availability of serum estrogens in breast cancer: a new hypothesis. In: Pike MC, Siiteri PK, Welsch GW eds. *Bambury Report 8*: *Hormones and Cancer*. Cold Spring Harbor Laboratory Press; 1981; 87-106.

[10] Siiteri, PK; Simberg ,NH; et al. Estrogens and breast cancer. *Ann. NY Acad. Sci.,* 1986 464, 138-151.

[11] Selby, C. Sex hormone binding globulin: origin, function and clinical significance. *Ann. Clin. Biochem.*, 1990 27, 532-41. Review.

[12] Sherman, BM; Korenman, SG. Inadequate corpus luteum function: a pathophysiological interpretation of human breast cancer epidemiology. *Cancer*, 1974 33, 1306-12.

[13] Korenman, SG. Oestrogen window hypothesis of the aetiology of breast cancer. *Lancet,* 1980 1, 700-1.

[14] Grattarola, R. The premenstrual endometrial pattern of women with breast cancer. A study of progestational activity. *Cancer,* 1964 17, 1119-1122.

[15] Micheli, A; Muti, P; Secreto, G; Krogh, V; Meneghini, E; Venturelli, E; Sieri, S; Pala, V; Berrino, F. Endogenous sex hormones and subsequent breast cancer in premenopausal women. *Int. J. Cancer,* 2004 112, 312-8.

[16] Kaaks, R; Berrino, F; Key, T; Rinaldi, S; Dossus, L; Biessy, C; Secreto, G; Amiano, P; Bingham, S; Boeing, H; Bueno de Mesquita, HB; Chang-Claude, J; Clavel-Chapelon, F; Fournier, A; van Gils, CH; Gonzalez, CA; Gurrea, AB; Critselis, E; Khaw, KT; Krogh, V; Lahmann, PH; Nagel, G; Olsen, A; Onland-Moret, NC; Overvad, K; Palli, D; Panico, S; Peeters, P; Quiros, JR; Roddam, A; Thiebaut, A; Tjonneland, A; Chirlaque, MD; Trichopoulou, A; Trichopoulos, D; Tumino, R; Vineis, P; Norat, T;

Ferrari, P; Slimani, N; Riboli, E. Serum sex steroids in premenopausal women and breast cancer risk within the European Prospective Investigation into Cancer and Nutrition (EPIC). *J. Natl. Cancer Inst.*, 2005 97, 755-65.

[17] Grattarola, R. Urinary excretion of 11-deoxy-17-ketosteroids by patients with breast cancer with or without ovulatory cycles. *J. Endocrinol.,* 1967 38,77-78.

[18] Grattarola, R. The urinary androgen metabolites pattern in patients with atypical endometrial hyperplasia. *Int. J. Gynecol. Obstet,*. 1970 8,830-835.

[19] Grattarola, R. Androgens in breast cancer. I. Atypical endometrial hyperplasia and breast cancer in married premenopausal women. *Am. Obstet. Gynecol.* 1973 116, 423-428.

[20] Grattarola, R; Secreto, G; Recchione, C; Castellini, W. Androgens in breast cancer. II. Endometrial adenocarcinoma and breast cancer in married postmenopausal women. *Am. J. Obstet. Gynecol.,* 1973, 118, 173-178.

[21] Grattarola, R; Secreto, G; Recchione, C. Androgens in breast cancer. III. Breast cancer recurrences years after mastectomy and increased androgenic activity. *A. J. Obstet. Gynecol.* 1974 121, 169-172.

[22] Grattarola, R. Misdiagnosis of endometrial adenocarcinoma in young women with polycistic ovarian disease. *Am. J. Obstet. Gynecol.,* 1969 105, 498-502.

[23] Grattarola, R. Misdiagnosis of endometrial adenoachantoma in a 27 years-old woman with adrenocortical tumor. *Oncology* 1973 28, 246-252.

[24] Grattarola, R. Increased androgenic activity in well-differentiated endometrial adenocarcinoma. *Gynecol Oncol.,* 1982 14, 40-48.

[25] Grattarola, R. Ovariectomy alone or in combination with dexamethasone in patients with advanced breast cancer and high levels of testosterone excretion. *J. Natl. Cancer Inst.,* 1976 56, 11-16.

[26] Sommers, SC. Endocrine abnormality in women with breast cancer. *Lab. Invest.*, 1955 4, 160-174.

[27] Sommers ,SC and Teloh, HA. Ovarian stromal hyperplasia in breast cancer *Arch. Pathol.* 1952 53, 160-168.

[28] Rice, BP, Savard, K. Steroid hormone formation in the human ovary. IV. Ovarian stroma compartment: formation of radioactive steroids from acetate-I-C14 and action of gonadotropins. *J. Clin. Endocrinol. Metab.,* 1966 26, 593-609.

[29] Secreto, G; Recchione, C; Cavalleri, A; Miraglia, M; Dati, V. Circulating levels of testosterone, 17β-oestradiol, luteinising hormone and prolactin in postmenopausal breast cancer patients. *B. J. Cancer*, 1983 47, 269-275.

[30] Secreto, G; Toniolo, P; Berrino, F; Recchione, C; Di Pietro, S; Fariselli, G; Decarli A. Increased androgenic activity and breast cancer risk in premenopausal women. *Cancer Res.*, 1984 44, 5902-5905.

[31] Secreto, G; Toniolo, P; Pisani, P; Recchione, C; Cavalleri, A; Fariselli, Totis, A; Di Pietro, S; . Berrino, F. Androgens and breast cancer in premenopausal women. *Cancer Res*. 49, 471-476, 1989.

[32] Secreto, G; Toniolo, P; Berrino, F; Recchione, C; Cavalleri, A; Pisani, P; Totis, Fariselli, G; di Pietro, S. Serum and urinary androgens and risk of breast cancer in postmenopausal women. *Cancer Res.*, 1991 51, 2572-2576.

[33] Balen, A. Polycystic ovary syndrome and cancer. *Hum. Reprod. Update*, 2001 7, 522-5. Review.

[34] Anderson, KE; Sellers, TA; Chen, PL; Rich, SS; Hong, CP; Folsom, AR. Association of Stein-Leventhal syndrome with the incidence of postmenopausal breast carcinoma in a large prospective study of women in Iowa. *Cancer*, 1997 79, 494-9.

[35] Coulam, CB; Annegers, JF; Kranz, JS. Chronic anovulation syndrome and associated neoplasia. *Obstet. Gynecol.* 1983, 61, 403-7.

[36] Gonzalez, ER. Chronic anovulation may increase postmenopausal breast cancer risk. *JAMA*, 1983 249, 445-6.

[37] Pierpoint, T; McKeigue, PM; Isaacs, AJ; Wild, SH; Jacobs, HS. Mortality of women with polycystic ovary syndrome at long-term follow-up. *J. Clin. Epidemiol.*, 1998 51, 581-6.

[38] Gammon, MD; Thompson, WD. Polycystic ovaries and the risk of breast cancer. *Am. J. Epidemiol.*, 1991 134, 818-24.

[39] Hartmann, LC; Sellers, TA; Frost, MH; Lingle, WL; Degnim, AC; Ghosh, K; Vierkant, RA; Maloney, SD; Pankratz, VS; Hillman, DW; Suman, VJ; Johnson, J; Blake, C; Tlsty, T; Vachon, CM; Melton, LJ 3rd; Visscher, DW. Benign breast disease and the risk of breast cancer. *N. Engl. J. Med.*, 2005 353, 229-37.

[40] Fenig, J; Arlen, M; Livingstone, SF; Levowitz, BS. The potential for carcinoma existing synchronously on a microscopic level within the second breast. *Surg. Gynecol. Obstet.*, 1975 141, 394-396.

[41] Santen, RJ; Mansel, R. Benign breast disorders. *N. Engl. J. Med.* 2005 353, 275-85.

[42] Grattarola, R. Anovulation and increased androgenic activity as breast cancer risk in women with fibrocystic disease of the breast. *Cancer Res*, 1978 38, 3051-3054.

[43] Veronesi, U.; Pizzoccaro, G. Breast cancer in women subsequent to cystic disease of the breast. *Surg. Gynecol. Obstet*, 1968 126, 529-532.

[44] Secreto, G; Fariselli, G; Bandieramonte, G; Recchione, C; Di Pietro, S. Androgen excretion in women with a family history of breast cancer or with epithelial hyperplasia or cancer of the breast. *Eur. J. Cancer Clin. Oncol*, 1983 19, 5-10.

[45] Secreto, G; Recchione, C; Fariselli, G; Di Pietro, S. High testosterone and low progesterone circulating levels in premenopausal patients with hyperplasia and cancer of the breast. *Cancer Res.*, 1984 44, 841-844.

[46] Secreto, G; Oriana, S; Recchione, C. Ovariectomy alone or in combination with dexamethasone in patients with advanced breast cancer and high levels of testosterone or androstanediol secretion. *Endocrine-Related Cancer*, 1984 14, 55-58

[47] Preda, F; Pizzoccaro, G; Oriana, S; Ribaldi, G; Severini, A; Di Fronzo, G; Secreto, G; Grattarola, R. Correlation between clinical response to bilateral oophorectomy, estrogen receptors and urinary androgen excretion in 49 patients with advanced breast cancer. *Tumori*, 1979 65, 325-330.

[48] Oriana, S; Secreto, G; Severini, A; Di Fronzo, G; Di Giuseppe, M; Valagussa, P; Preda, F. Bilateral ovariectomy in premenopausal patients with advanced breast cancer, after the evaluation of estrogen receptors and urinary androgen excretion. *Breast Cancer Res. Treat*, 1982 2, 101-104.

[49] Oriana, S; Secreto, G; Di Fronzo, G; Torri, A. Urinary androgens and tumor estrogen receptor as predictors of oophorectomy response and of survival in advanced breast cancer. *Breast Cancer Res. Treat*, 1987 9, 201-5.

[50] Secreto, G; Zumoff, B. Paradoxical effects associated with supranormal urinary testosterone excretion in premenopausal women with breast cancer: increased risk of postmastectomy recurrence and higher remission rate after ovariectomy. *Cancer Res.*, 1983 43, 3408-3411.

[51] Ballerini, P; Oriana, S; Duca, P; Martinetti, A; Venturelli, E; Ferrari, L; Dolci, S; Secreto, G. Urinary testosterone as a marker of risk of recurrence in operable breast cancer. *Breast Cancer Res. Treat,* 1993 26, 1-6.

[52] Berrino, F; Pasanisi, P; Bellati, C; Venturelli, E; Krogh, V; Mastroianni, A; Berselli ,E; Muti, P; Secreto, G. Serum testosterone levels and breast cancer recurrence. *Int. J. Cancer,* 2005 113, 499-502.

[53] Veronesi, U; De Palo, G; Marubini, E; Costa, A; Formelli, F; Mariani, L; Decensi, A; Camerini, T; Del Turco, MR; Di Mauro, MG; Muraca, MG; Del Vecchio, M; Pinto, C; D'Aiuto, G; Boni, C; Campa, T; Magni, A; Miceli, R; Perloff, M; Malone, WF; Sporn, MB. Randomized trial of fenretinide to prevent second breast malignancy in women with early breast cancer. *J. Natl. Cancer Inst.,* 1999 91, 1847-56.

[54] Goldhirsch, A; Glick, JH; Gelber, RD; Coates, AS; Thurlimann, B; Senn, HJ; Panel members. Meeting highlights: international expert consensus on the primary therapy of early breast cancer 2005. *Ann. Oncol.*, 2005 16, 1569-83.

[55] Hackenberg, R; Turgetto, I; Filmer, A; Schulz, KD: Estrogen and androgen receptor mediated stimulation and inhibition of proliferation by androst-5-ene-3b-17b-diol in human mammary cancer cells. *J. Steroid Biochem. Molec. Biol.,* 1993 46, 597-603.

[56] Bryan, R.M.; Mercer, R.J.; Rennie, G.C.; Lie T.H. and Morgan F.J.: Androgen receptors in breast cancer. *Cancer,* 1984 54, 2436-2440.

[57] Isola, JJ. Immunohistochemical demonstration of androgen receptor in breast cancer and its relationship to other prognostic factors. *J. Pathol.* 1993 170, 31–35.

[58] Pasqualini, J.R. Role of androgens in breast cancer. *J. Steroid Biochem. Molec. Biol.*, 1993 45 , 167-172.

[59] Moinfar, F; Okcu, M; Tsybrovskyy, O; Regitnig, P; Lax, SF; Weybora, W; Ratschek, M; Tavassoli, FA; Denk, H. Androgen receptors frequently are expressed in breast carcinomas. *Cancer,* 2003 98, 703–711.

[60] Selim, A; El-Ayat, G; Wellis, A. Androgen receptor expression in ductal carcinoma in situ of the breast: relation to oestrogen and progesterone receptors. *J. Clin. Pathol.,* 2002 55,14–16.

[61] Agoff, SN; Swanson, PE; Linden, H; Hawes, SE; Lawton, TJ. Androgen receptor expression in estrogen receptor-negative breast cancer. Immunohistochemical, clinical, and prognostic associations. *Am. J. Clin. Pathol.,* 2003 120, 725–731.

[62] Schippinger, W; Regitnig, P; Dandachi, N; Wernecke, KD; Bauernhofer, T; Samonigg, H; Moinfar, F. Evaluation of the prognostic significance of androgen receptor expression in metastatic breast cancer. *Virchows Arch.*, 2006 449, 24-30.

[63] Miller, W.R.; Telfors, J.; Dixon, J.M; Hawkins, R.A. Androgen receptor activity in human breast cancer and its relationship with oestrogen and progestogen receptor activity. *Eur. J. Cancer Clin. Oncol.,* 1985 21, 539-542.
[64] Valyani, SH; Roberts, JV; Colletta, AA; Iqbal JM. Sex hormone receptors in human breast cancer. Incidence and interrelationship. *Anticancer Res.,* 1987 7, 1281-1284.
[65] Kuenen-Boumeester, V; Vanderkwast, TH; Van Putten ,WLJ; Claassen, C; Vanooijen, B; Henzenlogmans, SC. Immunohistochemical determination of androgen receptors in relation to oestrogen and progesterone receptors in female breast cancer. *Int. J. Cancer,* 1992 52, 581–584.
[66] Farmer P; Bonnefoi H; Becette V; Tubiana-Hulin M; Fumoleau P; Larsimont D; Macgrogan G; Bergh J; Cameron D; Goldstein D; Duss S; Nicoulaz AL; Brisken C; Fiche M; Delorenzi M; Iggo R. Identification of molecular apocrine breast tumours by microarray analysis. *Oncogene,* 2005 24, 4660-71.
[67] Doane, AS; Danso, M; Lal, P; Donaton, M; Zhang, L; Hudis, C; Gerald, WL. An estrogen receptor-negative breast cancer subset characterized by a hormonally regulated transcriptional program and response to androgen. *Oncogene,* 2006 25, 3994-4008.
[68] Menard, S; Pupa, SM; Campiglio, M; Tagliabue ,E. Biologic and therapeutic role of HER2 in cancer. *Oncogene,* 2003 22, 6570-8. Review.
[69] Howell, A; Dodwell, DJ; Anderson, H. New Endocrine Approaches to Breast Cancer. In: Bailliere's Clinical Endocrinology and Metabolism. London: *Vol. 4: Endocrine Aspects of Malignancy*, SM Shalet Ed. Bailliere Tindall; 1990; 67-84.
[70] Lippman, ME; Dickson, RB; Bates, CH et al. Autocrine and paracrine growth regulation of human breast cancer. *Breast Cancer Res. Treat,* 1986 7, 59-70.
[71] Borellini, F; Oka, T. Growth control and differentiation in mammary epithelial cells. *Envirnmental Health Perspectives,* 1989 80, 85-899.
[72] Barthe, PL; Bullock, LP; Mowszowicz, I; Bardin, CW; Orth, DN. Submaxillary gland epidermal growth factor: a sensitive index of biologic androgen activity. *Endocrinol,* 1974 95, 1019-1025.
[73] Perheentupa, J; Hoath, SB; Fisher, DA. Hormonal modulation of mouse plasma concentration of epidermal growth factor. *Acta Endocrinol.,* 1984 107, 571-576.
[74] Wales, NAM; Ebling, FJ. The control of the apocrine glands of the rabbit by steroid hormones. *J. Endocrinol.,* 1971 51, 763-770.
[75] Zagorianakou, P; Zagorianakou, N; Stefanou, D; Makrydimas, G; Agnantis, NJ. The enigmatic nature of apocrine breast lesions. *Virchows Arch.* 2006 Mar 29. (Epub ahead of print).
[76] Labows, JN; Petri ,G; Hoelze, E; Leyden, J; Klingman, A. Steroid analysis of human apocrine secretion. *Steroids,* 1979 34, 249-258.
[77] Mazoujian, G; Pinkus, GS; Haagensen, DE. Immunochemistry of a gross cystic disease fluid protein (GCDFP-15) of the breast. A marker of apocrine epithelium and breast carcinomas with apocrine features. *Am. J. Pathol.,* 1983 110, 105-112.
[78] Dixon, JM; Lumdsen, AB; Miller, WR The relationship of cyst type to risk factors for breast cancer and the subsequent development of breast cancer in patients with breast cystic disease. *Eur. J. Clin. Oncol.,* 1985 21, 1047-1050.

[79] Boccardo, F; Valenti, G; Zanardi, S; Cerruti, G; Fassio, T; Bruzzi, P; De Franchis, V; Barreca, A; Del Monte, P; Minuto, F. Epidermal growth factor in breast cyst fluid: relationship with intracystic cation and androgen coniugate content. *Cancer Res.,* 1988 48, 5860-5863.
[80] Lai, LC; Ghilchik, MW; Shaikh, NA; Reed, MJ; James, VHT. Relationship between epidermal growth factor and dehydroepiandrosterone and its sulphate in breast cyst fluid. *Br J Cancer,* 1989 60, 320-323.
[81] Fisher, DA; Lakshmanan, J. Metabolism and effects of epidermal growth factor and related growth factors in mammals. *Endocrine Rev.,* 1990 11, 418-442.
[82] Van Landeghem, AA.; Poortman, J; Nabuurs, M; Thijssen, JHH. Endogenous concentration and subcellular distribution of estrogens in normal and malignant human breast tissue. *Cancer Res.,* 1985 45, 2900-2906.
[83] Vermeulen, A.; Deslypere, JP.; Paridaens, R.; Leclercq, G.; Roy, F; Heuson, JC. Aromatase, 17β-hydroxysteroid dehydrogenase and intratissular sex hormone concentrations in cancerous and normal glandular breast tissue in postmenopausal women. *Eur. J. Cancer Clin. Oncol,* 1986 22, 515-525.
[84] Santen, RJ. Determination of tissue oestradiol in human breast cancer. *Cancer Surveys,* 1986 5, 597-616.
[85] Thijssen, JHH; Blankenstein, MA. Endogenous oestrogens and androgens in normal and malignant endometrial and mammary tissues. *Eur. J. Cancer Clin. Oncol.,* 1989 25, 1953-1959.
[86] Blankestein, MA; Maitimu-Smeele, I; Donker, GH; Daroszewski, J; Milewicz, A; Thijssen, JHH: Tissue androgen and the endocrine autonomy of breast cancer. *J. Steroid Biochem Mol. Biol.,* 1992 43, 167-171.
[87] Mistry, P; Griffiths, K; Maynard, PV. Endogenous C19-steroids and oestradiol levels in human primary breast tumour tissues and their correlation with androgen and oestrogen receptors. *J Steroid Biochem,* 1986 24, 1117-1125.
[88] Recchione, C; Venturelli, E, ,; Cavalleri, A; Martinetti, A; Secreto, G. Testosterone, dihydrotestosterone and oestradiol levels in postmenopausal breast cancer tissues. *J. Steroid Biochem. Molec. Biol.,* 1995 52, 541-546.
[89] Secreto, G; Venturelli, E; Bucci, A; Piromalli, D; Fariselli, G; Galante, E. Intratumour amount of sex steroids in elderly breast cancer patients. An approach to the biological characterization of mammary tumours in the elderly. *J. Steroid Biochem. Mol. Biol.,* 1996 58, 557-61.
[90] Liao, DJ; Dickson, RB. Roles of androgens in the development, growth, and carcinogenesis of the mammary gland. *J Steroid Biochem Mol Biol,* 2002 80, 175-89. Review.
[91] Secreto, G; Zumoff, B. Abnormal production of androgens in women with breast cancer. *Anticancer Res.*, 1988 14,2113-2118.
[92] Hill, P; Garbaczewski, L; Kasumi, F. Plasma testosterone and breast cancer. *Eur. J. Cancer Clin. Oncol.,* 1985 21, 1265-1266.
[93] Key, TJ; Chen, J; Wang, DY; Pike, MC; Boreham, J. Sex hormones in women in rural China and in Britain. *Br. J. Cancer,* 1990 62, 631-636.

[94] Wang, DY; Key, TJ; Pike, MC; Boreham, J; Chen, J. Serum hormone levels in British and rural Chinese females. *Breast Cancer Res. Treat,* 1991 18, S41-S45.

[95] Secreto, G; Recchione, C; Grignolio, E; Cavalleri, A. Increased urinary androgen excretion is a hormonal abnormality detectable before the clinical onset of breast cancer. *Cancer Detection and Prevention,* 1983 6, 435-438.

[96] The Endogenous Hormones and Breast Cancer Collaborative Group: Endogenous sex hormones and breast cancer in postmenopausal women: reanalysis of nine prospective studies. *J. Nat. Cancer Inst.*, 2002 94, 606-616.

[97] Kaaks, R; Rinaldi, S; Key, TJ; Berrino, F; Peeters, PH; Biessy, C; Dossus, L; Lukanova, A; Bingham, S; Khaw, KT; Allen, NE; Bueno-de-Mesquita, HB; van Gils, CH; Grobbee, D; Boeing, H; Lahmann, PH; Nagel, G; Chang-Claude, J; Clavel-Chapelon, F; Fournier, A; Thiebaut, A; Gonzalez, CA; Quiros, JR; Tormo, MJ; Ardanaz, E; Amiano, P; Krogh, V; Palli, D; Panico, S; Tumino, R; Vineis, P; Trichopoulou, A; Kalapothaki, V; Trichopoulos, D; Ferrari, P; Norat, T; Saracci, R; Riboli, E. Postmenopausal serum androgens, oestrogens and breast cancer risk: the European prospective investigation into cancer and nutrition. *Endocr. Relat. Cancer,* 2005 12, 1071-82.

[98] Tamimi, RM; Hankinson, SE; Chen, WY; Rosner, B; Colditz, GA. Combined estrogen and testosterone use and risk of breast cancer in postmenopausal women. *Arch. Intern. Med.* 2006 166, 1483-9.

[99] Fournier, A; Berrino, F; Riboli, E; Avenel, V; Clavel-Chapelon, F. Breast cancer risk in relation to different types of hormone replacement therapy in the E3N-EPIC cohort. *Int J Cancer*. 2005 114, 448-54.

[100] Travis, RC; Key, TJ. Oestrogen exposure and breast cancer risk. *Breast Cancer Res.,* 2003 5, 239-247.

[101] Verheus, M; Peeters, PH; Rinaldi, S; Dossus, L; Biessy, C; Olsen, A; Tjonneland, A; Overvad, K; Jeppesen, M; Clavel-Chapelon, F; Tehard, B; Nagel, G; Linseisen, J; Boeing, H; Lahmann, PH; Arvaniti, A; Psaltopoulou, T; Trichopoulou, A; Palli, D; Tumino, R; Panico S; Sacerdote, C; Sieri, S; van Gils, CH; Bueno-de-Mesquita, BH; Gonzalez, CA; Ardanaz, E; Larranaga, N; Garcia, CM; Navarro, C; Quiros, JR; Key, T; Allen, N; Bingham, S; Khaw, KT; Slimani, N; Riboli, E; Kaaks, R. Serum C-peptide levels and breast cancer risk: Results from the European prospective investigation into cancer and nutrition (EPIC). *Int. J. Cancer,* 2006 119, 659-67.

[102] Goodwin, PJ; Ennis, M; Pritchard, KI; Trudeau, ME; Koo, J; Madarnas, Y; Hartwick, W; Hoffman, B; Hood, N. Fasting insulin and outcome in early-stage breast cancer: results of a prospective cohort study. *J Clin Oncol,* 2002 20, 42–51

[103] Rose, DP; Komninou, D; Stephenson, GD. Obesity, adipocytokines, and insulin resistance in breast cancer. *Obes. Rev.*, 2004 5, 153-65. Review.

[104] Rinaldi, S; Peeters, PH; Berrino, F; Dossus, L; Biessy, C; Olsen, A; Tjonneland, A; Overvad, K; Clavel-Chapelon, F; Boutron-Ruault, MC; Tehard, B; Nagel, G; Linseisen, J; Boeing, H; Lahmann, PH; Trichopoulou, A; Trichopoulos, D; Koliva, M; Palli, D; Panico, S; Tumino, R; Sacerdote, C; van Gils, CH; van Noord, P; Grobbee, DE; Bueno-de-Mesquita, HB; Gonzalez, CA; Agudo, A; Chirlaque, MD; Barricarte, A; Larranaga, N; Quiros, JR; Bingham, S; Khaw, KT; Key, T; Allen, NE; Lukanova, A; Slimani, N;

Saracci, R; Riboli, E; Kaaks, R. IGF-I, IGFBP-3 and breast cancer risk in women: The European Prospective Investigation into Cancer and Nutrition (EPIC). *Endocr. Relat. Cancer*, 2006 13, 593-605.

[105] Muti, P; Quattrin, T; Grant, BJ; Krogh, V; Micheli, A; Schunemann, HJ; Ram, M; Freudenheim, JL; Sieri, S; Trevisan, M; Berrino, F. Fasting glucose is a risk factor for breast cancer: A prospective study. *Cancer Epidemiol. Biomarkers Prev.*, 2002 11, 1361-1368.

[106] Hankinson, SE; Willett, WC; Colditz, GA; Hunter, DJ; Michaud, DS; Deroo, B; Rosner, B; Speizer, FE; Pollak, M. Circulating concentrations of insulin-like growth factor-I and risk of breast cancer. *Lancet,* 1998 351, 1393-1396.

[107] Toniolo, P; Bruning, PF; Akhmedkhanov, A; Bonfrer, JM; Koenig, KL; Lukanova, A; Shore, RE; Zeleniuch-Jacquotte, A. Serum insulin-like growth factor-I and breast cancer. 2000 *Int. J. Cancer,* 88, 828-832.

[108] Allen, NE; Roddam, AW; Allen, DS; Fentiman, IS; Dos SSI; Peto, J; Holly, JM; Key, TJ. A prospective study of serum insulin-like growth factor-I (IGF-I), IGF-II, IGF-binding protein-3 and breast cancer risk. 2005 *Br. J. Cancer* 92, 1283-1287.

[109] Lahmann, PH; Hoffmann, K; Allen, N; van Gil,s CH; Khaw, KT; Tehard, B; Berrino, F; Tjonneland, A; Bigaard, J; Olsen, A; Overvad, K; Clavel-Chapelon, F; Nagel, G; Boeing, H; Trichopoulos, D; Economou, G; Bellos, G; Palli, D; Tumino, R; Panico, S; Sacerdote, C; Krogh, V; Peeters, PH; Bueno-de-Mesquita, HB; Lund, E; Ardanaz, E; Amiano, P; Pera, G; Quiros, JR; Martinez, C; Tormo, MJ; Wirfalt, E; Berglund, G; Hallmans, G; Key, TJ; Reeves, G; Bingham, S; Norat, T; Biessy, C; Kaaks, R; Riboli, E. Body size and breast cancer risk: findings from the European Prospective Investigation into Cancer And Nutrition (EPIC). *Int. J. Cancer,* 2004 111, 762-71.

[110] Stephenson, GD; Rose, DP. Breast cancer and obesity: an update. *Nutr. Cancer*, 2003 45, 1–16.

[111] Kaaks, R. Nutrition, hormones, and breast cancer: is insulin the missing link? *Cancer Causes Control*, 1996 7, 605-25. Review.

[112] Hill, DJ; Milner, RD. Insulin as a growth factor. *Pediatr Res*, 1985 19, 879-86. Review.

[113] Straus, DS. Growth-stimulatory actions of insulin in vitro and in vivo. *Endocr. Rev.*, 1984 5, 356-69. Review.

[114] Conover, CA; Hintz RL, Rosenfeld RG. Comparative effects of somatomedin C and insulin on the metabolism and growth of cultured human fibroblasts. *J. Cell Physiol*, 1985 122, 133-141.

[115] Baxter, RC. Insulin-like growth factor (IGF)-binding proteins: interactions with IGFs and intrinsic bioactivities. *Am. J. Physiol. Endocrinol. Metab.*, 2000 278, E967-76.

[116] Rollison, DE; Newschaffer, CJ; Tao, Y; Pollak, M; Helzlsouer, KJ. Premenopausal levels of circulating insulin-like growth factor I and the risk of postmenopausal breast cancer. *Int. J. Cancer,* 2006 118, 1279-1284.

[117] Rinaldi S; Peeters PH; Berrino F; Dossus L; Biessy C; Olsen A; Tjonneland A; Overvad K; Clavel-Chapelon F; Boutron-Ruault MC; Tehard B; Nagel G; Linseisen J; Boeing H, Lahmann PH; Trichopoulou A; Trichopoulos D; Koliva M; Palli D; Panico S; Tumino R; Sacerdote C; van Gils CH; van Noord P; Grobbee DE; Bueno-de-Mesquita HB; Gonzalez CA; Agudo A; Chirlaque MD; Barricarte A; Larranaga N;

Quiros JR; Bingham S; Khaw KT; Key T; Allen NE; Lukanova A; Slimani N; Saracci R; Riboli E; Kaaks R. IGF-I, IGFBP-3 and breast cancer risk in women: The European Prospective Investigation into Cancer and Nutrition (EPIC). *Endocr. Relat. Cancer,* 2006 13,593-605.

[118] Hall, WD; Watkins, LO; Wright, JT Jr; Wenger, NK; Kumanyika, SK; Gavin, JR 3rd; Ferdinand, KC; Watson, K; Clark, LT; Flack, JM; Reed, JW; Horton, EW; Saunders E. The metabolic syndrome: recognition and management. *Dis. Manag.*, 2006 9, 16-33. Review.

[119] Largent, JA; McEligot, AJ; Ziogas, A; Reid, C; Hess, J; Leighton, N; Peel, D; Anton-Culver, H. Hypertension, diuretics and breast cancer risk. *J. Hum. Hypertens*, 2006 [Epub ahead of print].

[120] Soler, M; Chatenoud, L; Negri, E; Parazzini, F; Franceschi, S; La Vecchia, C. Hypertension and hormone-related neoplasms in women. *Hypertension*, 1999 34, 320-5.

[121] Furberg, AS; Veierod, MB; Wilsgaard, T; Bernstein, L; Thune, I. Serum high-density lipoprotein cholesterol, metabolic profile, and breast cancer risk. *J Natl Cancer Inst*, 2004 96, 1152-60.

[122] Han, C; Zhang, HT; Du, L; Liu, X; Jing, J; Zhao, X; Yang, X; Tian, B. Serum levels of leptin, insulin, and lipids in relation to breast cancer in china. *Endocrine*, 2005 26, 19-24.

[123] Mady, EA. Association between estradiol, estrogen receptors, total lipids, triglycerides, and cholesterol in patients with benign and malignant breast tumours. *Steroid. Biochem. Mol. Biol.*, 2000 75, 323-8.

[124] Potischman, N; McCulloch, CE; Byers, T; Houghton, L; Nemoto, T; Graham, S; Campbell, TC. Associations between breast cancer, plasma triglycerides, and cholesterol. *Nutr. Cancer,* 1991 15, 205-215.

[125] Berrino, F; Bellati, C; Secreto, G; Camerini, E; Pala, V; Panico, S; Allegro, G; Kaaks, R: Reducing bioavailable sex hormones through a comprehensive change in diet: the Diet and Androgens (DIANA) randomized trial. *Cancer Epidemiol. Biomarkers Prev.,* 2001 10, 25-33.

[126] Berrino, F; Bellati, C; Oldani, S; Mastroianni, A; Allegro, G; Berselli, E; Venturelli, E; Cavalleri, A; Cambie, M; Pala, V; Pasanisi, P; Secreto, G: DIANA trials on diet and endogenous hormones. *IARC Sci Publ*, 2002 156, 439-44.

[127] Kaaks, R; Bellati, C; Venturelli, E; Rinaldi, S; Secreto, G; Biessy, C; Pala, V; Sieri, S; Berrino, F. Effects of dietary intervention on IGF-I and IGF-binding proteins, and related alterations in sex steroid metabolism: the Diet and Androgens (DIANA) Randomised Trial. *Eur. J. Clin. Nutr.*, 2003 57, 1079-88.

[128] Pasanisi, P; Berrino, F; De Petris, M; Venturelli, E; Mastroianni A; Panico, S. Metabolic syndrome as a prognostic factor for breast cancer recurrences. *Int. J. Cancer*, 2006 119, 236-8.

[129] McPherson, K; Steel, CM; Dixon, JM. ABC of breast diseases. Breast cancer-epidemiology, risk factors, and genetics. *BMJ*, 2000 321, 624-8. Review.

[130] Kirschner, MA; Samojlik, E; Drejka, M; Szmal, E; Schneider, G; Ertel, N. Androgen-estrogen metabolism in women with upper body versus lower body obesity. *J. Clin. Endocrinol Metab.*, 1990 70, 473-9.

[131] Rosmond, R. Androgen excess in women - A health hazard? *Med. Hypotheses.*, 2006 67, 229-34.

[132] von Minckwitz, G; Graf, E; Geberth, M; Eiermann, W; Jonat, W; Conrad, B; Brunnert, K; Gerber, B; Vescia, S; Wollert, J; Kaufmann, M. CMF versus goserelin as adjuvant therapy for node-negative, hormone-receptor-positive breast cancer in premenopausal patients: A randomised trial (GABG trial IV-A-93). *Eur. J. Cancer*. 2006 Jun 8. (Epub ahead of print).

[133] Early Breast Cancer Trialist's Collaborative Group. Effects of chemotherapy and hormonal therapy for early breast cancer on recurrence and 15-year survival: an overview of the randomised trials. *Lancet,* 2005 365, 1687–717.

[134] Jonat, W; Kaufmann, M; Sauerbrei, W; Blamey, R; Cuzick, J; Namer, M; Fogelman, I; de Haes, JC; de Matteis, A; Stewart, A; Eiermann, W; Szakolczai, I; Palmer, M; Schumacher, M; Geberth, M; Lisboa ,B; Zoladex Early Breast Cancer Research Association Study. Goserelin versus cyclophosphamide, methotrexate, and fluorouracil as adjuvant therapy in premenopausal patients with node-positive breast cancer: the Zoladex Early Breast Cancer Research Association Study, *J. Clin. Oncol.,* 2002 20, 4628–4635.

[135] Castiglione-Gertsch, M; O'Neill, A; Price, KN; Goldhirsch, A; Coates, AS; Colleoni, M; Nasi, ML; Bonetti, M; Gelber, RD; International Breast Cancer Study Group. Adjuvant chemotherapy followed by goserelin versus either modality alone for premenopausal lymph node-negative breast cancer: a randomised trial, *J. Natl. Cancer Inst,*(2003, 95, 1833–1846.

[136] Diamanti-Kandarakis, E; Baillargeon, JP; Iuorno, MJ; Jakubowicz, DJ; Nestler JE. A modern medical quandary: polycystic ovary syndrome, insulin resistance, and oral contraceptive pills. *J Clin Endocrinol Metab*, 2003 88, 1927-32. Review.

[137] Gambineri, A; Pelusi, C; Genghini, S; Morselli-Labate, AM; Cacciari, M; Pagotto, U; Pasquali, R. Effect of flutamide and metformin administered alone or in combination in dieting obese women with polycystic ovary syndrome. *Clin. Endocrinol.*, 2004 60, 241-9.

[138] Ibanez, L; Valls, C; Cabre, S; De Zegher, F. Flutamide-metformin plus ethinylestradiol-drospirenone for lipolysis and antiatherogenesis in young women with ovarian hyperandrogenism: the key role of early, low-dose flutamide. *J. Clin. Endocrinol. Metab.*, 2004 89, 4716-20.

In: Frontiers in Breast Cancer Research
Editor: Louis P. Fortugno, pp. 71-97
ISBN: 978-1-60021-671-8

Chapter III

DNA Methylation and Epigenetic Gene Silencing in Breast Cancer

Qifeng Yang[1,*], Guohong Hu[2], Zhigang Yu[3], Jingzhong Sun[4], Goro Yoshimura[5] and Kennichi Kakudo[6]

[1] The Cancer Institute of New Jersey, New Brunswick, NJ
[2] Princeton University, Princeton, NJ
[1,3,4] Qilu Hospital of Shandong University, Ji'nan, P.R. China
[1,5] Affiliated Kihoku Hospital of Wakayama Medical University, Japan
[1,6] Wakayama Medical University, Japan

Abstract

Of all epigenetic modifications, hypermethylation is commonly considered as a critical causal event in silencing important classes of genes in cancer. In breast cancer, a series of tumor suppressor or related genes are frequently hypermethylated and which is associated with silencing of these genes. We now understand that DNA methylation mechanisms might include a number of DNA methyltransferases, proteins that direct DNA methyltransferases to specific promoters, chromatin modifying enzymes as well as demethylases. There are also data to suggest that pharmacological down regulation of some members of the DNA methylation machinery could inhibit cancer in vitro, in vivo and in clinical trials. The use of the methylation status of certain genes as a marker of cancer or cancerous conditions provides an additional weapon in early detection and prognosis of breast cancers. We describe the techniques used to decipher the complement of methylation-inactivated genes, discuss the epigenetic regulation of certain critical tumor suppressor and growth regulatory genes implicated in breast cancer and its relevance to breast cancer development, progression and therapy.

[*] Address correspondence to Qifeng Yang, M.D. Ph.D., The Cancer Institute of New Jersey, 195 Little Albany St., New Brunswick, NJ 08903-2681, USA, e-mail: yang-qf@mail.wakayama-med.ac.jp

Introduction

Breast cancer is the most common cancer among women, besides skin cancer. It is the second leading cause of cancer death in women, after lung cancer. About 211,240 women in the United States will developp invasive breast cancer in 2005. Although breast cancer mortality has begun to decline because of improved screening techniques, About 40,410 women will die from the disease this year. The transformation of normal cells into cancer cells involves multiple etiologic pathways and, at the very least, is a genetic, epigenetic and cytogenetic process. The genetic route to tumorigenesis has been studied extensively, and epigenetics is now coming of age. The genetic and epigenetic alterations that initiate and drive tumorigenesis are promising targets for early detection because they may precede clinically obvious cancers, can be detected at sensitive levels, may be specific to tumor cells, and can potentially provide information about the prognosis and treatment of the disease [1, 2].

The term "epigenetics" defines all meiotically and mitotically heritable changes in gene expression that are not coded in the DNA sequence itself. Three systems, including DNA methylation, histone modification and RNA-associated silencing, are used to initiate and sustain epigenetic silencing. DNA methylation is the only commonly occurring modification of human DNA [3]. Histone modification includes acetylation and methylation of conserved lysine residues on the amino-terminal tail domains. The acetylation of histones marks active, transcriptionally competent regions, whereas hypoacetylated histones are found in transcriptionally inactive euchromatic or heterochromatic regions. Histone methylaiton can be a marker for both active and inactive regions of chromatin. Antisense transcripts, noncoding RNAs (such as Xist) or RNA interference (RNAi), can also lead to mitotically heritable transcriptional silencing by the formation of heterochromatin. The major form of epigenetic information in mammalian cells is DNA methylation, or the covalent addition of a methyl group to the 5-position of cytosine predominantly within the CpG islands. DNA methylation has been shown by several lines of evidence to play a role in gene activity, cell differentiation, tumorogenesis, X-chromosome inactivation, genomic imprinting and other major biological processes. DNA hypermethylation has been used as a biomarker for breast cancer risk, classification and prognosis, and it is also a new target for breast cancer treatment.

Methyltransferase, Methylation and Gene Transcription

DNMTs and Methylation

The major form of epigenetic information in mammalian cells is DNA methylation, or the covalent addition of a methyl group to the 5-position of cytosine predominantly within the CpG islands. CpG islands are regions of more than 500 base pairs in size and with a GC content greater than 55% [4], CpG islands have been conversed during evolution because they are normally kept free of methylation. CpG islands are located within the promoter regions of about 40% of mammalian genes and, when methylated, cause stable heritable transcriptional silencing. Aberrant *de novo* methylation of CpG islands is a hallmark of human cancers and is found early during carcinogenesis.

DNA methylation is accomplished through the activity of specific enzymes, the DNA methyltransferases (DNMT's). The DNMTs known to date are DNMT1, DNMT1b, DNMT1o, DNMT1p, DNMT2, DNMT3A, DNMT3B with its isoforms, and DNMT3L[5]. Methylation can be *de novo* (when CpG dinucleotides on both DNA stands are unmethylated) or maintenance (when CpG dinucleotides on one strand are methylated). DNMT1 has *de novo* as well as maintenance methyltransferase activity, and DNMT3A and DNMT3B are powerful *de novo* methyltransferases [6]. DNMT2 has been cloned and characterized but catalytic activity of this enzyme has yet to be demonstrated *in vitro* or *in vivo* [7], but its catalytic domain lacks DNMT activity in the human.

DNMT1, the first methyltransferase, was discovered by Bestor et al [8]. The DNMT1 gene is located at human chromosome 19p13.2 and encodes a 200 kDa protein whose methyltransferase catalytic domain is located at the C-terminus of the protein. The generation of DNMT1-knockout mice has revealed that DNMT1 is required for proper embryonic development, imprinting, and X-inactivation. Mice deficient for DNMT1 show arrested development prior to the 8 somite stage and a nearly 70% reduction in their genomic 5-methylcytosine content. A research group at Johns Hopkins University [9] reported that DNMT1 expression is dysregulated in breast cancer. The elevated protein levels are not a result of increased mRNA levels, but rather an increase in protein half-life. They found that DNMT1 protein levels were elevated in breast cancer tissues and in MCF-7 breast cancer cells relative to normal Human Mammary Epithelial Cells (HMECs) without a concomitant increase in DNMT1 mRNA or proliferative fraction. While DNMT1 mRNA levels were properly S-phase regulated in both cell types, DNMT1 protein levels did not follow S-phase fraction in MCF-7 cells. Rather, an increase in DNMT1 protein stability was found for MCF-7 cells relative to HMECs, and a destruction domain was mapped to the N-terminal 120 amino acids of DNMT1 which was required for its proper ubiquitination and degradation in HMECs. Furthermore, overexpression of DNMT1 with this deleted destruction domain in HMECs resulted in significantly increased genomic 5-methylcytosine levels relative to overexpression of the full-length protein. The regulation of DNMT1 destruction via this domain may be dysfunctional in cancer cells leading to subsequent cytosine hypermethylation in the genome. Okano *et al* first described the characterization of the DNMT3 family of methyltransferases [10]. DNMT3 family members share some structural similarities with DNMT1 with a catalytic C-terminal region responsible for DNA methylation and a N-terminal region regulatory domain. They methylate CpG dinucleotides of unmethylated and hemimethylated DNA *in vitro*. The two genes are expressed at high levels in ES cells and relatively low levels in adult somatic tissues. Human DNMT3A has been mapped to chromosome 2p23 whereas DNMT3B maps to chromosome 20q11.2 [11]. Human DNMT3A is ubiquitously expressed but DNMT3B is expressed at low levels except in testis, thyroid and bone marrow. Overexpression of both DNMT3B and DNMT3A appears to characterize multiple types of human tumors [12]. A specific function for Dnmt3b, revealed by the mouse knockout experiments, is maintenance of DNA methylation of the minor satellite repeats adjacent to entromeres [13, 14]. The specific function for DNMT3A was not detectable with the knockout model but studies using the various DNMT-knockout ES cells in addition to transgenic Drosophila melanogaster expressing DNMT3A revealed that this enzyme may be specialized to methylate non-CpG sequences like CpA, and CpT although the function of non-CpG methylation in ES cells is unknown [15]. The catalytic activity of DNMT3A and 3B are much lower than that of DNMT1 [10]. DNMT1 is mainly responsible for maintenance of DNA methylation, whereas DNMT3A and DNMT3B have been shown to methylate hemimethylated and unmethylated DNA with equal efficiencies [13]. Overexpression of DNMT1 as well as the DNMT3 mRNAs has been reported in human tumors [11, 16], but this phenomenon is probably only partially responsible for the observed methylation changes.

Null mutations of the mammalian DNMTs are lethal at different stages, either prenatally and postnatally. ES cells homozygous for DNMT1 mutation are viable, with no growth or retain the 30% of genomic methylation. Some studies on cells with total or partial loss of DNMT1 function revealed abnormalities in transcriptional silencing of specific imprinted genes and the Xist allele on the chromosome [17]. Mice lacking DNMT3A die postnatally, whereas those lacking DNMT3B develop normally until E9.5, then die prior to term. Double mutants already show abnormality at E8.5, then die prior to E11.5. Specific DNMT isoforms, such the DNMT1o, oocyte-specific seem to play specific roles in the physiology of genomic methylation [18].

Methylation and Gene Transcription

The link between methylation and gene expression was revealed more than two decades ago when a mouse-human somatic cell hybrid clone was isolated [19], however, evidence directly connecting the two events has only recently been obtained [20].

The first mechanism suggested that the suppression of transcription by DNA methylation proposed direct inhibition of transcription factor binding. The active recruitment of methyl-CpG binding activities appears to be the dominant mechanism of methylation-dependent repression. MeCP1 and MeCP2 were the first two methyl-CpG binding activities to be described [21]. MeCP1 was originally identified as a large multi-protein complex, MeCP2 is a single polypeptide with an affinity for a single methylated CpG. MeCP2 germline mutations are responsible for the mental retardation disease Rett syndrome, and the absence of a functional MeCP2 in these patients causes specific dysregulation of the gene expression. Additional proteins harbouring the methyl-CpG binding domain (MBD), namely MBD1, MBD2, MBD3, and MBD4 have also been identified [22]. The first molecular evidence concerning the role of methyl-CpG binding proteins in repressing aberrantly methylated genes in cancer arose from the demonstration that methylation of a construct containing part of the 5’ BRCA1 CpG island inhibited gene expression in the presence of MeCP2 [23]. Recently, the presence of MBD proteins has been demonstrated to be a major hallmark of tumor suppressor genes hypermethylated and silenced in cancer [24].

Methylation might also influence transcription indirectly through chromatin condensation, which is the packing of DNA into high-order three-dimensional protein-nucleic acid structures, often associated with gene inactivity. The connection between DNA methylation and transcriptional repression by the modification of chromatin was first revealed in 1997 [20, 25]. Chromatin research has resulted in the description of a variety of histone modifications and the specificity of certain modifications under particular physiological conditions. Most histone modifications occur in their protruding N-terminal tails. It is hypothesized that histone modifications act sequentially or in combination to form a code that may be read by nuclear factors [26]. There are several modifications that are compatible with gene silencing. In general, histone deacetylation leads to gene silencing, whilst histone acetylation leads to gene activation. Although cytosine methylation can directly inhibit the binding of certain transcription factors, methylated DNA is recognized by different methyl-DNA binding proteins, such as MeCP2 and MBD2. It is widely accepted that methylated DNA binding proteins such as MeCP2 target methylated DNA. MeCP2 recruits co-repressor complexes and histone deacetylases and histone methyltransferases to the methylated gene precipitating an inactive chromatin structure [20, 25, 27]. Another important issue is that histone acetyl transferases and deacetylaces remodel chromatin by increasing or decreasing the net charge of the histones themselves, thus altering their affinity for negatively charged DNA. This process could alter gene expression by making DNA either more or less accessible to transcriptional activators or repressors.

Epigenetic modification may be found on the DNA primary sequence (e.g., cytosine methylation) or on the associated histones (lysine or arginine acetylation, serine phosphorylation), which determine the balance between chromatin activation or inactivation. Although it is now accepted that DNA methylation causes histone deacetylation, it is still not clear if histone acetylation can cause local DNA demethylation. DNA methylation could drive heterochromatin formation through other pathways independent of histone deacetylation. Recently, it was discovered that all three DNA methyltransferases interact directly with histone deacetylases HDAC1 and HDAC2 [28], inducing herochromatin formation and repressing transcription, bypassing cytosine methylation [29]. On the other hand, genes without a CpG island in their promoter cannot be efficiently silenced by methylation, but their transcription correlates with levels of histone acetylation in their promoters.

Short interfering RNAs (siRNAs) may play a critical role in gene silencing in the nucleus. SiRNAs are small duplex RNA molecules with a 2-bp 3' overhang, which have long been known to plant geneticists as mediators of post-transcriptional gene silencing (PTGS). PTGS, also known as 'RNA interference (RNAi)', consists of degradation of mRNAs homologous to the siRNAs [30]. SiRNA are able to induce heterochromatinization of homologous DNA stretches by directing DNA methylation and/or other chromatin modifications. One such modification is the methylation of histone H3 K9 residue. Recently, Kawasaki *et al.* [31] indicated that RNAi can cause transcriptional gene-silencing by RNA-directed promoter methylation in human breast cancer and in non-transformed breast epithelial cells. They presented evidence that siRNAs targeting CpG islands in the E-cadherin promoter increased methylation in MCF7 breast cancer cells, and they showed this was an RNAi sequence-specific event, and that a similar process could be induced in normal breast epithelial cells. Notably, histones can also be methylated by these RNAi sequences. The concentration of E-cadherin mRNA is decreased by using several siRNAs, and this siRNA-induced methylation was mediated by DNA methylases 1 and 3B. Although much work remains to be done in order to characterize naturally occurring short RNAs, antisense transcripts, and proteins interacting with short RNAs, it is clear that RNA plays a critical role in directing the epigenetic status of the genome.

Aberrant Methylation, Chromosome Instability and Mismatch Repair

Two kinds of changes in the DNA methylation pattern occur in breast cancer, regional hypermethylation of certain genes [32] and global hypomethylation [33, 34]. The exact nature of the defect in the cellular methylation machinery in tumor cells remains unknown. The global hypomethylation in cancer can not result from lack of DNMT activity or lack of methyl donors since many genes are hypermethylated and there is no evidence that DNMT levels are decreased in cancer, on the contrary several reports show elevated and deregulated levels of DNMT1 in cancer [35, 36]. Another hypothesis is that there is a global increase in demethylation activity in cancer cells, which drives global hypomethylation [37]. It is important to stress that tumors exhibit a global defect in the DNA methylation system with hypo- and hypermethylation events occurring in the same cells. DNA methylation changes may ultimately lead to the genetic instability characteristic of cancer in several ways.

First, 5-methylcytosine (5meC) serves as site of transition mutation by the hydrolytic deamination of 5meC to thymine. This phenomenon was used to explain the high incidence of CpG to TpG transition mutations observed in the p53 tumor suppressor gene. Such mutation frequently occurs in the well-known p53 tumor suppressor gene [38] and has also been reported in several other important genes like Rb, and c-H-ras-1 [39]. The relative importance of spontaneous deamination of 5-methylcytosine and carcinogen adduct formation at CpG sites in producing mutations remains to be clarified. Secondly, hypermethylation of certain critical genes in cancer by promoter methylation may predispose to genetic instability. Methylation of the mismatch repair gene (MLH1) is thought to be functionally linked with microsatellite instability (MSI) [40]. Mice knockouts of MLH1 show increased spontaneous mutations and cancer risk [41]. A close correlation between mismatch repair, genetic instability and methylation capacity has been reported in colon cancer cell models [42] [43]. In addition, a p53-inducible gene, 14-3-3σ is methylated in many cancers including breast carcinoma. Its inactivation may also facilitate the accumulation of genetic damages [44]. Thirdly, hypomethylation of repetitive sequences may also predispose cells to chromosomal defects and rearrangements that result in genetic instability [45]. The loss of methylation in tumor cells may predispose them to genomic instability *via* the transcriptional activation and movement of parasitic elements, these elements also pose a significant threat to the genome as mediators of homologous recombination. The most direct evidence that DNA methylation suppresses homologous recombination has come from the work in Ascobolus, but several studies support a similar role in mammalian cells. For example, DNMT1 knockout ES cells exhibit a 10-fold increased mutation rate involving gene rearrangements [46], and individuals with ICF syndrome or cultured cells treated with demethylation agent show increased numbers of chromosomal translocations [47].

Epigenetic change can predispose critical genetic mutations often found in tumorigenesis [48]. Methylation-mediated silencing occurs before the genetic change that underlies the MSI phenotype in endometrial cancers [49]. In breast cancer, it is postulated that methylation-associated inactivation of GSTP1 can result in adenine or guanine mutation by estrogen metabolites-DNA adduct formation and lead to genetic instability [50]. Hypermethylation and hypomethylation events can occur concomitantly. Rearrangements in the centromere of chromosomes 1 and 16 are observed in Wilms tumors and are thought to contribute to disease progression [51]. In breast carcinoma, satellite 2 DNA exhibits decreased methylation whereas the E-cadherin promoter is hypermethylated [51]. It is assumed that DNA methylation may suppress homologous recombination *via* masking of the recombination initiation site, maintenance of a highly condensed chromatin structure through the recruitment of DNA organizing proteins, destabilization of the recombination intermediate, or interference with the assembly of the recombination machinery. Loss of DNA methylation from repetitive elements may occur early in tumor progression and may predispose cells to genome rearrangements *via* mitotic recombination which could inactivate critical growth regulatory genes or, aberrantly regulate tumor suppressor genes or oncogenes.

Methods for Studying DNA Methylation

Methylation can be monitored either by methods that require methylation-sensitive restriction enzymes, or by methods that rely on chemical modification of the DNA with sodium bisulfite. Restriction enzyme based methods are based on the inability of methylation sensitive restriction enzymes to cleave methylated cytosines in their recognition site (Figure 1). After cleavage, analysis of methylation patterns has traditionally been conducted by utilizing southern hybridization techniques or PCR and is based on the length of the digested DNA fragment. The inability to digest methylated sequences results in longer fragments, indicating a methylated CpG dinucleotide. Restriction enzyme based methods are simple and rapid, however, it is limited to specific restriction sites and a substantial amount of initial DNA is required. This technique is useful for genome-wide methylation analyses and marker discovery. False positive results may result from incomplete digestion by the enzymes. Chemical modification of the DNA with sodium bisulfite for methylation analysis was discovered by Frommer et al. in 1992 [52](Figure 2). Sodium bisulfite reacts with cytosines in a methylation-specific manner: unmethylated cytosines are converted to uracils and methylated cytosines are not (Figure 3). The difference in methylation status marked by bisulfite reactivity can be accurately determined by PCR, sequencing, array hybridization, etc. Sodium bisulfite based detection of DNA methylation can circumvent the problems associated with restriction enzyme analysis and is now used extensively.

Methylation-specific PCR (MSP) was introduced by Herman *et al.* [53]. MSP is based on the use of two distinct methylation specific primer sets for the sequence of interest. The primers must be specific for sodium bisulfite converted DNA and therefore have to contain a substantial number of both non-CpG and CpG cytosines in the original template. Both unmethylated (U) and methylated (M) primers are commonly designed for analysis. The U primer will only amplify sodium bisulfite converted DNA in an unmethylated condition, while the M primer is specific for sodium bisulfite converted methylated DNA. Software tools are available to support MSP primer design [54, 55].

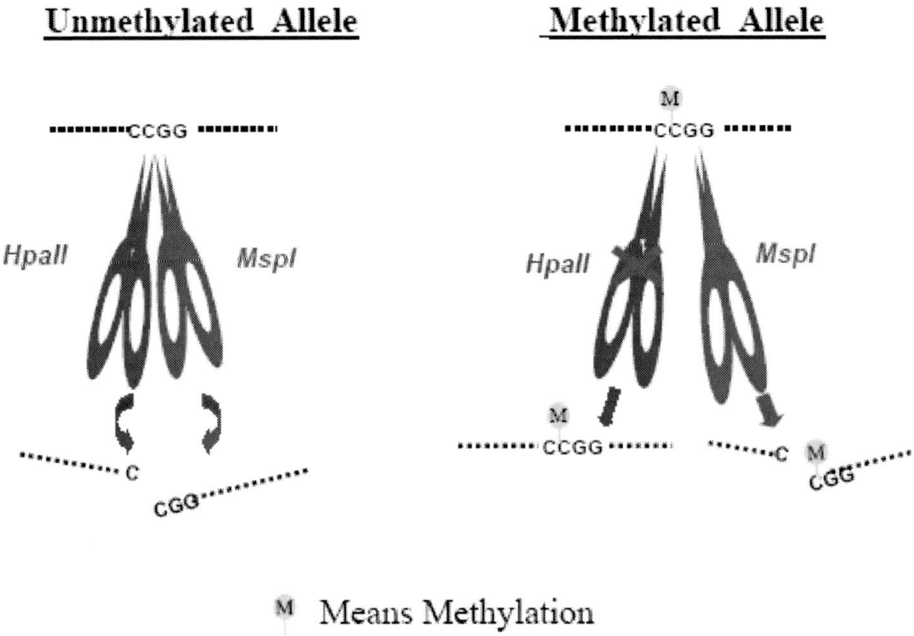

Figure 1. The cleavage of DNA by restriction endonucleases HpaII and MSPI. HapII is prevented by the presence of a 5-methyl group at the internal C residue of its recognition sequence CCGG. MspI cleaves DNA irrespective of the presence of a methyl group at this position.

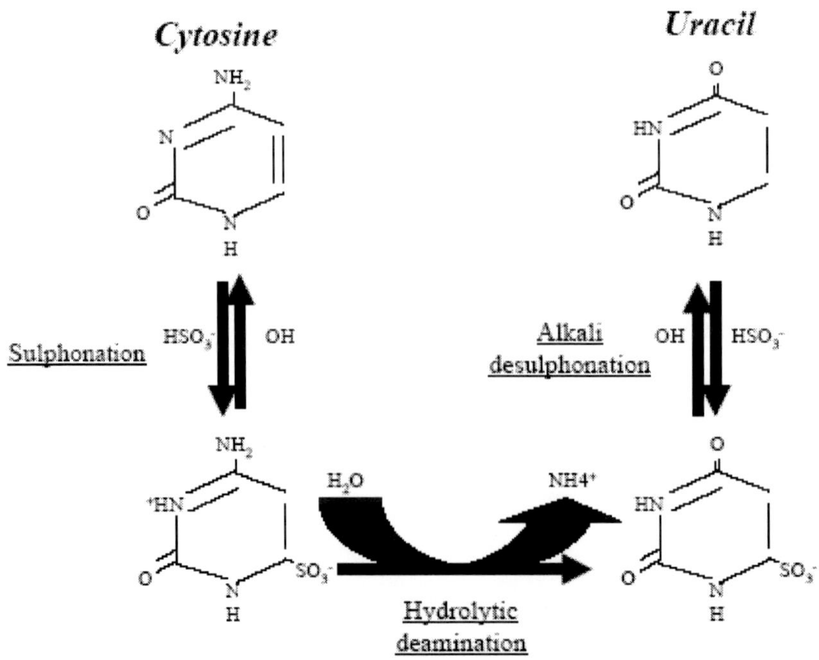

Figure 2. Bisulfite modifies cytosine to uracil.

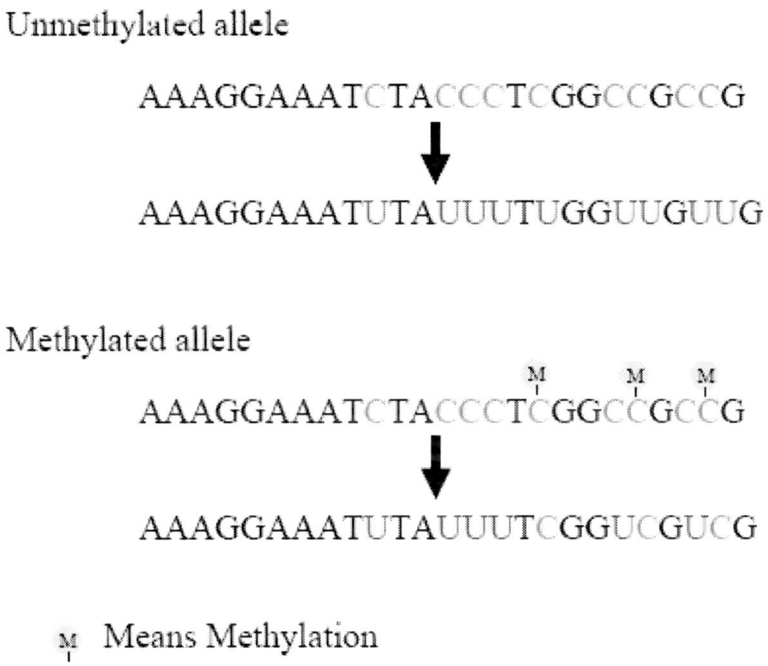

Figure 3. Sequence change with bisulfite treatment. In unmethylated allele, unmethylated cytosines are converted to uracils. In methylated allele, only unmethylated cytosines are converted to uracils.

MSP provides a sensitive and cost-effective test and makes it possible to analyze clinical samples with a limited amount of available template DNA. To increase the sensitivity of MSP for detection of methylated DNA in a background of unmethylated DNA, Palmisano *et al.* [56] developed a nested, two-round MSP. The first round primer is designed in regions flanking the MSP primers and harbouring a substantial number of cytoines but no CpG dinucleotides. In this way, the first round PCR should amplify both methylated and unmethylated alleles.

The first round PCR product is subjected to second round PCR reactions using U and M specific primers as described above. Using nested MSP, one methylated allele in >50000 unmethylated alleles is detectable. False positives for MSP analysis may be caused by the lack of the single-stranded conformation, renaturation and incomplete sodium bisulfite conversion [57-59]. Commercially available kits can improve the ease and robustness of bisulfite treatment (e.g., EZ DNA methylation kit by *Biocompare Inc.* [South San Francisco, CA] and *Zymco Research Corp.* [Orange, CA] CpGenome modification kit by *Chemicon International* [Temecula, CA] and *Intergen Co.* [Burlington, MA]. Nevertheless, when using bisulfite treatment, reaction conditions must be well controlled and controls must ensure that the treatment is complete but has not resulted in excessive degradation of DNA. Commercial and noncommercial software can help in the design of PCR primers for bisulfite-treated genomic DNA (e.g., CpGWARE primer design software by Chemicon International and Methprimer by the University of California, San Francisco Department of Urology, [available at www.urogene.org/methprimer/]). Finally, the amplification of bisulfite-treated DNA may result in preferential amplification of either the methylated or unmethylated alleles.

Quantitative MSP (Q-MSP) technology which takes advantage of the development of quantitative real-time PCR has been developed to exactly quantify the number of methylated alleles. A well-known assay is MethyLight [60]. This method relies on relative quantification against controls that are methylation insensitive, as well as a standard curve based on serial dilution of a control sample. A typical MethyLight reaction has two primers and a probe, each incorporating several CpGs so that the assay is specific. During the extension phase of the PCR, the 5' to 3' exonuclease activity of the TaqDNA Polymerase cleaves the reporter from the probe, releasing it from the quencher, resulting in an increase in fluorescence emission. Data are normalized to an internal reference gene, *e.g.* actin, which is designed in a region that does not contain any CpG nucleotides to allow an unbiased amplification. It should be noted that the quantitation provided is for the relative amounts of methylated DNA with a particular methylation pattern compared to some reference control gene. This quantitation may reflect actual changes in methylation density or differences in tumor DNA within a specific sample. To further increase the sensitivity of this technology, Fackler *et al.* [61] used a quantitative multiplex nested MSP (QM-MSP) strategy. External primers lacking CG nucleotides are used in the first round PCR reaction, therefore, both methylated and unmethylated alleles are amplified. In the second step, quantitative analysis of methylated and unmethylated DNA for each gene was performed separately with the primer pairs and probes. Q-MSP has been used for analyzing formalin-fixed, paraffin-embedded surgical samples even laser-assisted microdissected samples of breast tumors [62]. Other analytical methods include the use of methylation-specific restriction enzymes, methylation-specific single-base primer extension, arrays, or Sanger sequencing. The latter can be applied as direct genomic sequencing for semiquantitative analysis of multiple adjacent CpG sites, setting it apart from most methods, which generate data for an individual position per assay (i.e., primer). Pyrosequencing technology is a method for sequencing-by-synthesis in real time. It is based on an indirect bioluminometric assay of the pyrophosphate (PPi) that is released from each deoxynucleotide (dNTP) upon DNA-chain elongation. Pyrosequencing technology has a number of valuable attributes for methylation studies. This method provides internal controls to confirm the completeness of bisulfite treatment together with the ability to analyze several individual neighboring methylation sites. In addition, the surrounding sequence generated around the methylated areas provides control peaks that can be used to confirm the correct placement of the primer on the modified DNA template, which is now rich in adenine (A) and thymine (T).

HeavyMethyl assay [63] is another PCR-based technique for methylation detection. This kind of assay uses a blocker oligo to prevent priming of unmethylated DNA, therefore, a template with at least one methylated CpG in the blocking area and comethylation of the CpGs in the probe-binding region is required. Recently, the genome-wide methylation profiling microarray technique has been able to combine efficiently either the fragmentation by a methyl-sensitive restriction endonuclease followed by size fractionation [64] or the MSP methodology described above with the high density array method [65]. Different microarray-based strategies that have been used for methylation profiling have distinct features and provide different types of information. Ednonuclease cleavage combined with either size fractionation or PCR amplification typically has a mapping resolution of a few kilobases, without providing specific information about any individual methylated base. Therefore, cleavage-based methods are suitable for surveying gene-sized targets. One approach uses ligation-mediated PCR to preferentially amplify strongly methylated genomic regions [66]. The amplification of nonmethylated regions is suppressed by the digestion of the template DNA before PCR with the restriction enzymes BstUI and HpaII, which are blocked by cytosine methylation. A related method [67] uses digestion with SmaI, which cleaves the unmethylated sequence 5'-CCCGGG-3', followed by digestion with XmaI. The cleavage products of XmaI have 5' protruding ends, whereas SmaI leaves blunt ends. Following adaptors specific for the XmaI ends are ligated, PCR is performed using primers that are complementary to these adaptors. The PCR product should contain only genomic regions with methylated 5'-CCCGGG-3' sequences, could be hybridized to microarrays. In contrast, the bisulfite-based strategy, which has a single base pair resolution, provides only information about specific residues that have been chosen in advance as being informative. Therefore, the bisulfite-based methods may be used when particular sites have been identified and oligonucleotide pairs optimized.

Hypermethylation as Breast Cancer Biomarkers

DNA hypermethylation is the most common and best characterized epigenetic abnormality in human malignancies, including breast cancer. By searching the Medline database using query "breast AND hypermethylation", 222 records appeared on March 8, 2005. These genes include classic and putative tumor-suppressor genes and genes involved in a number of cellular pathways such as hormonal responses, tumor-cell invasion and/or tumor architecture, cell cycle control, and DNA damage repair. For many of these genes, promoter hypermethylation is often the main mechanism underlying the functional loss in breast cancer. Aberrant silencing of these genes can contribute to cancer initiation, progression, and metastasis. Hypermethylation of these genes in breast cancer can correlate with histological type, pathologic grade, clinical stage and prognosis.

Hypermethylation as a Marker for Predicting Breast Cancer Risk

To date, several studies have shown that methylation-associated silencing inactivates certain tumor suppressors as effectively as mutations and is one of the cancer-predisposing hits described in Knudson's two hit hypothesis. For some genes, an aberrant decrease or absence of expression may not be a consequence of somatic mutations or allele loss at all, DNA hypermethylation may be the primary mechanism of gene inactivation. One possibility is that hypermethylation could begin in a monoallelic form with subsequent expansion to both alleles of the gene and the resultant complete abrogation of gene function. Methylation may also function synergistically with genetic mutations to promote tumourigenesis in a more indirect fashion. In our previous study, we demonstrated that biallelic inactivation of the FHIT gene could result from either epigenetic inactivation of both parental alleles, or from epigenetic modification of one allele and deletion of the remaining allele [68]. A model for the biallelic inactivation of tumor suppressor genes by aberrant DNA methylation alone or in combination with mutations or deletions is shown in Figure 4.

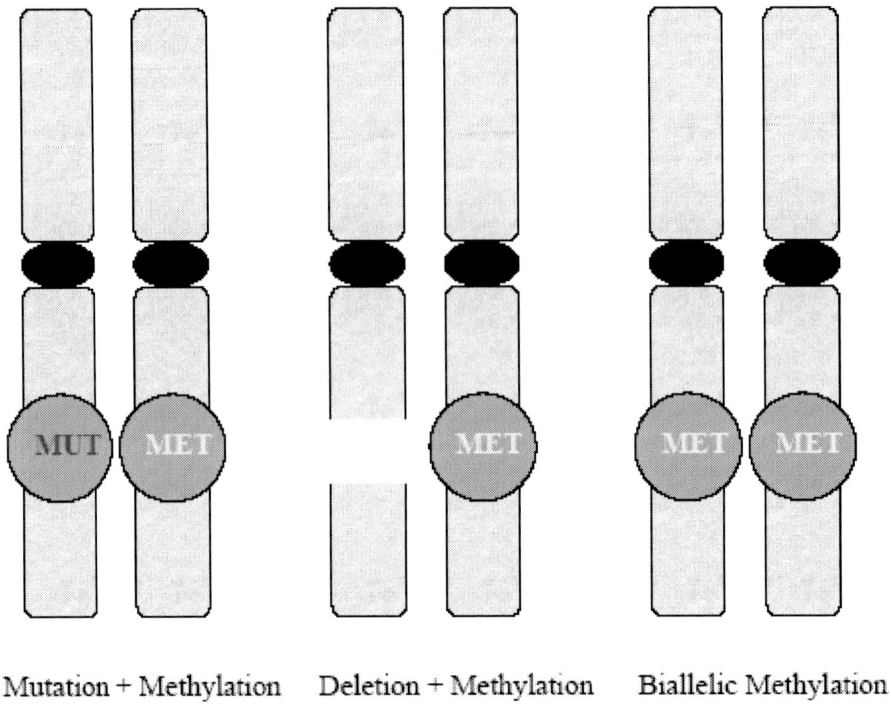

Figure 4. Schematic representation of tumor suppressor gene inactivation. Hypermethylation (METH) progresses in a monoallelic form and can expand to both alleles of the gene. Biallelic inactivation of tumor suppressor gene may be resulted from mutation (MUT) and hypermethylation, loss of heterozygosity (deletion) and hypermethylation, and biallelic hypermethylation.

Epidemiologic risk factors such as age, cancer family history, history of breast biopsies, and reproductive history have been combined in mathematical models that are useful for categorizing women as having a low, intermediate, or high risk for breast cancer. The tumor suppressor genes (TSGs) RASSF1A, APC, H-cadherin, RARβ2, and cyclin D2 are methylated more frequently in breast cancer than in adjacent benign tissue. These data suggest that methylation of certain TSGs may occur as a field change and may be associated with increased risk for malignant progression.

Lewis *et al.* [69] analyzed the methylation status of these five TSGs in benign and malignant breast cells to determine whether TSG methylation frequency in benign breast tissue is associated with epidemilogic markers of breast cancer risk. They found that cyclin D2 methylation seems to occur later in breast epithelial cell transformation and may be exploited in the future as a marker for the early detection of breast cancer, whereas RARβ2, APC, and RASSF1A promoter methylation occurs frequently in benign breast epithelium and is associated with epidemiologic markers of increased breast cancer risk. More specifically, RARβ2 methylation is correlated with a personal history of breast cancer, whereas APC and RASSF1A methylation is associated with calculated breast cancer risk particularly in women with prior benign breast biopsies. This may suggest a field change in benign breast epithelium that could be exploited for tissue-based individualized breast cancer risk stratification.

Hypermethylation as a Marker for Cancer Detection

Detection of breast cancer at an early stage is the key to successful treatment and outcome. Despite the availability of mammography and prevalence of self-examination, there is still additional benefit to be gained from additional screening methodologies. Novel approaches to early detection of breast neoplasia therefore merit examination. The genetic and epigenetic alterations that initiate and drive tumorigenesis are promising targets for early detection because they may precede clinically obvious cancer, can be detected at sensitive levels, may be specific to tumor cells, and can potentially provide information about the prognosis and treatment of the disease.

Currently, fine needle aspiration (FNA) cytology is an integral part of the diagnostic evaluation of suspicious breast lesions. However, because morphological features of malignancy are more ambiguous in small tumors and premalignant lesions, this procedure is prone to challenge the cytopathologist, and renders a diagnosis that is highly dependent on the proficiency of the performer. Nipple aspiration is a noninvasive technique that provides a fluid sample containing both cells shed from the breast duct lining and proteins secreted and concentrated into the duct lumen. FNA washings from breast lesions and nipple aspiration are suitable clinical samples for DNA-based detection of breast cancer. Detection of hypermethylation offers several advantages. A major one is that abnormal promoter hypermethylation profiling of cancer-associated genes may be a tumor-specific marker, and this alteration is often enhanced during disease progression, thus making it readily detectable in clinical specimens. In addition, hypermethylation constitutes a positively detectable signal with a very high degree of specificity, even in presence of a vast excess of unmethylated DNA. Detection of TSG hypermethylation has been detected in nipple aspirate [70] as well as in ductal lavage [71]. Jeronimo *et al.* [72] demonstrated that detection of gene hypermethylation in FNA washings by MSP is feasible. It is important that the target epigenetic alteration is cancer-specific and not present in normal or benign cells. Krassenstein *et al.* [70] using a hypermethylation panel of 6 genes (GSTP1, RARβ2, p16, p14, RASSF1A, and death-associated protein kinase) provided 100% coverage in nipple aspirate fluid samples. Jeronimo *et al.* did not select the cancer-specific targets, the methylated gene pattern could not discriminate between benign and malignant breast lesions in their study [72].

Serum or plasma is a more readily accessible bodily fluid, and provision of a specimen does not require the presence of a specialist. DNA is known to be released into serum/plasma, which is enriched from tumor DNA in cancer patients [73]. Importantly, tumor cell-specific DNA alterations in serum were not limited to patients with metastatic ancer but were also present in serum from patients with early or organ-confined tumors. Neoplastic DNA in the serum most likely arises from cells that have left the site of the primary lesion and have invaded the circulatory system but lack he capacity of metastasis to new organs or may be released from the primary tumor as free DNA from nonviable (apoptotic) neoplastic cells [1, 74]. Dulaimi *et al.* demonstrated tumor cell specific promoter hypermethylation of APC,

RASSF1A, and DAP-kinase is present in ductal carcinoma *in situ*, lobular carcinoma *in situ*, and all grades and stages of invasive breast cancer. Hypermethylation can be detected by MSP analysis in serum DNA from patients with preinvasive and early-stage breast cancer amenable to cure.

Hypermethylation as a Marker for Histological Classification

According to the World Health Organization Classification, invasive breast carcinoma is subclassified as invasive ductal carcinoma, invasive lobular carcinoma and other special types. Ductal (over 80%) and lobular (about 10%) cancers are the two largest morphological subgroups of invasive breast cancer. Special subtypes include medullary carcinoma, mucinous carcinoma, papillary carcinoma, tubular carcinoma, adenoid cystic carcinoma, apocrine carcinoma, carcinoma with metaplasia, squamous type, spindle-cell type, cartilaginous and osseous type, mixed type, and others [75]. Because conventional histological behavior of specific cancers could not predict biological behavior, classifying cancers on a molecular level is urgently needed. Some researchers addressed the question whether different histological subtypes of cancer originating in the same organ differ in the epigenetic inactivation of essential genes.

Osada *et al.* [76] discovered a strong association between small lung cell cancer and 14-3-3δ hypermethylation, which was rarely found in non-small cell lung cancer. Graff *et al.* [77] found different methylation frequencies for the E-cadherin gene in different subtypes of thyroid carcinoma. Plachot *et al.* [78] investigated the effect of DNA methylation on the regulation of mammary acinar differention. They found that acinar morphogenesis was accompanied with chromatin remodeling, as shown by alterations in histone 4 acetylation, heterozhromatin 1 protein, and histone 3 methylated on lysine 9, and with an increase in expression of MeCP2. The results indicate that DNA methylation may act at least on two critical aspects of mammary epithelial differentiation, including tissue polarity and also potentially progenitor capabilities. Therefore, methylation pattern may be related with morphological phenotype in breast cancer.

Lehmann *et al.* [79] demonstrated that promoter hypermethylation of death-associated protein (DAP) kinase was found to be significantly higher in invasive lobular carcinoma compared to invasive ductal carcinoma. Fackler *et al.* [80] reported that Twist was hypermethylated less often in invasive lobular carcinoma than in invasive ductal carcinoma. Bae *et al.* [81] evaluated methylation status of 12 different genes in a series of 109 invasive breast tumors representing the ductal, lobular, and mucinous histologic subtypes using MSP. The selected genes include 10 genes that are commonly methylated in breast cancer (RASSF1A, HIN1, Twist, Cyclin D2, RARβ2, THRβ, E-cadherin, ER, BRCA1, and GSTP1), as well as two genes that are infrequently methylated in breast cancer (BAX and RB). As the results, lobular cancers and mucious cancers, which often have relatively low levels of chromosomal changes, have higher overall frequencies of hypermethylation than ductal cancers (49% in lobular and mucinous versus 40% in ductal), but there is a relatively unimodal distribution of methylation frequency of all three histologic types. Only BRCA1 shows a frequency of methylation that is significantly different among the various histologic categories, which is consistent an earlier report [53]. These findings suggest that methylation patterns of selected genes could contribute to the molecular classification of breast cancer. Differential methylation hybridization methods, including CpG island microarrays [66, 82, 83] are available to do epigenome-wide analysis. Analysis of more breast cancer cases and consideration of large amount of genes could help to define classes of breast cancer based on patterns of aberrant gene promoter methylation.

Hypermethylation as a Marker for Progression Evaluation

Another potential use of DNA methylation is in the classification of tumors depending on their methylation status. Such classification might be of use in determining patient prognosis. LATS1 and LATS2 are tumor suppressor genes implicated in the regulation of cell cycle. Hypermethylation of the promoter regions of LATS1 and LATS2 likely plays an important role in the down-regulation of their mRNA levels in breast cancers, and breast cancers with a decreased expression of LATS1 or LATS2 mRNA levels have a biologically aggressive phenotype [84]. Huang *et al.* developed an array-based methylation detection technology, called differential methylation hybridization (DMH), allowing for genome-wide screening of CpG island hypermethylation in breast cancer cell lines [82] and primary tumors [85]. Using DMH, they found that poorly differentiated tumors appeared to exhibit more hypermethylated CpG islands than their moderately or well-differentiated counterparts [85].

Systematic analysis of laser-microdissected ductal carcinoma *in situ* (DCIS) as well as epithelial hyperplasia and intraductal papillomas was performed by Lehamann *et al.* [62]. Four growth regulatory genes, p16, RASSF1, cyclin D2 and 14-3-3δ were investigated. They found that aberrant promoter methylation was already prevalent in pure intraductal carcinoma with different frequencies and different methylation levels for the four genes analyzed. RASSF1A and 14-3-3δ promoter methylation was also demonstrated in epithelial hyperplasia and intraductal papillomas. However, aberrant methylation of cyclinD2 and p16 was restricted to cancerous epithelium, and increased methylation of the cyclinD2 gene was significantly associated with a higher van Nuys grade.

The estrogen receptor (ER) gene and E-cadherin gene have been implicated frequently in the initiation and/or progression of human breast cancer. Loss of expression of either gene has been associated with poorly differentiated tumors and poorer prognosis [86, 87]. Loss of ER expression, as well as loss of E-cadherin expression, has been associated with aberrant 5'CpG methylation in breast cancers [88, 89]. Nass et al. [90] have surveyed 111 breast ductal carcinomas for aberrant methylation of ER and E-cadherin 5' CpG islands. Hypermethylation of either CpG island was evident prior to invasion in 30% of ductal carcinoma *in situ* lesions and increased significantly to nearly 60% in metastatic lesions. Coincident methylation of both CpG islands also increased significantly from 20% in ductal carcinoma *in situ* to nearly 50% in metastatic lesions. The increase in the coincident methylation of both CpG islands suggests that malignant progression of human breast cancer involves an accumulation of epigenetic events. The transcription factor activator protein-2α (AP-2α) is a tumor suppressor protein that can be lost during tumor progression. Recently, Douglas *et al.* [91] found that hypermethylation of a small CpG-rich region correlates with loss of AP-2α expression during progression of breast cancer. ER and E-cadherin are the down-stream factors of AP-2α, loss of AP-2α function might jield only a partial loss of tumor suppressor function for the ER and E-cadherin genes. Since ER and E-cadherin could also be attacked directly by local promoter change, coincident methylation of AP-2α, ER and E-cadherin may drive cancer invasion and progression.

The presence of methylation in certain genes within a tumour might be useful to identify more aggressive subtypes of cells. Such patterns of methylation in breast tumours may finally provide vital information for the individualisation of treatment. In addition, DNA methylation could be detected in bloodstream of breast cancer patients. Muller *et al.* [92] addressed whether DNA methylation in serum could be used as prognostic marker for breast cancer patients. Five genes (ESR1, APC, HSD17B4, HIC1, and RASSF1A) were selected to be candidate prognostic factors for breast cancer using a high-throughput MethyLight assay. Multivariate analysis showed methylated RASSF1A and/or APC serum DNA are independently associated with poor outcome.

Because neoadjuvant therapy has become increasingly popular as primary medical treatment of breast cancer, much attraction is focused on grading tumors on FNA cytology. Such grading would allow assessment of the tumor *in situ*, so the most-suitable treatment could be selected before primary surgery, and morbidity associated with overtreatment of low-grade tumors could be avoided. We developed a semiquatitative grading system for invasive ductal carcinoma on FNAC recently [93]. Without our method, tumor differentiation and progression could be evaluated preoperatively (Figure 5. Using FNA samples, combined analysis of cytological grading with certain genes methylation pattern may contribute to defined evaluation of tumor progression before operation.

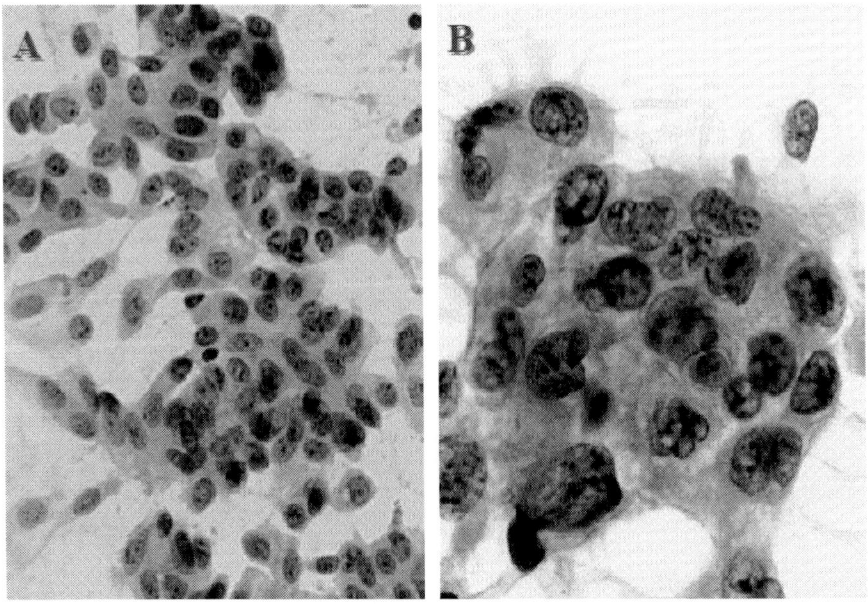

Figure 5. Cytological smear of invasive ductal carcinoma (Papanicolaou stain x40). (A) a well differentiated ductal carcinoma. (B) a poorly differentiated ductal carcinoma.

Hypermethylation as a Predictor of Response to Treatment

The presence of estrogen receptor (ER) and/or progesterone receptor (PR) is an important diagnostic feature of breast cancer, and reflective of disease etiology. Over the three decades, the estrogen receptor antagonist tamoxifen has been mainstay of hormonal therapy, approximately 30% of patients treated with this agent still die within 10 years of follow-up treatment, and relapses can occur for more than 20 years following therapy [94]. The cause of treatment failure in many breast cancer patients receiving tamoxifen is resistance to it. Hormone receptor (HR) status, defined as ER and/or PR positivity, has been shown to predict response to tamoxifen treatment [95]. ERs comprose two subtypes, ER α and ER β. ER β was often coexpressed with ER α and sometimes inversely correlated PR. Recent studies have shown that hypermethylation appears to play a role in inactivation of these genes. Southern blot and MSP analyses revealed that ER α was unmethylated in normal breast tissue and ER-positive tumor cell lines, such as MCF-7, T47-D and ZR75-1; it is methylated in about 50% of unselected primary breast cancers and most ER-negative cancer cell lines, *e.g.* MDA-MB-231, MDA-MB-435, MDA-MB-468, Hs578t and MCF-7/Adr. The ER α island methylation is associated with reduced or absent ER mRNA expression. PR gene methylation has been demonstrated by Southern analysis in about 40% of PR-negative breast tumors and several PR-negative breast cancer cell lines such as MDA-MB-231, MDA-MB-468, MDA-MB-435 and Hs578t. Chang *et al.* [96] investigated the methylation patterns of the ER genes in the tamoxifen-resistant tumors. They used bisulfite genomic sequencing and reverse transcriptase PCR to determine the methylation patterns and mRNA expression of the two ER genes, α and β, from control and tamoxifen-resistant tissues chosen by an age-matched sampling method. The methylation rate of the ER β but not the ER α in the control group was significantly higher than in its counterpart. Among the methylated tumors mean methylation density of ER α and ER β in the resistant cases was significantly elevated. The tamoxifen-resistant tumors showed more dense methylation of the ER β gene than control tumors.

Rectinoic acid receptor β is also a member of the nuclear receptor superfamily. Loss of RAR β2 has been observed in solid tumor cells, including lung carcinoma, squamous cell carcinoma, and breast cancer. These findings suggest that the specific loss of RAR β2 expression may be an important event during tumorigenesis. This hypothesis is supported by the observation that introduction of RAR β into retinoic acid-insensitive breast cancer cell lines restored retinoic acid responsiveness to growth inhibition and induction of apoptosis. To further examine the hypothesis that the chemopreventive effects of retinoids are due to RAR β2 induction, Sun *et al.* [97] blocked ATRA-induced RAR β expression in H157 cells using a retroviral vector harboring multiple copies of antisense RAR β2 sequences. Antisense RAR β-transfected cells shows not only decreased expression of ATRA-induced RAR β protein but also reduced ATRA-induced RARE binding activity and transactivation. Importantly, all antisense RAR β transfectants of H157 cells were less responsive than vector-retinoids ATRA and Ch55 *in vitro*. These results demonstrated that RAR β induction might play an important role in mediating growth inhibitory effects of retinoids in cancer cells. DNA methylation of the RAR β2 has been demonstrated in human cancer cell lines and tumors [98, 99], methylation assay of RAR β2 may provide critical information for retinoid response in breast cancer.

Combined use of epigenetic drugs with agents that target reactivated genes—in effect using epigenetic drugs as cellular sensitizers is a promising strategy for cancer treatment. Restoration of response to retinoid signaling using this approach has been observed in acute myeloid leukemia and in colon and breast cancers [100-102]. This approach could be used to reactivate other genes silenced in precancerous tissues that are targets for established chemopreventive agents such as ER gene described above. Recently, Fiegl et al. [103] analyzed *RASSF1A* DNA methylation in pretherapeutic sera and serum samples collected 1 year after surgery from 148 patients with breast cancer who were receiving adjuvant tamoxifen; 19.6% and 22.3% of patients with breast cancer showed *RASSF1A* DNA methylation in their pretherapeutic and 1-year-after serum samples, respectively. *RASSF1A* methylation 1 year after primary surgery (and during adjuvant tamoxifen therapy) was an independent predictor of poor outcome. Based on their findings, measurement of serum DNA methylation allows adjuvant systemic treatment to be monitored for efficacy: disappearance of *RASSF1A* DNA methylation in serum throughout treatment with tamoxifen indicates a response, whereas persistence or new appearance means resistance to adjuvant tamoxifen treatment. Therefore, serum DNA methylation such as *RASSF1A* is an easy means of detecting patients undergoing adjuvant treatment who need advanced treatment.

Epigenetic Modulators for Breast Cancer Treatment

Unlike genetic alterations such as mutations, epigenetic changes such as DNA methylation are potentially reversible. Methylation causes the inactivation of numerous genes that are important in the development of most tumor types including breast cancer, therefore, epigenetic changes are attractive target for cancer therapy. 5-Azacytidine and 5-aza-2'-deoxycytidine (5-Aza-CdR) (Figure 6), nucleoside analog inhibitors of DNMTs, have been widely used to reverse abnormal DNA hypermethylation and restore silenced gene expression. In one of our previous studies [104], the effect of 5-Aza-CdR RAR β2 restoration was investigated in the MRK-nu-1 human female breast cancer cell line. Changes of the RAR β2 methylation status were assessed by MSP. Reverse transcription PCR was used to evaluate RAR β2 restoration. Cell cycling and growth inhibition were studied using flow cytometric analysis of DNA content and CellTiter 96 AQueous non-radioactive cell proliferation assay, respectively. 5-Aza-CdR treatment resulted in complete demethylation of the RAR β2 gene. RAR β2 restoration was accompanied by cell cycle arrest (increase in the G0/G1- and decrease in the S- and G2/M-phases) and time-dependent growth inhibition. Nucleoside analog inhibitors of DNMTs have many potential side effects, such as myelotoxicity, mutagenesis, and tumorigenesis. A few non-nucleoside inhibitors of DNA methyltransferases have been reported, including the anti-arrhythmia drug, procainamide. Following this need to find new demethylating agents, Villar-Garea *et al.* [105] have tested the potential use of procaine, an anesthetic drug related to procainamide. Using the MCF-7 breast cancer cell line, they found that procaine is a DNA-demethylating agent that produces a 40% reduction in 5-methylcytosine DNA content as determined by high-performance capillary electrophoresis or total DNA enzyme digestion.

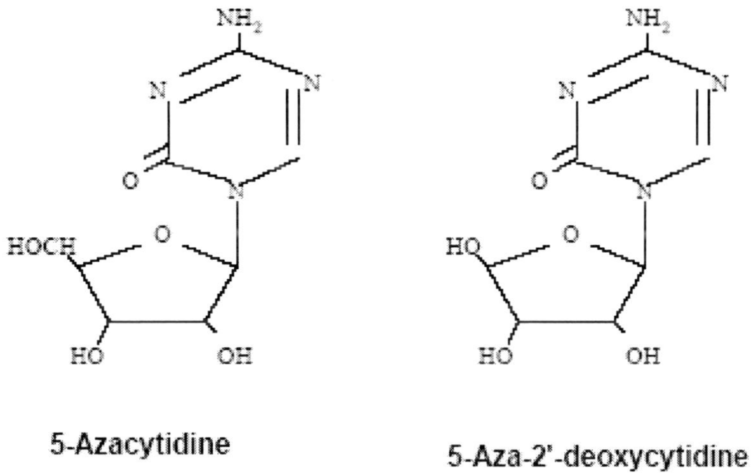

Figure 6. Structure of 5-Azacytidine and 5-Aza-2'-deoxycytidine.

Procaine can also demethylate densely hypermethylated CpG islands, such as those located in the promoter region of the RAR β2 gene, restoring gene expression of epigenetically silenced genes. Non-nucleoside analog DNA methyltransferase inhibitors such as procainamide are attractive alternative for possible clinical use. Very recently, Grunt et al.[106] reported that other reagents may also have demethylation activity. They demonstrated that the EGFR inhibitor PD153035 not only blocked activation of EGFR and inhibited cell growth, but also stimulated RAR-beta expression in MDA-MB-468 breast and OVCAR-3 ovarian carcinoma cells. Upregulation of RAR-beta by PD153035 was confirmed by real-time reverse transcription-polymerase chain reaction. In contrast, expression of other retinoid receptors and of estrogen receptor-alpha was not affected. PD153035-mediated re-induction of RAR-beta was associated with demethylation of the RAR-beta2 gene promoter P2 as demonstrated by methylation-specific polymerase chain reaction. These novel results on the ErbB/retinoid receptor cross-talk may be useful for designing future anticancer combination regimens.

As described above, histone deacetylase activity is important in the transcriptional repression of methylated sequences. Histone deacetylase inhibitors induce cell-cycle arrest, apoptosis, and/or differentiation in transformed cells *in vitro* and suppress the growth of a wide variety of solid tumor xenografts with minimal toxicity. Several structural classes of histone deacetylase inhibitors have been identified, including short-chain fatty acids (butyric and valproic acids), hydroxamic acids (suberoylanilide hydroxamic acid, *m*-carboxycinnamic acid bishydroxamide, trichostatin A, oxamflatin, and pyroxamide), tetrapeptides (depsipeptide), and benzamides (MS-275, which stands for *N*-(2-aminophenyl)-4-[*N*-(pyridin-3-yl-methoxycarbonyl)aminomethyl]benzamide and CI-994, which stands for *N*-acetyldinaline). Keen *et al.* [107] demonstrated that combining treatment with 5-aza-2'-deoxycytidine and the histone deacetylase (HDAC) inhibitor resulted in expression of functional ER mRNA and protein. Suberoylanilide hydroxamic acid decreased the incidence and multiplicity of *N*-methyl-*N*-nitrosourea-induced rat mammary tumors; unlike 5-aza-2'-deoxycytidine, inhibitory effects were manifest at stages after initiation. Suberoylanilide hydroxamic acid also inhibited hyperplastic nodule formation in response to 7,12-

dimethylbenz[*a*]anthracene treatment in mouse mammary gland organ culture and the multiplicity of carcinogen-induced lung tumors in mice [108]. Very recently, Sharma *et al.* [109] demonstrated that inhibitors of DNA DNMT and histone deacetylases (HDAC) synergistically activate the methylated ER gene promoter in ER negative MDA-MB-231 human breast cancer cells. Chromatin immunoprecipitation (ChIP) was used to examine the chromatin status and repressor complex associated with silenced ER and changes in the key regulatory factors during reactivation by inhibitors of DNMT (5-aza-2'deoxycytidine or 5-aza-dC) and HDAC (trichostatin A or TSA). The silencing of ER due to CpG hypermethylation correlates with binding of specific methyl-binding proteins, DNA methyltransferases and HDAC proteins. Inhibition of HDAC activity by TSA results in the accumulation of hyperacetylated core histones. The activation of ER gene expression by 5aza-dC also involves the release of the repressor complex involving various methyl binding proteins, DNMTs, and HDAC1. HDAC and DNMT inhibitors modulate histone methylation at H3-K9 and H3-K4 to form a more open chromatin structure necessary for reactivation of silenced ER transcription. Combining demethylating agents and histone deacetylase inhibitors may provide a means to reduce the side effects associated with the former drugs. Synergy between 5-aza-2'-deoxycytidine and trichostatin A has been achieved in reactivating methylation-silenced tumor suppressor genes [110].

Conclusion

DNA methylation is an epigenetic modification with an important role in the control of gene expression in human cancer. Within the past few years, the number of known DNMT enzymes, the number of genes known to be targeted by methylation have increased significantly and the mechanisms by which DNA methylation leads to transcriptional inactivation have been greatly elucidated. Aberrant promoter methylation of cancer-related genes are not randomly distributed in breast cancers [111], therefore, breast cancer could be grouped based on methylation pattern. DNMTs such as DNMT1, 3A, 3B are differentially distributed in breast cancer [112], the relative roles of the individual DNMTs in individual gene expression remain unclear. The reason that hypomethylation and hypermethylation co-exist in breast cancer tumors need further research. Breast cancer cells typically contain somatically altered nucleic acid, characterized by mutation, amplification, or deletion of critical genes. In addition, the nucleic acid from breast cancer cells often displays epigenetic changes, e.g. DNA methylation. Currently, there is a lack of both evidence and consensus with regard to the timing of genetic versus epigenetic perturbations in tumorigenesis and plausible non-mutually exclusive mechanisms can be proposed in either case. The timing of the methylation and gene inactivation process with respect to tumor formation remains to be properly defined.

DNA methylation detection can serve as a promising tumor biomarker of early diagnosis. Diagnostic approaches based on identification of epigenetic changes in specific genes are likely to allow implementation of early detection strategies and novel therapeutic approaches. Targeting these early changes might lead to more effective cancer treatment. However, very few markers have been demonstrated with high sensitivity and specificity. Identifying new aberrantly methylated genes using high-throughput microarray technology should be performed toward tumor marker selection. Increased interests are focused on using novel approaches to reversing tumor-specific methylation.

Combining demethylating agents and histone deacetylase inhibitors may provide a means to reduce the side effects associated with the former drugs. Synergy between 5-aza-2'-deoxycytidine and trichostatin A has been achieved in reactivating methylation-silenced tumor suppressor genes[110]. Other promising strategies include the use of the combined use of epigenetic drugs with agents that target reactivated genes, in this way, epigenetic drugs are used as cellular sensitizers. Restoration of response to retinoid signaling using this approach has been observed in many tumor types including breast cancer [102, 113, 114]. In addition, a combination of DNMT inhibitors and histone deacetylation inhibitors may be an alterative attractive strategy for the treatment of breast cancer patients.

References

[1] Sidransky, D., Emerging molecular markers of cancer. *Nat. Rev. Cancer*, 2002. *2*(3): p. 210-9.

[2] Laird, P.W., The power and the promise of DNA methylation markers. *Nat. Rev. Cancer*, 2003. *3*(4): p. 253-66.

[3] Ballestar, E. and M. Esteller, The impact of chromatin in human cancer: linking DNA methylation to gene silencing. *Carcinogenesis*, 2002. *23*(7): p. 1103-9.

[4] Takai, D. and P.A. Jones, Comprehensive analysis of CpG islands in human chromosomes 21 and 22. *Proc. Natl. Acad. Sci. USA*, 2002. *99*(6): p. 3740-5.

[5] Robertson, K.D., *DNA* methylation and chromatin - unraveling the tangled web. *Oncogene*, 2002. *21*(35): p. 5361-79.

[6] Costello, J.F. and C. Plass, Methylation matters. *J. Med. Genet*, 2001. *38*(5): p. 285-303.

[7] Yoder, J.A. and T.H. Bestor, A candidate mammalian DNA methyltransferase related to pmt1p of fission yeast. *Hum. Mol. Genet,* 1998. *7*(2): p. 279-84.

[8] Bestor, T., et al., Cloning and sequencing of a cDNA encoding DNA methyltransferase of mouse cells. The carboxyl-terminal domain of the mammalian enzymes is related to bacterial restriction methyltransferases. *J. Mol. Biol.*, 1988. *203*(4): p. 971-83.

[9] Agoston, A.T., et al., Increased protein stability causes DNA methyltransferase 1 dysregulation in breast cancer. *J. Biol. Chem.*, 2005.

[10] Okano, M., S. Xie, and E. Li, Cloning and characterization of a family of novel mammalian DNA (cytosine-5) methyltransferases. *Nat. Genet.*, 1998. *19*(3): p. 219-20.

[11] Robertson, K.D., et al., The human DNA methyltransferases (DNMTs) 1, 3a and 3b: coordinate mRNA expression in normal tissues and overexpression in tumors. *Nucleic. Acids Res.*, 1999. *27*(11): p. 2291-8.

[12] Xie, S., et al., Cloning, expression and chromosome locations of the human DNMT3 gene family. *Gene*, 1999. *236*(1): p. 87-95.

[13] Okano, M., et al., DNA methyltransferases Dnmt3a and Dnmt3b are essential for de novo methylation and mammalian development. *Cell*, 1999. *99*(3): p. 247-57.

[14] Xu, G.L., et al., Chromosome instability and immunodeficiency syndrome caused by mutations in a DNA methyltransferase gene. *Nature*, 1999. *402*(6758): p. 187-91.
[15] Ramsahoye, B.H., et al., Non-CpG methylation is prevalent in embryonic stem cells and may be mediated by DNA methyltransferase 3a. *Proc. Natl. Acad. Sci. USA*, 2000. *97*(10): p. 5237-42.
[16] Mizuno, S., et al., Expression of DNA methyltransferases DNMT1, 3A, and 3B in normal hematopoiesis and in acute and chronic myelogenous leukemia. *Blood*, 2001. *97*(5): p. 1172-9.
[17] Ordway, J.M. and T. Curran, Methylation matters: modeling a manageable genome. *Cell Growth Differ*, 2002. *13*(4): p. 149-62.
[18] Howell, C.Y., et al., Genomic imprinting disrupted by a maternal effect mutation in the Dnmt1 gene. *Cell,* 2001. *104*(6): p. 829-38.
[19] Mohandas, T., R.S. Sparkes, and L.J. Shapiro, Reactivation of an inactive human X chromosome: evidence for X inactivation by DNA methylation. *Science*, 1981. *211*(4480): p. 393-6.
[20] Nan, X., et al., Transcriptional repression by the methyl-CpG-binding protein MeCP2 involves a histone deacetylase complex. *Nature*, 1998. *393*(6683): p. 386-9.
[21] Lewis, J.D., et al., Purification, sequence, and cellular localization of a novel chromosomal protein that binds to methylated DNA. *Cell,* 1992. *69*(6): p. 905-14.
[22] Hendrich, B. and A. Bird, Identification and characterization of a family of mammalian methyl-CpG binding proteins. *Mol. Cell Biol.*, 1998. *18*(11): p. 6538-47.
[23] Magdinier, F., et al., Regional methylation of the 5' end CpG island of BRCA1 is associated with reduced gene expression in human somatic cells. *Faseb J.*, 2000. *14*(11): p. 1585-94.
[24] Ballestar, E., et al., Methyl-CpG binding proteins identify novel sites of epigenetic inactivation in human cancer. *Embo J.*, 2003. *22*(23): p. 6335-45.
[25] Jones, P.L., et al., Methylated DNA and MeCP2 recruit histone deacetylase to repress transcription. *Nat. Genet*, 1998. *19*(2): p. 187-91.
[26] Turner, B.M., Cellular memory and the histone code. *Cell,* 2002. *111*(3): p. 285-91.
[27] Fuks, F., et al., The methyl-CpG-binding protein MeCP2 links DNA methylation to histone methylation. *J. Biol. Chem.*, 2003. *278*(6): p. 4035-40.
[28] Robertson, K.D., et al., DNMT1 forms a complex with Rb, E2F1 and HDAC1 and represses transcription from E2F-responsive promoters. *Nat. Genet*, 2000. *25*(3): p. 338-42.
[29] Burgers, W.A., F. Fuks, and T. Kouzarides, DNA methyltransferases get connected to chromatin. *Trends Genet*, 2002. *18*(6): p. 275-7.
[30] Matzke, M., A.J. Matzke, and J.M. Kooter, RNA: guiding gene silencing. *Science*, 2001. *293*(5532): p. 1080-3.
[31] Kawasaki, H. and K. Taira, Induction of DNA methylation and gene silencing by short interfering RNAs in human cells. *Nature*, 2004. *431*(7005): p. 211-7.
[32] Baylin, S.B., et al., Aberrant patterns of DNA methylation, chromatin formation and gene expression in cancer. *Hum. Mol. Genet*, 2001. *10*(7): p. 687-92.
[33] Feinberg, A.P., et al., Reduced genomic 5-methylcytosine content in human colonic neoplasia. *Cancer Res.*, 1988. *48*(5): p. 1159-61.

[34] Narayan, A., et al., Hypomethylation of pericentromeric DNA in breast adenocarcinomas. *Int. J. Cancer*, 1998. *77*(6): p. 833-8.
[35] Nass, S.J., et al., Expression of DNA methyl-transferase (DMT) and the cell cycle in human breast cancer cells. *Oncogene*, 1999. *18*(52): p. 7453-61.
[36] De Marzo, A.M., et al., Abnormal regulation of DNA methyltransferase expression during colorectal carcinogenesis. *Cancer Res.*, 1999. *59*(16): p. 3855-60.
[37] Szyf, M., Targeting DNA methylation in cancer. *Ageing Res. Rev.*, 2003. *2*(3): p. 299-328.
[38] Magewu, A.N. and P.A. Jones, Ubiquitous and tenacious methylation of the CpG site in codon 248 of the p53 gene may explain its frequent appearance as a mutational hot spot in human cancer. *Mol. Cell Biol.*, 1994. *14*(6): p. 4225-32.
[39] Ghazi, H., et al., Changes in the allelic methylation patterns of c-H-ras-1, insulin and retinoblastoma genes in human development. *Dev. Suppl.*, 1990: p. 115-23.
[40] Strand, M., et al., Destabilization of tracts of simple repetitive DNA in yeast by mutations affecting DNA mismatch repair. *Nature*, 1993. *365*(6443): p. 274-6.
[41] Prolla, T.A., et al., Tumour susceptibility and spontaneous mutation in mice deficient in Mlh1, Pms1 and Pms2 DNA mismatch repair. *Nat. Genet*, 1998. *18*(3): p. 276-9.
[42] Lengauer, C., K.W. Kinzler, and B. Vogelstein, Genetic instability in colorectal cancers. *Nature*, 1997. *386*(6625): p. 623-7.
[43] Lengauer, C., K.W. Kinzler, and B. Vogelstein, Genetic instabilities in human cancers. *Nature*, 1998. *396*(6712): p. 643-9.
[44] Ferguson, A.T., et al., High frequency of hypermethylation at the 14-3-3 sigma locus leads to gene silencing in breast cancer. *Proc. Natl. Acad. Sci. USA*, 2000. *97*(11): p. 6049-54.
[45] Almeida, A., et al., Hypomethylation of classical satellite DNA and chromosome instability in lymphoblastoid cell lines. *Hum. Genet*, 1993. *91*(6): p. 538-46.
[46] Chen, R.Z., et al., DNA hypomethylation leads to elevated mutation rates. *Nature*, 1998. *395*(6697): p. 89-93.
[47] Ji, W., et al., DNA demethylation and pericentromeric rearrangements of chromosome *1. Mutat Res.*, 1997. *379*(1): p. 33-41.
[48] Kane, M.F., et al., *Methylation of the hMLH1 promoter correlates with lack of expression of hMLH1 in sporadic colon tumors and mismatch repair-defective human tumor cell lines.*, 1997. *57*(5): p. 808-11.
[49] Esteller, M., et al., hMLH1 promoter hypermethylation is an early event in human endometrial tumorigenesis. *Am. J. Pathol.*, 1999. *155*(5): p. 1767-72.
[50] Cavalieri, E.L., et al., Molecular origin of cancer: catechol estrogen-3,4-quinones as endogenous tumor initiators. *Proc. Natl. Acad. Sc.i USA*, 1997. *94*(20): p. 10937-42.
[51] Qu, G.Z., et al., Frequent hypomethylation in Wilms tumors of pericentromeric DNA in chromosomes 1 and 16. *Cancer Genet Cytogenet*, 1999. *109*(1): p. 34-9.
[52] Frommer, M., et al., A genomic sequencing protocol that yields a positive display of 5-methylcytosine residues in individual DNA strands. *Proc. Natl. Acad. Sci. USA*, 1992. *89*(5): p. 1827-31.
[53] Herman, J.G., et al., Methylation-specific PCR: a novel PCR assay for methylation status of CpG islands. *Proc. Natl. Acad. Sci. USA*, 1996. *93*(18): p. 9821-6.

[54] Li, L.C. and R. Dahiya, MethPrimer: designing primers for methylation PCRs. *Bioinformatics*, 2002. *18*(11): p. 1427-31.
[55] Rozen, S. and H. Skaletsky, Primer3 on the WWW for general users and for biologist programmers. *Methods Mol. Biol.*, 2000. *132*: p. 365-86.
[56] Palmisano, W.A., et al., Predicting lung cancer by detecting aberrant promoter methylation in sputum. *Cancer Res.*, 2000. *60*(21): p. 5954-8.
[57] Fraga, M.F. and M. Esteller, DNA methylation: a profile of methods and applications. *Biotechniques*, 2002. *33*(3): p. 632, 634, 636-49.
[58] Harrison, J., C. Stirzaker, and S.J. Clark, Cytosines adjacent to methylated CpG sites can be partially resistant to conversion in genomic bisulfite sequencing leading to methylation artifacts. *Anal. Biochem.*, 1998. *264*(1): p. 129-32.
[59] Rein, T., et al., Absence of an unusual "densely methylated island" at the hamster dhfr ori-beta. *J. Biol. Chem.*, 1997. *272*(15): p. 10021-9.
[60] Eads, C.A., et al., MethyLight: a high-throughput assay to measure DNA methylation. *Nucleic Acids Res.*, 2000. *28*(8): p. E32.
[61] Fackler, M.J., et al., Quantitative multiplex methylation-specific PCR assay for the detection of promoter hypermethylation in multiple genes in breast cancer. *Cancer Res.*, 2004. *64*(13): p. 4442-52.
[62] Lehmann, U., et al., Quantitative assessment of promoter hypermethylation during breast cancer development. *Am. J. Pathol.*, 2002. *160*(2): p. 605-12.
[63] Cottrell, S.E. and P.W. Laird, Sensitive detection of DNA methylation. *Ann. NY Acad. Sci.*, 2003. *983*: p. 120-30.
[64] Tompa, R., et al., Genome-wide profiling of DNA methylation reveals transposon targets of CHROMOMETHYLASE3. *Curr. Biol.*, 2002. *12*(1): p. 65-8.
[65] Gitan, R.S., et al., Methylation-specific oligonucleotide microarray: a new potential for high-throughput methylation analysis. *Genome Res.*, 2002. *12*(1): p. 158-64.
[66] Yan, P.S., et al., Dissecting complex epigenetic alterations in breast cancer using CpG island microarrays. *Cancer Res.*, 2001. *61*(23): p. 8375-80.
[67] Hatada, I., et al., A microarray-based method for detecting methylated loci. *J. Hum. Genet*, 2002. *47*(8): p. 448-51.
[68] Yang, Q., et al., Two-hit inactivation of FHIT by loss of heterozygosity and hypermethylation in breast cancer. *Clin. Cancer Res.*, 2002. *8*(9): p. 2890-3.
[69] Lewis, C.M., et al., Promoter hypermethylation in benign breast epithelium in relation to predicted breast cancer risk. *Clin. Cancer Res.*, 2005. *11*(1): p. 166-72.
[70] Krassenstein, R., et al., Detection of breast cancer in nipple aspirate fluid by CpG island hypermethylation. *Clin. Cancer Res.*, 2004. *10*(1 Pt 1): p. 28-32.
[71] Evron, E., et al., Detection of breast cancer cells in ductal lavage fluid by methylation-specific PCR. *Lancet*, 2001. *357*(9265): p. 1335-6.
[72] Jeronimo, C., et al., Detection of gene promoter hypermethylation in fine needle washings from breast lesions. *Clin. Cancer Res.*, 2003. *9*(9): p. 3413-7.
[73] Leon, S.A., et al., Free DNA in the serum of cancer patients and the effect of therapy. *Cancer Res.*, 1977. *37*(3): p. 646-50.
[74] Dulaimi, E., et al., Tumor suppressor gene promoter hypermethylation in serum of breast cancer patients. *Clin. Cancer Res.*, 2004. *10*(18 Pt 1): p. 6189-93.

[75] Berg, J.W. and R.V. Hutter, Breast cancer. *Cancer*, 1995. *75*(1 Suppl): p. 257-69.
[76] Osada, H., et al., Frequent and histological type-specific inactivation of 14-3-3sigma in human lung cancers. *Oncogene*, 2002. *21*(15): p. 2418-24.
[77] Graff, J.R., et al., Distinct patterns of E-cadherin CpG island methylation in papillary, follicular, Hurthle's cell, and poorly differentiated human thyroid carcinoma. *Cancer Res.*, 1998. *58*(10): p. 2063-6.
[78] Plachot, C. and S.A. Lelievre, DNA methylation control of tissue polarity and cellular differentiation in the mammary epithelium. *Exp. Cell Res.*, 2004. *298*(1): p. 122-32.
[79] Lehmann, U., et al., Promoter hypermethylation of the death-associated protein kinase gene in breast cancer is associated with the invasive lobular subtype. *Cancer Res.*, 2002. *62*(22): p. 6634-8.
[80] Fackler, M.J., et al., DNA methylation of RASSF1A, HIN-1, RAR-beta, Cyclin D2 and Twist in in situ and invasive lobular breast carcinoma. *Int. J. Cancer*, 2003. *107*(6): p. 970-5.
[81] Bae, Y.K., et al., Hypermethylation in histologically distinct classes of breast cancer. *Clin. Cancer Res.*, 2004. *10*(18 Pt 1): p. 5998-6005.
[82] Huang, T.H., M.R. Perry, and D.E. Laux, Methylation profiling of CpG islands in human breast cancer cells. *Hum. Mol. Genet*, 1999. *8*(3): p. 459-70.
[83] Shi, H., et al., Expressed CpG island sequence tag microarray for dual screening of DNA hypermethylation and gene silencing in cancer cells. *Cancer Res.*, 2002. *62*(11): p. 3214-20.
[84] Takahashi, Y., et al., Down-regulation of LATS1 and LATS2 mRNA expression by promoter hypermethylation and its association with biologically aggressive phenotype in human breast cancers. *Clin Cancer Res.*, 2005. *11*(4): p. 1380-5.
[85] Huang, S., et al., Characterization of the human and mouse WRN 3'-->5' exonuclease. *Nucleic Acids Res.*, 2000. *28*(12): p. 2396-405.
[86] McGuire, W.L., Hormone receptors: their role in predicting prognosis and response to endocrine therapy. *Semin Oncol*, 1978. *5*(4): p. 428-33.
[87] Siitonen, S.M., et al., Reduced E-cadherin expression is associated with invasiveness and unfavorable prognosis in breast cancer. *Am. J. Clin. Pathol.*, 1996. *105*(4): p. 394-402.
[88] Lapidus, R.G., et al., Methylation of estrogen and progesterone receptor gene 5' CpG islands correlates with lack of estrogen and progesterone receptor gene expression in breast tumors. *Clin. Cancer Res.*, 1996. *2*(5): p. 805-10.
[89] Graff, J.R., et al., E-cadherin expression is silenced by DNA hypermethylation in human breast and prostate carcinomas. *Cancer Res.*, 1995. *55*(22): p. 5195-9.
[90] Nass, S.J., et al., Aberrant methylation of the estrogen receptor and E-cadherin 5' CpG islands increases with malignant progression in human breast cancer. *Cancer Res.*, 2000. *60*(16): p. 4346-8.
[91] Douglas, D.B., et al., Hypermethylation of a small CpGuanine-rich region correlates with loss of activator protein-2alpha expression during progression of breast cancer. *Cancer Res.*, 2004. *64*(5): p. 1611-20.
[92] Muller, H.M., et al., DNA methylation in serum of breast cancer patients: an independent prognostic marker. *Cancer Res.*, 2003. *63*(22): p. 7641-5.

[93] Taniguchi, E., et al., Cytologic grading of invasive breast carcinoma. Correlation with clinicopathologic variables and predictive value of nodal metastasis. *Acta Cytol.*, 2000. *44*(4): p. 587-91.
[94] Eiermann, W., et al., Preoperative treatment of postmenopausal breast cancer patients with letrozole: A randomized double-blind multicenter study. *Ann. Oncol.*, 2001. *12*(11): p. 1527-32.
[95] Bardou, V.J., et al., Progesterone receptor status significantly improves outcome prediction over estrogen receptor status alone for adjuvant endocrine therapy in two large breast cancer databases. *J. Clin. Oncol.*, 2003. *21*(10): p. 1973-9.
[96] Chang, H.G., et al., Tamoxifen-resistant breast cancers show less frequent methylation of the estrogen receptor beta but not the estrogen receptor alpha gene. *J. Mol. Med.*, 2005. *83*(2): p. 132-9.
[97] Sun, S.Y., et al., Evidence that retinoic acid receptor beta induction by retinoids is important for tumor cell growth inhibition. *J. Biol. Chem.*, 2000. *275*(22): p. 17149-53.
[98] Yang, Q., T. Sakurai, and K. Kakudo, Retinoid, retinoic acid receptor beta and breast cancer. *Breast Cancer Res. Treat*, 2002. *76*(2): p. 167-73.
[99] Yang, Q., et al., Biallelic inactivation of retinoic acid receptor beta2 gene by epigenetic change in breast cancer. *Am J Pathol*, 2001. *158*(1): p. 299-303.
[100] Ferrara, F.F., et al., Histone deacetylase-targeted treatment restores retinoic acid signaling and differentiation in acute myeloid leukemia. *Cancer Res.*, 2001. *61*(1): p. 2-7.
[101] Cote, S. and R.L. Momparler, Activation of the retinoic acid receptor beta gene by 5-aza-2'-deoxycytidine in human DLD-1 colon carcinoma cells. *Anticancer Drugs*, 1997. *8*(1): p. 56-61.
[102] Widschwendter, M., et al., Methylation and silencing of the retinoic acid receptor-beta2 gene in breast cancer. *J. Natl. Cancer Inst.*, 2000. *92*(10): p. 826-32.
[103] Fiegl, H., et al., Circulating tumor-specific DNA: a marker for monitoring efficacy of adjuvant therapy in cancer patients. *Cancer Res.*, 2005. *65*(4): p. 1141-5.
[104] Yang, Q., et al., 5-aza-2'-deoxycytidine induces retinoic acid receptor beta 2 demethylation, cell cycle arrest and growth inhibition in breast carcinoma cells. *Anticancer Res*, 2002. *22*(5): p. 2753-6.
[105] Villar-Garea, A., et al., Procaine is a DNA-demethylating agent with growth-inhibitory effects in human cancer cells. *Cancer Res.*, 2003. *63*(16): p. 4984-9.
[106] Grunt, T.W., et al., An EGF receptor inhibitor induces RAR-beta expression in breast and ovarian cancer cells. *Biochem Biophys Res. Commun*, 2005. *329*(4): p. 1253-9.
[107] Keen, J.C., et al., A novel histone deacetylase inhibitor, scriptaid, enhances expression of functional estrogen receptor alpha (ER) in ER negative human breast cancer cells in combination with 5-aza 2'-deoxycytidine. *Breast Cancer Res. Treat*, 2003. *81*(3): p. 177-86.
[108] Desai, D., et al., Chemopreventive efficacy of suberoylanilide hydroxamic acid (SAHA) against 4-(methylnitrosamino)-1-(3-pyridyl)-1-butanone (NNK)-induced lung tumorigenesis in female A/J mice. *Anticancer Res.*, 2003. *23*(1A): p. 499-503.

[109] Sharma, D., et al., Release of Methyl CpG Binding Proteins and Histone Deacetylase 1 from the Estrogen Receptor Alpha (ER) Promoter upon Reactivation in ER-negative Human Breast Cancer Cells. *Mol. Endocrinol.*, 2005.

[110] Cameron, E.E., et al., Synergy of demethylation and histone deacetylase inhibition in the re-expression of genes silenced in cancer. *Nat. Genet.*, 1999. *21*(1): p. 103-7.

[111] Parrella, P., et al., Nonrandom distribution of aberrant promoter methylation of cancer-related genes in sporadic breast tumors. *Clin. Cancer Res.*, 2004. *10*(16): p. 5349-54.

[112] Girault, I., et al., Expression analysis of DNA methyltransferases 1, 3A, and 3B in sporadic breast carcinomas. *Clin. Cancer Res.*, 2003. *9*(12): p. 4415-22.

[113] Sirchia, S.M., et al., Evidence of epigenetic changes affecting the chromatin state of the retinoic acid receptor beta2 promoter in breast cancer cells. *Oncogene*, 2000. *19*(12): p. 1556-63.

[114] Sirchia, S.M., et al., Endogenous reactivation of the RARbeta2 tumor suppressor gene epigenetically silenced in breast cancer. *Cancer Res.*, 2002. *62*(9): p. 2455-61.

In: Frontiers in Breast Cancer Research
Editor: Louis P. Fortugno, pp. 99-117
ISBN: 978-1-60021-671-8

Chapter IV

Racial Disparities in the Medical Care of Women with Breast Cancer

M. S. Simon*[*1,2,3], N. Petrucelli[1,3] and T. L. Albrecht[1,4]
[1] Division of Hematology and Oncology, Karmanos Cancer Institute at Wayne State University, Detroit, MI
[2] Population Studies and Prevention Program, Karmanos Cancer Institute at Wayne State University, Detroit, MI
[3] Cancer Genetic Counseling Service, Karmanos Cancer Institute at Wayne State University, Detroit, MI
[4] Communication and Behavioral Oncology Program, Karmanos Cancer Institute at Wayne State University, Detroit, MI

Abstract

Breast cancer incidence rates are higher among white than African-American (AA) women in the USA, although mortality rates from breast cancer are higher among AA women. Many published studies have shown trends towards younger age at diagnosis, worse prognostic features and lower survival rates for AA and other ethnic minority women with breast cancer compared with white women. Other studies have reported on racial and ethnic differences in patterns of care for women with breast cancer, suggesting that unequal access to care may in part explain the noted disparity in survival. While debate continues as to the relative degree in which tumor biology vs. socioeconomic factors influence racial differences in survival, cultural and behavioral differences play at least some role, and can partially explain the noted disparity in breast cancer survival seen among different racial and ethnic groups. Approximately 5 to 10% of all breast cancer in this country is associated with known hereditary mutations in the *BRCA1* and *BRCA2* genes, meaning nearly 22,000 breast cancer cases diagnosed per year are due to mutations in these cancer susceptibility genes. Hereditary breast cancer is more common

* Address correspondence to: Michael S. Simon, M.D., MPH, Professor of Medicine and Oncology Barbara Ann Karmanos Cancer Institute, Room 4221 HWCRC, 4100 John R. Detroit MI, 48201. office: (313) 576-8727; fax: (313) 576-8764; E-mail: Simonm@karmanos.org

among women with early age at diagnosis and is also more common among certain ethnic groups. While AA women are more likely to develop breast cancer at a younger age than white women, cancer risk assessment and testing for hereditary breast cancer syndromes is underutilized among AA women compared to non-minority women. It is incumbent on health care professionals to help develop solutions to the inequities in access to medical care for women with breast cancer in order to decrease the gap in breast cancer outcomes seen in this country. One way to achieve this is to improve access to screening and cancer risk assessment for all eligible women, and to make state of the art cancer treatment available for all women affected with breast cancer.

Introduction

Compared to whites, at every point of their life-span, AAs have greater morbidity and mortality from all causes of disease [1-7]. Cancer is a significant cause of morbidity and mortality in the AA population with AAs sharing a disproportionate share of the cancer burden in this country [5;8;9]. Recent statistics show higher death rates among AA men and women for the four major causes of cancer compared to any other racial or ethnic group studied [10].

Breast cancer is the most common cause of cancer among women in the US. While breast cancer incidence is higher among white than AA women, mortality due to breast cancer is higher among AA women [10;11]. Many published reports have shown trends towards younger age at diagnosis, worse prognostic features and lower survival rates for AA women with breast cancer compared with white women [12]. Other reports have documented racial and ethnic differences in patterns of care, suggesting that unequal access may in part explain the noted disparity in survival [13]. While debate continues as to the relative degree in which tumor biology vs. socioeconomic factors influence survival differences, cultural and behavioral differences play at least some role in access to care, and can partially explain the noted racial disparity in breast cancer survival. For society as a whole, health inequalities are a leading indicator of worsening social and economic quality of life, suggesting that racial disparities in breast cancer treatment and survival should be a matter of high priority for the public health agenda in this country [14].

The Effect of Race and Age on Breast Cancer Incidence and Mortality

According to the American Cancer Society (ACS) 1 in 3 women in the US will develop cancer sometime during their lifetime [15]. In 2005 there were an estimated 211,240 newly diagnosed cases of invasive female breast cancer, and 40,410 deaths from breast cancer in the US, making breast cancer the most common cause of cancer, and second leading cause of cancer related death among women [16]. As reported in the National Cancer Institute's (NCI) Surveillance Epidemiology and End Results (SEER) Program, there are noted racial differences in breast cancer rates, with higher incidence seen among white women, and higher mortality among AA women [17]. Between 1996 and 2000, age-adjusted breast cancer incidence rates (per 100,000 women) were 140.8 for white women and 121.7 for AA women, resulting in a 14 percent higher overall incidence among white women. During the same time period, age adjusted mortality rates (per 100,000 women) were 27.2 for white women compared to 35.9 for AA women resulting in a 25 percent greater mortality from breast cancer among AA women [18].

According to the SEER data, between 1990 and 2002, there were no significant changes in breast cancer incidence rates for both white and AA women, and for the same time period, mortality rates have dropped presumably due to improvements in available treatments. On closer evaluation though, the gap in mortality for white and AA women has widened over time, and higher mortality rates first seen among AA women in the early 1980's, have increased for the subsequent two decades. From 1990 through 2002 mortality due to breast cancer had dropped by 2.4 percent among white women, and only by 1.0 percent among AA women [15;19]. This racial discrepancy in mortality was also seen in a study of women treated in the US Department of Defense Healthcare system [20].

While mortality from breast cancer is higher among AA women for all reported age groups, there is a reversal in incidence rates by race beginning at about age 40, with incidence slightly higher among AA than white women younger than age 35 at diagnosis, and increasingly higher for white than AA women after age 40 [17]. This cross-over in incidence in the mid-to late 30's was also seen in reports of breast cancer risk based on data from two large case-control studies [21;22]. It is unclear why an age-related cross-over in incidence occurs. Possible explanations include age related differences in childbearing [23], other risk factor patterns related to age [24;25] or other socio-cultural influences [26]. In an analysis of risk-factor patterns among white and AA participants in the population based Carolina Breast Cancer Study, multiparity was associated with an increased risk of cancer among younger AA women but not younger white women. There was also noted to be racial variability in the presence of other reproductive variables (age at first full-term pregnancy and nulliparity) both of which have an influence on breast cancer risk [24].

Based on SEER data collected between 2000 and 2002, a woman's estimated lifetime risk of developing invasive breast cancer through age 80 is 13.2 percent or 1 in 8 [15]. Gail et al utilized data collected through the Breast Cancer Detection and Demonstration Project and computed lifetime breast risk estimates based on age, family history, prior breast biopsies and reproductive history initially only for white women [27;28], and later expanded to include AA women [29]. Claus et al utilized data from the Cancer and Steroid Hormone (CASH) Study to estimate lifetime breast cancer risks for both white and AA women with a family history of breast cancer [22]. These risk estimates were based on family history information collected from a population that consisted of female relatives of index cases diagnosed between the ages 20 and 54 years of whom only 10% (490) were AA. From a genetic analysis of the CASH data based on white participants [30], Claus et al. published lifetime breast cancer risk estimates stratified by the number and types of affected relatives and ages at diagnosis of those relatives [31]. More recently cancer risk estimates for both white and AA women with a family history of breast cancer were analyzed using information derived from the National Institute of Child Health and Human Development's (NICHD) Women's Contraceptive and Reproductive Experiences (CARE) Study [21]. This population-based case-control study was conducted among women aged 35 to 64 years and over-sampled AA women in order to permit sufficient numbers to address race-specific questions (30% AA). Based on CARE data, white women with a family history of breast cancer have a cumulative life-time risk of 22.4% (S.E. 1.25) compared to 14.5% (1.45) for AA women. These statistics highlight the importance of understanding differences in the etiology of breast cancer by race.

The Impact of Race on Breast Cancer Survival

A number of population-based studies using SEER data [32-45] as well as studies of smaller populations from hospitals and/or other health care systems [20;46-51] and data from randomized controlled trials [52], have revealed worse prognostic features and lower survival rates for AA and other ethnic minority women with breast cancer compared with white women. A recent meta-analysis of 20 studies all which utilized some measure of socioeconomic status (SES) in their analytic models, found that AA women with breast cancer had a considerably significant excess risk of overall death (mortality hazard, 1.27; 95% CI, 1.18 to 1.38) and death due to breast cancer (mortality hazard, 1.18; 95% CI, 1.19 to 1.29) [12]. According to SEER, overall survival trends for women with breast cancer have slowly improved over the past several decades, although disparities by race remain, with recent 5-year adjusted survival for AA women with breast cancer reported as 76 percent, compared to 90 percent for white women [17]. The degree to which racial differences in survival are due to inherent biologic and/or genetic differences, versus social economic differences and/or factors related to quality of medical care received remains to be determined [53].

The majority of reports which have evaluated breast cancer survival indicate that AA compared to white women are more likely to be diagnosed at a younger age, more advanced stage, and with prognostic features associated with more aggressive disease [33-39;41-43;47;54] [20;45;48-52;55]. As reported in an analysis of 9,321 incident cases of female invasive breast cancer diagnosed between 1988 and 1992 in the Detroit Metropolitan Area [33], AA women were more likely than white women to be diagnosed at a younger age (33% of AA women diagnosed at age 50 or less, compared to 24% of white women ($p< 0.001$)), to have larger diameter tumors at the time of diagnosis (almost twice as many AA vs. white women had tumors greater than 5 cm in greatest diameter, $p< 0.001$) and to present with tumor involvement of the axillary lymph nodes (36% of AA compared with 31% of white women, $p< 0.001$). AA women were also more likely than white women to have poorly differentiated tumors (26% vs. 16% $p< 0.001$), ER negative tumors (17% vs. 9% $p< 0.001$) and PR negative tumors (20% vs. 14% $p< 0.001$).

A number of studies have reported on racial differences in the patterns of care received among women with breast cancer [33;35;38;39;42;43;45;48;51;52;54;56;57] [13]. In the analysis conducted among women diagnosed in the Detroit metropolitan area [33], AA women were more likely than white women to undergo mastectomy (69% of AA women compared to 66% of white women $p<0.001$) and less likely to have gone through breast conserving surgery (29% of AA women had lumpectomy vs. 32% of white women $p<0.001$). Only 18% of the AA women underwent lumpectomy followed by radiation compared to 22% of white women ($p < 0.001$). Other reports have shown similar findings. Li et al [42] reported that AA and other ethnic minority women were less likely than white women to receive a first course of surgical and radiation treatment that met current standards of care. In another SEER based analysis, AA women were similarly less likely to receive breast radiotherapy [38]. In two prior reports of treatment utilization in the Detroit Metropolitan area, AA women were less likely to undergo lumpectomy and radiation therapy [57], or lumpectomy alone [56]. These findings suggest that AA women are more likely than white women to receive more aggressive treatment (i.e. mastectomy), and less likely to receive lumpectomy or radiation following lumpectomy.

Other studies have evaluated the effect of various measures of socioeconomic differences among women with breast cancer [21;35;43;45;48;50-52;54] [58]. In the context of a population based study, SES is generally not available on an individual basis, but rather a measure of SES is derived for a particular geographic region and used as a proxy for individual-specific SES. One methodology used to develop an aggregate SES measure is to utilize a person's address at the time of diagnosis to derive a SES Group variable. This methodology involves a geo-coding process that first assigns each individual in the study to a census block-group number [55;59].

Variables which have been used to estimate SES Groups include occupation, poverty status, educational attainment and age. The U.S. Census Bureau utilized 13 occupational categories of which 5 are defined as "professional" and the remaining 8 identified as "working class". Professional block-groups are defined as those geographic areas where 34% or more of employed persons have supervisory or executive positions. Working-class block-groups are defined as those areas in which 66% or more of employed persons report a working class occupation, such as administrative support or laborer. In regards to poverty status, poor block-groups are defined as those in which 20% or more of the population is below the poverty level. The poverty level in 1990 (corresponding to the 1990 census) is defined as an income of $12,674 for family of four. Educational attainment is stratified into educated vs. undereducated block groups. An educated block group is defined as a geographic region where at least 75% of residents age 25 and older have completed ast least a high school education vs. undereducated block groups defined as those where < 75% completed high school.

In the Detroit SEER study [33], the SES Groups used for analysis were computed for each individual woman according to the method of Krieger et al [60]. Women were assigned to one of four SES Groups which included: 1) Working, Poor (WP); 2) Working, Non-poor, Undereducated (WNP-UE); 3) Working, Non-poor, Educated (WNP-E); and 4) Professional (P). This analysis revealed that AA women were more likely to reside in a census area that had a higher proportion of individuals categorized as WP and a lower proportion categorized as P (62% of AA women resided in a WP census block and 19% resided in P census block). In contrast, 8% of CA women resided in a WP census block, and 46% resided in a P census block ($p < 0.001$). While grouped census data only serves as a proxy for individual SES, others have argued that neighborhood SES also functions as a predictor of access to care [61].

In the Detroit analysis [33], utilizing SEER staging categories, the unadjusted HR (95% CI) of death for AA compared to white women with breast cancer was 1.28 (1.15-1.44) for local, and 1.45 (1.30-1.61) for regional stage disease. After taking into account age, tumor size, axillary lymph node involvement, SES, and treatment, the multivariable adjusted HR (95% CI) of death for AA vs. white women was not significantly different for women with local stage breast cancer 1.07 (0.90-1.27), and was still greater but attenuated for AA vs. white women with regional stage disease 1.27 (1.10-1.46). Of note, women who lived in a census block group ranked as WP or WNP-UE compared to women who resided in a P census block group had the greater risk of death (HR (95% CI) 1.34 (1.13-1.6) and 1.18 (1.03-1.35) respectively for local stage disease, and 1.24 (1.06-1.45) and 1.20 (1.05-1.36) respectively for regional stage disease.

Other investigators have also found that access to care and other socio-demographic factors account for a large component of the survival differences seen among AA and white women with breast cancer. Chu et.al. found racial differences in survival for younger women compared with women aged 65 and older, concluding that access to Medicare allowed for better survival among older women with breast cancer [39]. Other studies have shown that adjustment for prior mammography use [47], treatment [38] or SES [32;35;44;45;50;52] account for a significant component of the racial or ethnic differences in survival. Because SES is known to be a significant predictor of stage at diagnosis [55], and stage at diagnosis is a strong predictor of survival, it is not surprising that the results of survival studies have found an attenuation of racial differences in survival after adjustment for SES. These results suggest that known prognostic and predictive factors as well as SES account for at least some of the racial differences in survival.

In order to evaluate racial differences in treatment and survival among a group of women who because of where they were treated, should have all had equal access to state of the art medical care, patterns of care and outcomes were evaluated among women with breast cancer treated at a single large NCI funded Comprehensive Cancer Center [54]. The results of this analysis showed no racial differences in treatment utilization as assessed by the use of surgery, radiation therapy, chemotherapy, hormonal therapy, or in the overall costs of treatment. In this data set AA women were actually slightly more likely than white women to undergo lumpectomy. After adjustment for age, stage and hormone receptor status, and the presence of other co-morbid conditions, there were no significant racial differences in breast cancer survival. These results suggest that equal access to care results in comparable survival outcomes. Improvement in screening, early detection and access to good medical care can have a significant on survival among women with breast cancer. Further research is needed to better quantify the impact of SES on breast cancer survival and to evaluate interventions at the community level which could potentially impact racial differences in cancer mortality.

Hereditary Breast and Ovarian Cancer: Racial Differences in Utilization of Genetic Counseling and Testing

Estimates from population-based studies suggest that in 5% to 10% of women with breast cancer, and 10% to 15% of women with ovarian cancer, cancer risk is associated with germ line mutations in highly penetrant susceptibility genes such as *BRCA1* (breast cancer gene 1) and *BRCA2* (breast cancer gene 2). Inherited mutations in *BRCA1* or *BRCA2* confer a significantly increased risk of both breast and ovarian cancer. Women harboring a mutation in either gene have up to an 87% lifetime risk of developing breast cancer, and a 44% lifetime risk of ovarian cancer for *BRCA1* mutation carriers, and greater than 20% lifetime risk for *BRCA2* carriers [62]. In addition, breast cancer survivors with an inherited mutation in *BRCA1/2* are at a substantial risk to develop a second breast cancer, as well as an ovarian cancer and other types of cancer. Men who carry *BRCA1/2* mutations are at increased risk to develop breast, prostate, and pancreatic cancer [63-65].

Genetic testing to identify deleterious *BRCA1* and *BRCA2* mutations became available in 1996, and can provide individual information about breast and ovarian cancer risk, and thus can influence decisions about risk reduction strategies. For example, prophylactic mastectomy has been demonstrated to reduce the risk of breast cancer, by more than 90 percent [66]. It has also been shown that prophylactic oophorectomy in *BRCA1/2* carriers reduces the risk of ovarian cancer by as much as 96%, and if performed pre-menopausally reduces the risk of breast cancer risk by 53% [67]. Prophylactic oophorectomy has also been shown to extend life expectancy by more than 3 years, and has been found to be widely acceptable to women with *BRCA1/2* mutations who have completed childbearing [68;69]. In addition to medical management implications for the individual undergoing genetic testing, the identification of a *BRCA1/2* mutation within a family enables other family members to better define their own cancer risk secondary to the autosomal dominant fashion in which these mutations are inherited.

Predictive genetic testing for hereditary breast and ovarian cancer is not without risks or limitations. Mutations in the *BRCA1/2* genes are rare and explain only about 7 to 10 percent of all cases of breast and ovarian cancer. While the presence of a *BRCA1/2* mutation does not guarantee that an individual will develop cancer, it is impossible to predict if and/or when cancer will develop. Moreover, testing is expensive and therefore, may be inaccessible to individuals with few financial resources. Concerns about genetic discrimination exist however there are no well-documented cases of genetic discrimination in regards to cancer genetic testing [70]. Finally, the psychosocial ramifications of genetic testing have been recognized, in both the genetics and oncology communities. Accordingly, not all women with a family history of breast and/or ovarian cancer will choose to undergo genetic counseling to discuss the risks, benefits, and limitations of *BRCA1/2* testing.

Genetic counseling and testing may be especially beneficial for AA women who are at a greater risk of developing early-onset breast cancer and have higher breast cancer mortality rates when compared to their white counterparts [71]. This may result in added benefits from prevention and early detection in the AA community. Thus, there is no clear clinical rationale why utilization of genetic counseling and testing should differ for AA and white women with a family history of breast or ovarian cancer. Furthermore, although the published data are sparse, several studies have suggested that the prevalence of *BRCA1/2* mutations in AA hereditary breast cancer families may be similar to that in white hereditary breast cancer families [72]. Therefore, racial differences in the use of *BRCA1/2* counseling and testing cannot be directly attributed to differences in the clinical utility of testing.

Little is known about the determinants of the use of genetic testing in the general population, including racial differences and disparities in interest and utilization. To assess the association between race and use of genetic counseling for *BRCA1/2* testing among women at risk of carrying a *BRCA1/2* mutation, Armstrong et al conducted a case-control study of 408 women with a family history of breast or ovarian cancer [73]. It was found that white women had almost 5 times the chance of undergoing *BRCA1/2* cancer genetic counseling as AA women. The noted disparity in utilization of counseling was not explained by differences in a woman's predicted probability of carrying a *BRCA1/2* mutation, SES, cancer risk perception and worry, attitudes about the risks and benefits of *BRCA1/2* testing, or primary care physician discussions regarding *BRCA1/2* testing. Other studies have demonstrated racial differences in attitudes about genetic testing, as well as racial differences in cancer risk perception, and interest in education and counseling about *BRCA1/2* testing in a research setting [74-77]. A number of studies have reported that AA women have more concerns about the limitations and risks of testing compared to white women, with a greater proportion of AA women reporting worry that testing would be too difficult to handle emotionally and might have a significant effect on family members [74] [78]. Other studies have found that AA women had more concerns regarding confidentiality of test results [78;79]. There is evidence that AA women who declined *BRCA1/2* counseling were more likely to anticipate that they would feel ashamed, singled out, and that others would view them negatively if they were found to carry a *BRCA1/2* mutation, compared to women who accepted counseling [80]. The Armstrong study; however, provides some of the first empirical evidence of a racial disparity in utilization of genetic testing in clinical practice, but the authors conclude that other variables may be contributing to this disparity.

There are several empiric reasons to believe that racial disparities in the use of predictive genetic testing are likely to exist. Disparities have been demonstrated in many areas of health care and may be most significant when new technologies such as genetic testing are being considered. In a report entitled "*Unequal Treatment: Understanding Racial and Ethnic Disparities in Health Care*" published by the Institute of Medicine [81], the authors emphasize that the advent of new technologies has the potential to increase health care disparities even more than what already exists. The use of genetic counseling and testing for primary cancer prevention is yet another area of health care in which racial and ethnic disparities may be predicted to intensify.

Health care related-distrust has been demonstrated to be higher among AA than white women and may serve as a major barrier to use of medical care. As an example, AA men and women have been the targets of selective testing for genetic traits such as mass screening for sickle cell trait as part of the National Sickle Cell Anemia Control Act of 1972 [82] [83]. While this legislation was originally intended to increase the availability of medical services to AAs who carry this trait, this mass screening program has resulted in further discrimination and reinforcement of unfavorable racial stereotypes resulting in insurance and job discrimination. This historical legacy may at least partially contribute to trepidation experienced among AA women with a family history of breast or ovarian cancer in regards to genetic technology, even when a better understanding of hereditary cancer risk may have significant health implications.

Some populations may be particularly likely to distrust genetic testing because of prior attempts to label certain racial groups as genetically inferior. Others may feel that the assessment of genetic risk may defy one's basic religious belief that medical conditions or predispositions are viewed as part of "God's plan" and that new technology may disrupt this plan [82]. There is evidence that when queried, AA compared to white women are more likely to agree that genetic testing is used to show that their ethnic group is not as good as others, to interfere with the way God meant for people to be, and to interfere with the natural order of life [84]. These same women were more likely compared to white women to agree that genetic testing allows scientists and doctors to "play God". The impact of religious beliefs on the utilization of genetic services is an area which needs further exploration.

Racial disparities in the use of *BRCA1/2* counseling and testing may also reflect differences in the characteristics of the primary care physicians who take care of AA and white women rather than differences in the characteristics of the women themselves. It has been shown that AAs are less likely to be cared for by primary care physicians that are board certified and are more likely to be cared for by physicians that report difficulty in their ability to deliver high quality medical care [85]. In a recent study Freedman et al [86] found that 51% of 1,251 physicians in the USA felt qualified to recommend genetic counseling to their patients. Among primary care physicians, only 40% felt qualified to recommend genetic counseling. Therefore, the role of the physician in identifying and referring high-risk women for cancer genetic counseling and testing cannot be underestimated.

Explanations for racial disparities in the use of cancer genetic testing may be further explained by the results of the 2000 National Health Interview Survey [87]. The results indicated that in regards to their perceived risk of breast cancer and ovarian cancer, that AA controls had consistently lower scores than their white counterparts indicating that a greater proportion reported "less than average" risk. In the National Health Interview Survey, investigators found that 49.9% of white women had reported that they had ever heard of genetic testing for cancer susceptibility compared to only 32.9% of AA participants. These findings suggest that the average AA woman underestimates her risk of breast cancer and are generally less aware of genetic testing technology as a way of assessing personal risk.

In a focus group session conducted at the University of Chicago, Matthews AK et al [88] found that virtually half (48%) of their AA participants with a strong family history of cancer reported rarely discussing cancer-related issues with their family members, and that none had prior awareness of breast cancer genetics, genetic counseling, or of the *BRCA1/2* genes. These findings of poor personal knowledge of risk, and limited information regarding cancer genetics are likely related to the lower utilization of genetic services by AAs. Until efforts are made to improve the racial, ethnic, and socioeconomic disparities that contribute to unequal access and utility of preventive medical care, the benefits gained from cancer risk assessment, genetic counseling and testing will not be fully realized. Only by advancing our ability to identify and characterize cancer risk in all Americans can steps be taken to effectively reduce racial disparities in health outcomes.

Sociodemographic Influences on Racial Disparities

Low rates of participation in cancer screening and treatment protocols including early termination of chemotherapy by the patients themselves [89] contribute directly to health disparities experienced by urban AAs, particularly those aged 55 and older, as does lack of access to newer medical treatments [90]. This group is characterized by relatively higher rates of poverty and co-morbid medical conditions as well as lower overall SES [91]. AA women are also less likely to engage in primary prevention behaviors such as exercise, smoking cessation, and maintaining a healthy weight [92], important because smoking and lack of physical activity are both associated with cancer risk [93]. Relative to whites, AAs take greater risks with their health [94]. AA breast cancer patients are also less likely to seek cancer related information from sources such as the Internet [95].

Disparities also exist among women who survive breast cancer. AA breast cancer survivors report significantly more pain, other symptomotology, and basic functional difficulties [96]. AA women with invasive breast cancer still have significantly lower survivorship rates even when they report having access to care and adequate insurance [97]. Genetic testing for breast cancer among AA relatives poses further difficulties. Families, though large, are often geographically separated and attitudes, beliefs and lack of social support mitigate against the motivation to undergo genetic testing and obtain information about genetic predisposition [98]. As a result of poorer health care across a lifetime, combined with documented and perceived barriers to care, older AA women and men distrust much of the health system. This lack of trust directly affects rates of participation in health research, including community screening and treatment. Specifically, AAs are more suspicious about medical testing [77], and are more likely to harbor misconceptions about medical treatments, and procedures [99].

Racial Disparities in Mammography Screening

Studies show that active and sustained engagement in screening programs appears to occur as part of a set of preferred health practices for healthy AA and healthy white women alike. Having recent contact with a physician and participation in other secondary prevention activities (e.g., pap smears, dental checkups) together with the belief that annual breast screening for early detection improves health status was associated with maintaining a schedule for routine mammograms [90]. Conversely, lack of screening has been correlated with self-reported poor health [90], lack of access to health insurance [100], fear of mastectomy [101], fatalism or belief that a breast cancer diagnosis inevitably results in death, as well as drug and domestic abuse [102;103] [104].

Church-based education programs have been touted as economically effective for increasing mammography usage among rural AA women, given that barriers to mammography reported by this group of women included lack of a perceived need for early detection, a view of mammography as "embarrassing", and religious beliefs related to mortality and "God's Will" [105]. Religious beliefs also accounts for the past refusal by AA women to participate in a breast cancer prevention trial, asserting that faith was more important for preventing cancer than taking drugs [106]. Finally, under-representation of AA women in mammography screening programs is a factor in disparities regarding late stage at diagnoses. The fact that race was found to be a significant and independent predictor of the lack of medical follow-up after an abnormal screening result is particularly disturbing [107].

Racial Disparities in Regards to Provider-Patient Communications

A more complicated and controversial source of health disparities is based in the breadth and quality of interactions between AA breast cancer patients and their physicians or other health providers. The disparate treatment accorded patients may range from a relatively straightforward question of whether or not the physician is recommending screening, to the extent to which providers are reassuring survivors in ways that enhance their cognitive and emotional well being, to dynamics that involve stereotyping or other biases that result in unequal treatment [108] [109].

Physician recommendations are known to influence behavior, whether it concerns screening, treatment, or accrual to clinical trials [110;111]. A recent study by Garber and Chiasson [112] showed that AA women who reported receiving a recommendation from their physician for breast cancer screening were eight times more likely to have actually obtained a mammogram. However, the investigators also found that U.S.-born AA women as opposed to those born in the Caribbean were more likely to report receiving a recommendation, clearly a potential source of disparity.

The reason for health disparities across diseases that was given the most attention in the report of the Study Committee of the Institute of Medicine (IOM) [109] was that quality of health care provided to AA and other racial/ethnic minorities is inferior to that provided to white patients. The conclusion in the report was that "in almost every identifiable respect the quality of health care provided to ethnic minorities was poorer and less effective than that provided to the European-American majority". The Committee argued that one way this was manifested was that providers may be treating "majority group" and "minority group" patients differently, with minorities disadvantaged in the level of health care received.

The Committee identified ways in which providers' can engage in "discriminatory patterns of healthcare." These include holding biases against minorities, and engaging in stereotypes about the behavior or health of minorities. Health providers may react differently to AA and white patients, according to the report [113]. Cline and McKenzie [114] reviewed the literature on physician-patient communication and strongly suggested that this occurs in physician-patient interactions. For example, van Ryn and Burke [115] found that physicians believe AA are less likely to comply with treatment recommendations and more likely to behave in ways that will interfere with their recovery.

To the extent that these processes are implicit or explicit in patient-provider encounters is likely a fundamental source of breast cancer disparities. Interactions with providers span the spectrum of women's health, including primary prevention (physical activity, diet), secondary prevention (routine and regular breast exams and mammography) to diagnostic follow-up, treatment decision making, medical care, and survivorship. If any or all of these points of contact are disrupted, particularly for AA women, either by lack of communication, system breakdowns, or interpersonal biases/stereotypes, it is clear that affected patients will disproportionately suffer.

Conclusions

Although breast cancer is more common among white than AA women, AA women are more likely to die as a result of breast cancer and are somewhat more likely to develop breast cancer at a younger age. AA women are more likely than white women to present with more aggressive and more advanced stage breast cancer and despite adjustment for stage, survival rates are generally worse among AA women. Much of the disparities in survival are due to lack of access to necessary health care resources. Genetic counseling and genetic testing for hereditary breast and ovarian cancer has the potential to identify individuals at higher risk for both breast and ovarian cancer, although these services are underutilized in the AA community in part due to lack of trust in the health care system. Much of the work in health care disparities centers on socioeconomic differences and the lack of availability of adequate resources. Central to the proper care of women with breast is the relationship between provider and patient. To the extent that miscommunication based on ethnic differences may disrupt this relationship, there may be a major impact on how medical care is delivered. Further work is needed to have a better understanding of how health care providers can decrease disparities experienced by women with breast cancer who come from different ethnic or racial backgrounds.

References

[1] *Health issues in the black community*. San Francisco: Jossey-Bass, 2006.

[2] Freeman VL, Durazo-Arvizu R, Keys LC, Johnson MP, Schafernak K, Patel VK. Racial differences in survival among men with prostate cancer and comorbidity at time of diagnosis. *Am. J. Public Health* 2004; 94(5):803-808.

[3] *Life in black America*. Newbury Park: Sage Publications, 1991.

[4] Jackson JS, Sellers S. African American health over the life course: A multidimensional framework. In: Kato PM, Mann T, editors. *Handbook of diversity issues in health psychology*. New York: Plenum Press, 1996: 301-317.

[5] LaVeist TA. African Americans and health policy: Strategies for a multiethnic society. In: Jackson JS, editor. *New directions: African Americans in a diversifying nation*. Washington, DC: National Policy Association, 2000: 144-161.

[6] Rauscher GH, Earp JA, O'Malley M. Relation between intervention exposures, changes in attitudes, and mammography use in the North Carolina Breast Cancer Screening Program. *Cancer Epidemiol Biomarkers Prev*. 2004; 13(5):741-747.

[7] Yabroff KR, Breen N, Vernon SW, Meissner HI, Freedman AN, Ballard-Barbash R. What factors are associated with diagnostic follow-up after abnormal mammograms? Findings from a U.S. National Survey. *Cancer Epidemiol Biomarkers Prev*. 2004; 13(5):723-732.

[8] Merrill RM, Weed DL. Measuring the public health burden of cancer in the United States through lifetime and age-conditional risk estimates. *Ann. Epidemiol*. 2001; 11(8):547-553.

[9] Glanz K, Croyle RT, Chollette VY, Pinn VW. Cancer-related health disparities in women. *Am. J. Public Health* 2003; 93(2):292-298.

[10] Weir HK, Thun MJ, Hankey BF, Ries LA, Howe HL, Wingo PA et al. Annual report to the nation on the status of cancer, 1975-2000, featuring the uses of surveillance data for cancer prevention and control. *J. Natl. Cancer Inst.* 2003; 95(17):1276-1299.

[11] Gloeckler Ries LA, Reichman ME, Lewis DR, Hankey BF, Edwards BK. Cancer survival and incidence from the Surveillance, Epidemiology, and End Results (SEER) program. *Oncologist* 2003; 8(6):541-552.

[12] Newman LA, Griffith KA, Jatoi I, Simon MS, Crowe JP, Colditz GA. Meta-analysis of survival in African American and white American patients with breast cancer: ethnicity compared with socioeconomic status. *J. Clin Oncol.* 2006; 24(9):1342-1349.

[13] Shavers VL, Brown ML. Racial and ethnic disparities in the receipt of cancer treatment. *J. Natl. Cancer Inst.* 2002; 94(5):334-357.

[14] Miringoff M, Miringoff ML. The social health of the nation: How American is really doing. New York: Oxford University Press, 1999.

[15] American Cancer Society. *Breast Cancer Facts and Figures 2005-2006*. 3. 2005. Atlanta, Georgia, American Cancer Society Inc. Ref. Type: Report.

[16] Jemal A, Murray T, Ward E, Samuels A, Tiwari RC, Ghafoor A et al. Cancer statistics, 2005. *CA Cancer J. Clin.* 2005; 55(1):10-30.

[17] SEER *Cancer Statistics Review*, 1975-2002. Ries LAG, Eisner MP, Kosary CL, editors. 2005. Bethesda, MD, National Cancer Institute. Ref Type: Report.

[18] Ries LAG, Reichman ME, Lewis DR, Hankey BF, Edwards BK. Cancer survival and incidence from the Surveillance, Epidemiology, and End Results (SEER) program. *Oncologist* 2003; 8(6):541-552.

[19] Surveillance, Epidemiology, and End Results (SEER) Program (www.seer.cancer.gov) SEER*Stat Database: Mortality-All COD, public-Use with State, total U.S. for expanded races (1990-2002). 2005. National Cancer Institute, DCCPS, Surveillance Research PRogram, *Cancer Statistics Branch.* Ref Type: Report

[20] Jatoi I, Becher H, Leake CR. Widening disparity in survival between white and African-American patients with breast carcinoma treated in the U. S. Department of Defense Healthcare system. *Cancer* 2003; 98(5):894-899.

[21] Simon MS, Korczak JF, Yee CL, Malone K, Ursin G, Bernstein L et al. Breast cancer risk estimates for relatives of Caucasian and African American women with breast cancer in the Women's Contraceptive and Reproductive Experiences (CARE) Study. *J. Clin. Oncol.* 2006; 24(16):2498-2504.

[22] Claus EB, Risch NJ, Thompson WD. Age at onset as an indicator of familial risk of breast cancer. *Am. J. Epidemiol.* 1990; 131(6):961-972.

[23] Palmer JR, Wise LA, Horton NJ, Adams-Campbell LL, Rosenberg L. Dual effect of parity on breast cancer risk in African-American women. *J. Natl. Cancer Inst.* 2003; 95(6):478-483.

[24] Hall IJ, Moorman PG, Millikan RC, Newman B. Comparative analysis of breast cancer risk factors among African-American women and White women. *Am. J. Epidemiol.* 2005; 161(1):40-51.

[25] Mayberry RM. Age-specific patterns of association between breast cancer and risk factors in black women, ages 20 to 39 and 40 to 54. *Ann. Epidemiol.* 1994; 4(3):205-213.

[26] Krieger N. Social class and the black/white crossover in the age-specific incidence of breast cancer: a study linking census-derived data to population-based registry records. *Am. J. Epidemiol.* 1990; 131(5):804-814.

[27] Gail MH, Brinton LA, Byar DP, Corle DK, Green SB, Schairer C et al. Projecting individualized probabilities of developing breast cancer for white females who are being examined annually. *J. Natl. Cancer Inst.* 1989; 81(24):1879-1886.

[28] Benichou J, Gail MH, Mulvihill JJ. Graphs to estimate an individualized risk of breast cancer. *J. Clin. Oncol.* 1996; 14(1):103-110.

[29] Euhus DM. Understanding mathematical models for breast cancer risk assessment and counseling. *Breast J.* 2001; 7(4):224-232.

[30] Claus EB, Risch N, Thompson WD. Genetic analysis of breast cancer in the cancer and steroid hormone study. *Am. J. Hum. Genet.* 1991; 48(2):232-242.

[31] Claus EB, Risch N, Thompson WD. Autosomal dominant inheritance of early-onset breast cancer. Implications for risk prediction. *Cancer* 1994; 73(3):643-651.

[32] Simon MS, Severson RK. Racial differences in survival of female breast cancer in the Detroit metropolitan area. *Cancer* 1996; 77(2):308-314.

[33] Simon MS, Banerjee M, Crossley-May H, Vigneau FD, Noone A, Schwartz K. Racial differences in breast cancer survival in the Detroit Metropolitan area. *Breast Cancer Res. Treat* 2005.

[34] Edwards MJ, Gamel JW, Vaughan WP, Wrightson WR. Infiltrating ductal carcinoma of the breast: the survival impact of race. *J. Clin. Oncol.* 1998; 16(8):2693-2699.

[35] O'Malley CD, Le GM, Glaser SL, Shema SJ, West DW. Socioeconomic status and breast carcinoma survival in four racial/ethnic groups: a population-based study. *Cancer* 2003; 97(5):1303-1311.

[36] Clegg LX, Li FP, Hankey BF, Chu K, Edwards BK. Cancer survival among US whites and minorities: a SEER (Surveillance, Epidemiology, and End Results) Program population-based study. *Arch. Intern. Med.* 2002; 162(17):1985-1993.

[37] Shavers VL, Harlan LC, Stevens JL. Racial/ethnic variation in clinical presentation, treatment, and survival among breast cancer patients under age 35. *Cancer* 2003; 97(1):134-147.

[38] Joslyn SA. Racial differences in treatment and survival from early-stage breast carcinoma. *Cancer* 2002; 95(8):1759-1766.

[39] Chu KC, Lamar CA, Freeman HP. Racial disparities in breast carcinoma survival rates: seperating factors that affect diagnosis from factors that affect treatment. *Cancer* 2003; 97(11):2853-2860.

[40] Joslyn SA. Hormone receptors in breast cancer: racial differences in distribution and survival. *Breast Cancer Res. Treat* 2002; 73(1):45-59.

[41] Joslyn SA, West MM. Racial differences in breast carcinoma survival. *Cancer* 2000; 88(1):114-123.

[42] Li CI, Malone KE, Daling JR. Differences in breast cancer stage, treatment, and survival by race and ethnicity. *Arch. Intern. Med.* 2003; 163(1):49-56.

[43] Grann V, Troxel AB, Zojwalla N, Hershman D, Glied SA, Jacobson JS. Regional and racial disparities in breast cancer-specific mortality. *Soc. Sci. Med.* 2005.

[44] Delgado DJ, Lin WY, Coffey M. The role of Hispanic race/ethnicity and poverty in breast cancer survival. *P. R. Health Sci. J.* 1995; 14(2):103-116.

[45] Bradley CJ, Given CW, Roberts C. Race, socioeconomic status, and breast cancer treatment and survival. *J. Natl. Cancer Inst.* 2002; 94(7):490-496.

[46] Du W, Simon MS. Racial disparities in treatment and survival of women with stage I-III reast cancer at a large academic medical center in Metropolitan Detroit. *Breast Cancer Res. Treat* 2005.

[47] Wojcik BE, Spinks MK, Stein CR. Effects of screening mammography on the comparative survival rates of African American, white, and Hispanic beneficiaries of a comprehensive health care system. *Breast J.* 2003; 9(3):175-183.

[48] Gwyn K, Bondy ML, Cohen DS, Lund MJ, Liff JM, Flagg EW et al. Racial differences in diagnosis, treatment, and clinical delays in a population-based study of patients with newly diagnosed breast carcinoma. *Cancer* 2004; 100(8):1595-1604.

[49] Mancino AT, Rubio IT, Henry-Tillman R, Smith LF, Landes R, Spencer HJ et al. Racial differences in breast cancer survival: the effect of residual disease. *J. Surg. Res.* 2001; 100(2):161-165.

[50] Yood MU, Johnson CC, Blount A, Abrams J, Wolman E, McCarthy BD et al. Race and differences in breast cancer survival in a managed care population. *J. Natl. Cancer Inst.* 1999; 91(17):1487-1491.

[51] Ansell D, Whitman S, Lipton R, Cooper R. Race, income, and survival from breast cancer at two public hospitals. *Cancer* 1993; 72(10):2974-2978.

[52] Gordon NH, Crowe JP, Brumberg DJ, Berger NA. Socioeconomic factors and race in breast cancer recurrence and survival. *Am. J. Epidemiol.* 1992; 135(6):609-618.

[53] Jones BA, Kasl SV, Howe CL, Lachman M, Dubrow R, Curnen MM et al. African-American/White differences in breast carcinoma: p53 alterations and other tumor characteristics. *Cancer* 2004; 101(6):1293-1301.

[54] Du W, Simon MS. Racial disparities in treatment and survival of women with stage I-III breast cancer at a large academic medical center in metropolitan Detroit. *Breast Cancer Res. Treat* 2005; 91(3):243-248.

[55] Schwartz KL, Crossley-May H, Vigneau FD, Brown K, Banerjee M. Race, socioeconomic status and stage at diagnosis for five common malignancies. *Cancer Causes Control* 2003; 14(8):761-766.

[56] Simon MS, Severson RK. Racial differences in breast cancer survival: the interaction of socioeconomic status and tumor biology. *Am. J. Obstet. Gynecol.* 1997; 176(6):S233-S239.

[57] Chuba PJ, Simon MS. Trends in primary surgical and radiation therapy for localized breast cancer in the Detroit Metropolitan area 1973-1992. *Int. J. Radiat. Oncol. Biol. Phys.* 1997; 38(1):103-107.

[58] Baquet CR, Commiskey P. Socioeconomic factors and breast carcinoma in multicultural women. *Cancer* 2000; 88(5 Suppl):1256-1264.

[59] US Census Bureau. Census of Population and Housing (1990) Summary Tape File 3 Technical Documentation. 1991. Washington DC, US Census Bureau. Ref Type: Report.

[60] Krieger N, Quesenberry C, Jr., Peng T, Horn-Ross P, Stewart S, Brown S et al. Social class, race/ethnicity, and incidence of breast, cervix, colon, lung, and prostate cancer among Asian, Black, Hispanic, and White residents of the San Francisco Bay Area, 1988-92 (United States). *Cancer Causes Control* 1999; 10(6):525-537.

[61] Diez-Roux AV, Kiefe CI, Jacobs DR, Jr., Haan M, Jackson SA, Nieto FJ et al. Area characteristics and individual-level socioeconomic position indicators in three population-based epidemiologic studies. *Ann. Epidemiol.* 2001; 11(6):395-405.

[62] Ford D, Easton DF, Stratton M, Narod S, Goldgar D, Devilee P et al. Genetic heterogeneity and penetrance analysis of the BRCA1 and BRCA2 genes in breast cancer families. The Breast Cancer Linkage Consortium. *Am J Hum Genet.* 1998; 62:676-689. .

[63] Ford D, Easton DF, Bishop DT, Narod SA, Goldgar DE. Risks of cancer in BRCA1-mutation carriers. Breast Cancer Linkage Consortium. *Lancet* 1994; 343(8899):692-695.

[64] Cancer risks in BRCA2 mutation carriers.The Breast Cancer Linkage Consortium. *J. Natl. Cancer Inst.* 1999; 91(15):1310-1316.

[65] Thompson D, Easton DF. Cancer Incidence in BRCA1 mutation carriers. *J. Natl. Cancer Inst*. 2002; 94(18):1358-1365.

[66] Rebbeck TR, Friebel T, Lynch HT, Neuhausen SL, van ', V, Garber JE et al. Bilateral prophylactic mastectomy reduces breast cancer risk in BRCA1 and BRCA2 mutation carriers: the PROSE Study Group. *J. Clin. Oncol*. 2004; 22(6):1055-1062.

[67] Rebbeck TR, Lynch HT, Neuhausen SL, Narod SA, Van't Veer L, Garber JE et al. Prophylactic oophorectomy in carriers of BRCA1 or BRCA2 mutations. *N. Engl. J. Med*. 2002; 346(21):1616-1622.

[68] Grann VR, Jacobson JS, Thomason D, Hershman D, Heitjan DF, Neugut AI. Effect of prevention strategies on survival and quality-adjusted survival of women with BRCA1/2 mutations: an updated decision analysis. *J. Clin. Oncol.* 2002; 20(10):2520-2529.

[69] Lerman C, Hughes C, Croyle RT, Main D, Durham C, Snyder C et al. Prophylactic surgery decisions and surveillance practices one year following BRCA1/2 testing. *Prev. Med*. 2000; 31(1):75-80.

[70] Hall MA, Rich SS. Laws restricting health insurers' use of genetic information: impact on genetic discrimination. *Am. J. Hum. Genet*. 2000; 66(1):293-307.

[71] Royak-Schaler R, deVellis BM, Sorenson JR, Wilson KR, Lannin DR, Emerson JA. Breast cancer in African-American families. Risk perception, cancer worry, and screening practices of first-degree relatives. A*nn. NY Acad. Sci.* 1995; 768:281-285.

[72] Olopade OI, Fackenthal JD, Dunston G, Tainsky MA, Collins F, Whitfield-Broome C. Breast cancer genetics in African Americans. *Cancer* 2003; 97(1 Suppl):236-245.

[73] Armstrong K, Micco E, Carney A, Stopfer J, Putt M. Racial differences in the use of BRCA1/2 testing among women with a family history of breast or ovarian cancer. *JAMA* 2005; 293(14):1729-1736.

[74] Hughes C, Gomez-Caminero A, Benkendorf J, Kerner J, Isaacs C, Barter J et al. Ethnic differences in knowledge and attitudes about BRCA1 testing in women at increased risk. *Patient Educ. Couns*. 1997; 32(1-2):51-62.

[75] Hughes C, Lerman C, Lustbader E. Ethnic differences in risk perception among women at increased risk for breast cancer. *Breast Cancer Res. Treat* 1996; 40(1):25-35.

[76] Lerman C, Hughes C, Benkendorf JL, Biesecker B, Kerner J, Willison J et al. Racial differences in testing motivation and psychological distress following pretest education for BRCA1 gene testing. *Cancer Epidemiol Biomarkers Prev*. 1999; 8(4 Pt 2):361-367.

[77] Peters N, Rose A, Armstrong K. The association between race and attitudes about predictive genetic testing. *Cancer Epidemiol Biomarkers Prev*. 2004; 13(3):361-365.

[78] Donovan KA, Tucker DC. Knowledge about genetic risk for breast cancer and perceptions of genetic testing in a sociodemographically diverse sample. *J. Behav. Med*. 2000; 23(1):15-36.

[79] Durfy SJ, Bowen DJ, McTiernan A, Sporleder J, Burke W. Attitudes and interest in genetic testing for breast and ovarian cancer susceptibility in diverse groups of women in western Washington. *Cancer Epidemiol Biomarkers Prev*. 1999; 8(4 Pt 2):369-375.

[80] Thompson HS, Valdimarsdottir HB, Duteau-Buck C, Guevarra J, Bovbjerg DH, Richmond-Avellaneda C et al. Psychosocial predictors of BRCA counseling and testing decisions among urban African-American women. *Cancer Epidemiol Biomarkers Prev*. 2002; 11(12):1579-1585.

[81] Unequal Treatment: Understanding Racial and Ethnic Disparities in Health Care. 2002. Institute of Medicine, The National Academic Press. Ref Type: Report.

[82] Telfair J, Nash KB. African American culture. In: Fisher NL, editor. *Cultural and ethnic diversity: a guide for genetic professionals*. Baltimore: The John Hopkins University Press, 2000: 37-59.

[83] Bowman JE. Technical, genetic, and ethical issues in screening and testing of African-Americans for hemochromatosis. *Genet. Test* 2000; 4(2):207-212.

[84] Thompson HS, Valdimarsdottir HB, Jandorf L, Redd W. Perceived disadvantages and concerns about abuses of genetic testing for cancer risk: differences across African American, Latina and Caucasian women. *Patient Educ. Couns*. 2003; 51(3):217-227.

[85] Bach PB, Pham HH, Schrag D, Tate RC, Hargraves JL. Primary care physicians who treat blacks and whites. *N. Engl. J. Med*. 2004; 351(6):575-584.

[86] Freedman AN, Wideroff L, Olson L, Davis W, Klabunde C, Srinath KP et al. US physicians' attitudes toward genetic testing for cancer susceptibility. *Am. J. Med. Genet*. 2003; 120(1):63-71.

[87] Wideroff L, Vadaparampil ST, Breen N, Croyle RT, Freedman AN. Awareness of genetic testing for increased cancer risk in the year 2000 National Health Interview Survey. *Community Genet*. 2003; 6(3):147-156.

[88] Matthews AK, Cummings S, Thompson S, Wohl V, List M, Olopade OI. Genetic testing of African Americans for susceptibility to inherited cancers: Use of focus groups to determine factors contributing to participation. *Journal of Psychosocial Oncology* 2000; 18(2):1-19.

[89] Hershman D, McBride R, Jacobson JS, Lamerato L, Roberts K, Grann VR et al. Racial disparities in treatment and survival among women with early-stage breast cancer. *J. Clin. Oncol.* 2005; 23(27):6639-6646.

[90] Jatoi I, Anderson WF, Rao SR, Devesa SS. Breast cancer trends among black and white women in the United States. *J. Clin. Oncol.* 2005; 23(31):7836-7841.

[91] Maloney N, Koch M, Erb D, Schneider H, Goffman T, Elkins D et al. Impact of race on breast cancer in lower socioeconomic status women. *Breast J.* 2006; 12(1):58-62.

[92] Dowda M, Ainsworth BE, Addy CL, Saunders R, Riner W. Correlates of physical activity among U.S. young adults, 18 to 30 years of age, from NHANES III. *Ann. Behav. Med.* 2003; 26(1):15-23.

[93] Bernstein L, Patel AV, Ursin G, Sullivan-Halley J, Press MF, Deapen D et al. Lifetime recreational exercise activity and breast cancer risk among black women and white women. *J. Natl. Cancer Inst.* 2005; 97(22):1671-1679.

[94] Rosen AB, Tsai JS, Downs SM. Variations in risk attitude across race, gender, and education. *Med. Decis. Making* 2003; 23(6):511-517.

[95] Talosig-Garcia M, Davis SW. Information-seeking behavior of minority breast cancer patients: an exploratory study. *J. Health Commun.* 2005; 10 Suppl 1:53-64.

[96] Deimling GT, Sterns S, Bowman KF, Kahana B. The health of older-adult, long-term cancer survivors. *Cancer Nurs.* 2005; 28(6):415-424.

[97] Field TS, Buist DS, Doubeni C, Enger S, Fouayzi H, Hart G et al. Disparities and survival among breast cancer patients. *J. Natl. Cancer Inst. Monogr.* 2005;(35):88-95.

[98] Lee R, Beattie M, Crawford B, Mak J, Stewart N, Komaromy M et al. Recruitment, genetic counseling, and BRCA testing for underserved women at a public hospital. *Genet. Test* 2005; 9(4):306-312.

[99] Margolis ML, Christie JD, Silvestri GA, Kaiser L, Santiago S, Hansen-Flaschen J. Racial differences pertaining to a belief about lung cancer surgery: results of a multicenter survey. *Ann. Intern. Med.* 2003; 139(7):558-563.

[100] Rosenberg L, Wise LA, Palmer JR, Horton NJ, Adams-Campbell LL. A multilevel study of socioeconomic predictors of regular mammography use among African-American women. *Cancer Epidemiol Biomarkers Prev.* 2005; 14(11 Pt 1):2628-2633.

[101] Fernandez ME, Palmer RC, Leong-Wu CA. Repeat mammography screening among low-income and minority women: a qualitative study. *Cancer Control 2005*; 12 Suppl 2:77-83.

[102] Green BL, Lewis RK, Wang MQ, Person S, Rivers B. Powerlessness, destiny, and control: the influence on health behaviors of African Americans. *J. Community Health* 2004; 29(1):15-27.

[103] Moy B, Park ER, Feibelmann S, Chiang S, Weissman JS. Barriers to repeat mammography: cultural perspectives of African-American, Asian, and Hispanic women. *Psychooncology* 2005.

[104] Russell KM, Perkins SM, Zollinger TW, Champion VL. Sociocultural context of mammography screening use. *Oncol. Nurs. Forum* 2006; 33(1):105-112.

[105] Husaini BA, Emerson JS, Hull PC, Sherkat DE, Levine RS, Cain VA. Rural-urban differences in breast cancer screening among African American women. *J. Health Care Poor Underserved 2005*; 16(4 Suppl A):1-10.

[106] Paternıti DA, Melnikow J, Nuovo J, Henderson S, DeGregorio M, Kuppermann M et al. "I'm going to die of something anyway": women's perceptions of tamoxifen for breast cancer risk reduction. *Ethn. Dis.* 2005; 15(3):365-372.
[107] Jones BA, Dailey A, Calvocoressi L, Reams K, Kasl SV, Lee C et al. Inadequate follow-up of abnormal screening mammograms: findings from the race differences in screening mammography process study (United States). *Cancer Causes Control* 2005; 16(7):809-821.
[108] Clayton MF, Mishel MH, Belyea M. Testing a model of symptoms, communication, uncertainty, and well-being, in older breast cancer survivors. *Res. Nurs. Health* 2006; 29(1):18-39.
[109] *Unequal treatment: Confronting racial and ethnic disparities in health care.* Washington, D.C.: The National Academies Press, 2002.
[110] Albrecht TL, Blanchard C, Ruckdeschel JC, Coovert M, Strongbow R. Strategic physician communication and oncology clinical trials. *J. Clin. Oncol.* 1999; 17(10):3324-3332.
[111] Katz SJ, Lantz PM, Janz NK, Fagerlin A, Schwartz K, Liu L et al. Patient involvement in surgery treatment decisions for breast cancer. *J. Clin. Oncol.* 2005; 23(24):5526-5533.
[112] Garbers S, Chiasson MA. Breast cancer screening and health behaviors among African American and Caribbean Women in New York City. *J. Health Care Poor Underserved 2006;* 17(1):37-46.
[113] Cooper LA, Roter DL. Patient-provider communication: The effect of race and ethnicity on process and outcomes of healthcare. In: Smedley BD, editor. *Unequal treatment: Confronting racial and ethnic disparities in health care*. Bethesda: Institute of Medicine, 2003: 552-593.
[114] Cline RJ, McKenzie NJ. The many cultures of health care: Taling social structures, talking medical outcomes. In: Jackson LD, Duffy BK, editors. *Health communication research: A guide for developments and direction.* Westport: Greenwood Publishing Company, 1998: 57-74.
[115] van Ryn M, Burke J. The effect of patient race and socio-economic status on physicians' perceptions of patients. *Soc. Sci. Med.* 2000; 50(6):813-828.

In: Frontiers in Breast Cancer Research
Editor: Louis P. Fortugno, pp. 119-139
ISBN: 978-1-60021-671-8

Chapter V

Genomic Instability in Breast Cancer

Sigurdur Ingvarsson*
Institute for Experimental Pathology
University of Iceland at Keldur

Abstract

The presence of numerical and structural chromosome aberrations is a common characteristic of tumor cells. Accumulation of these aberrations leads to dramatic changes within the genome. These changes have tumor type and stage specific pattern of segmental losses and gains, resulting in gene losses and gene copy number imbalances. Tumor development and progression is driven by sequential acquisition of specific gene alterations, and chromosome aberrations contribute to these processes. Genomic instability in tumors can be classified as chromosome instability (CIN) and microsatellite instability (MIN). MIN is in general less frequent in tumors than CIN, but is rather frequent in some tumors of the digestive tract. This is mainly due to germline mutations in mismatch repair genes associated with the HNPCC cancer syndrome, but can also be due to somatic mutations and epigenetic mechanism. While MIN is rare in breast tumors, CIN is demonstrated in the majority of breast tumors (about 70%) by aneuploidy, deletions, amplifications and rearrangements. Although the reasons for CIN in breast tumors are not well understood, explanations can partly be obtained from deficient control of genes controlling cell proliferation, apoptosis, DNA repair or chromosome segregation. Among these genes are TP53, MYC, AURKA, BRCA1 and BRCA2. TP53 is relatively well studied and is believed to be a guardian of genome integrity. Myc seems to affect tumor pathogenesis in several ways, including increased proliferation and immortalization of the cancer cells and induction of CIN. The STK15 gene encodes the aurora A kinase, which has been shown to bind to centrosomes and is important in controlling their number and the segregation of correct chromosomes to the daughter cells during mitosis. Genomic instability is high in some hereditary breast cancer, particularly in tumors of BRCA1 and BRCA2 mutation carriers, a finding which is in line with the role of the gene products in DNA repair. Some recent developments in drug

* Tel. 354-5855100; Fax: 354-5673979; Email: siguring@hi.is

therapy are based on molecular and genomic findings about breast cancer pathogenesis. Defects in checkpoint control generate CIN and are believed to facilitate tumorigenesis, but additional disabling of checkpoint signaling is a possible anticancer strategy.

Introduction

Breast cancer has all the hallmarks of a multigenic disease. Although germline mutations in several genes are well known to be involved in breast tumor progression, this is largely a consequence of somatic evolution. Tumors in the breast have, like most other cancer types, several characteristics of abnormal genome. The number of chromosomes is frequently abnormal, as is the amount of DNA.

Genetic instability is typically seen in cancerous cells, as predicted by Boveri, who theorized that tumors may become malignant as the result of abnormal chromosome numbers (Boveri 1914). Later it was postulated that tumor progression is facilitated by genomic instability, with 5-10 essential mutations to establish the malignant phenotype in most solid tumors (Hanahan and Weinberg 2000). It has been demonstrated that normal mutation rate is unable to allow for the accumulation of mutations essential for cancer progression, suggesting a need for genomic destabilization (Loeb et al. 2001). Therefore genomic instability can be considered to be the underlying mechanism of tumor evolution. It also provides a means to generate the heterogeneous subpopulation of cells that typifies many solid tumors. Such heterogeneous tumors can be subpopulations of biologically aggressive metastatic and therapy-resistant cancer cells, whose outgrowth can lead to poor clinical outcome. It has been pointed out that, for tumor progression, sufficient genomic instability is required, but it has to be within certain limits, since circumstances causing overwhelming genomic instability probably result in nonviable cells (Cahill et al. 1999). Hence "moderate" genomic instability facilitates tumor development.

The molecular basis of genomic instability in breast tumors is mostly unknown, but some recent developments cast light on some of the pathways and networks involved. The proteins involved participate in cell growth control, cell-cycle checkpoints and genome integrity. Various mechanisms have been described which lead to their deregulation or dysfunction. Defective DNA repair, that is unable to cope with normally occurring damage, provides an indirect means of generating genomic instability. This can arise from deficiencies in repair enzymes or from checkpoint defects, which fail to halt the cell cycle if DNA is damaged. Segregation of chromosomes to daughter cells provides a further opportunity for large losses and perturbations of genetic information. The spectrum of genetic alterations that occur in genetically unstable cells varies considerably. In this chapter on breast cancer progression and genomic instability, the focus will be on proteins involved in DNA repair, centrosome control and telomere maintenance (Table I).

Table I. Genes, proteins and dysfunctions involved in the progression of genomic instability in breast tumors

Gene	Protein function	Cellular function	Function in tumor progression	Abnormalities in breast cancer	Frequency (%)
ATM	Phosphatidyl inositol kinase	Response to DNA damage	Signaling to tumor suppressors	Germline variants	10
AURKA	Protein kinase	Chromosome separation in mitosis	Oncoprotein	Gene amplification	15
BRCA1	Multifunctional, including DNA repair	Genome integrity	Tumor suppressor	Mutation*, methylation	5, 15
BRCA2	Multifunctional, including DNA repair	Genome integrity	Tumor suppressor	Mutation*	5
MYC	Transcription factor	Cell turnover	Oncoprotein	Gene amplification	20
TERT	Telomerase reverse transcriptase	Telomere maintenance	Cell immortalization	Overexpression	70
TP53	Transcription factor	Genome integrity, cell turnover	Tumor suppressor	Mutation and other	30

*Germline mutations – somatic mutations are rare. See further details and references in the main text.

Chromosomal Instability

Genomic instability in tumors can be classified as chromosomal instability (CIN) or microsatellite instability (MIN). MIN is in general less frequent in tumors that CIN, but is rather frequent in some tumors of the digestive tract. A possible explanation for this is the special turnover of the cells in the digestive tract and also exposure to the "environment", i.e. food and food digestion. MIN is mainly due to germline mutations in mismatch repair genes associated with the HNPCC syndrome, but can also be due to somatic mutations and epigenetic mechanism. Frequent mutations are seen within short repetitive sequences in tumors with MIN, which can be within genes that may have a role in tumor progression (Johannsdottir et al. 2000). CIN phenotype is characterized by increased propensity for numerical chromosome aberrations.

CIN is demonstrated in the majority of breast tumors (70%) by aneuploidy, deletions, amplifications and rearrangements, while MIN is rare (Huiping et al. 1999a).

There is a difference in genomic alterations in the two histological types of breast cancer, ductal and lobular. In general the genome is more stable in lobular than ductal breast cancer, with the exception of loss at chromosome arm 16q, which is detected with higher loss in lobular breast cancer (Huiping et al. 1999b). This may be relevant with respect to the rather frequent mutation rate of E-cadherin in lobular breast cancer, not seen in ductal breast cancer.

Alterations at certain chromosome regions are frequently detected in breast tumors with an unstable genome, while alterations at other chromosomes seem to be unrelated to genomic instability. Frequent losses at certain chromosome regions not associated with genomic instability presumably involve a tumor suppressor gene, a loss which gives growth advantage to the cell, resulting in clonal expansion. When losses at certain chromosome regions are associated with genomic instability, a tumor suppressor gene involvement is not as suggestive. Loss at these chromosome regions could reflect the unstable nature of the breast cancer genome, and therefore these losses could serve as markers for genomic instability. But this does not exclude the possibility that the growth advantage of the breast tumor cells, due to tumor suppressor gene elision, may be of importance for the clonal selection of these chromosomal losses. We have shown that chromosome arms 3p, 6q and 8p are the regions most frequently altered in breast tumors with an unstable genome (Ingvarsson 2004). In contrast, loss at chromosome 16q is not associated with an unstable genome, even though this is the chromosome region most frequently altered in sporadic breast cancer (Skirnisdottir et al. 1995). Chromosome 16q loss also differs from chromosomal losses associated with genomic instability with regard to clinicopathological factors, i.e. while chromosome 3p, 6q and 8p losses are associated with aneuploidy, high S-phase and reduced patient survival, chromosome 16 loss does not show this association, and is in contrast associated with low S-phase and elevated patient survival (Bragadottir et al. 1995; Eiriksdottir et al. 1995; Hansen et al. 1998; Sigbjornsdottir et al. 2000; Skirnisdottir et al. 1995). No definitive answer has yet been found to the question of whether losses of 3p, 6q, 8q and some other chromosomes are only markers for genomic instability, or whether true tumor suppressor genes of importance for malignant progression of breast cancer are located there.

The 3p region is not only frequently altered in breast cancer, but is also among the most frequently lost regions in many types of cancer (Ingvarsson 2005). However, it has been a difficult region in which to find a definite tumor suppressor gene, and it has been hypothesized that combined functional loss of several tumor suppressor genes located at 3p contributes to tumor pathogenesis (Huebner 2001). The FHIT gene is located at the most common fragile site in the human genome at 3p14.2, FRA3B, and is frequently altered in breast cancer, particularly if it is of hereditary origin, where DNA repair genes are mutated (Ingvarsson et al. 1999a, 2001). This could merely reflect the unstable nature of the fragile site in the breast tumor cell, but it is also possible that FHIT plays a tumor suppressor role. Specific Fhit pathways have not been identified, but a recent study suggests a role in homologous recombination repair (Hu et al. 2005). The question may be asked, whether the fragile sites in the genome are more sensitive to alterations in a background of germline mutations where DNA repair is dysfunctional. This could be part of the story, but not the only explanation. When comparing losses from chromosomes that carry the most common fragile sites in the genome, FRA3B, FRA16D and FRA6E, only chromosomes 3p and 6q show elevated loss in hereditary tumors associated with DNA repair dysfunction, compared to sporadic breast tumors, but not chromosome 16q (Ingvarsson 2004). Also, there is higher loss at chromosome 8p in hereditary tumors with mutated repair genes, as against sporadic tumors, even though this chromosome region does not contain a defined fragile site (Sigbjornsdottir et al. 2000).

Centrosome Amplification

A defect in centrosome maturation has been described in several cancer types, including breast cancer (Pihan et al. 2003). Centrosome defects are believed to affect normal segregation of chromosomes and produce aneuploid cells. One of the contributing factors for CIN in breast cancer cells is the presence of more than two centrosomes during mitosis, usually called centrosome amplification. Breast cancer cells frequently display an excess number of centrosomes (D'Assoro et al. 2002, Lingle et al. 2002). Precisely two centrosomes are required for accurate chromosome segregation into daughter cells. Cells are equipped with a mechanism controlling the duplication of centrosomes and DNA in every single cell cycle, and these two events are coordinated, probably to ensure that these two cellular components duplicate only once. If proliferating cells fail to coordinate centrosome duplication with DNA replication, abnormal segregation of chromosomes is provoked. The coupling of the initiation of DNA and centrosome duplication is at least in part achieved by specific activation of cyclin-dependent kinases and their corresponding regulation partner, cyclins (Koff et al. 1992). It has been shown that centrosome amplification is an early event in the development of breast cancer, and amplification of centrosome size and number correlates with CIN (Lingle et al. 2002).

Centrosome amplification is seen in a subset of breast cancer cells harboring mutations in tumor suppressor proteins such as p53, Brca1 and Brca2 or overexpression of oncoproteins such as the aurora kinase A. Among the several centrosome-associated kinases and target substrates implicated in the regulation of centrosome duplication cycle that may become altered during the development of centrosome amplification in breast cancer, the best-documented evidence is for the role of aurora kinase A.

Additional proteins involved in mitotic checkpoints and possibly centrosome amplification are MAD1 and MAD2, both found to be mutated in breast cancer (Percy et al. 2000, Tsukasaki et al. 2001). Also, a recent study describes the prolyl isomerase Pin1, which is overexpressed in breast cancer, as a regulator of centrosome duplication (Suizu et al. 2006).

The Aurora Kinase A

The aurora kinase A is overexpressed in a subset of breast cancer (Courjal et al. 1996, Sen et al. 1997). This overexpression can partly be explained by gene amplification, but also by dysregulation at transcriptional or translational level (Bischoff et al. 1998, Jeng et al. 2003).

The aurora kinase A is important for cell-cycle regulation, in particular the passage from G2 to M, and is believed to be involved in a checkpoint network. The aurora kinase A contributes to ensuring that the two daughter cells receive identical copies of the genome in the cell-cycle progression. It is located at centrosomes and microtubules at the spindle poles, and the kinase activity is involved in maturation and separation of centrosomes and assembly and stability of the spindle (Kimura et al. 1997). The deregulation of aurora kinase A leads to defects in centrosome separation and spindle defects (Glover et al. 1996). It has been defined as an oncoprotein, based on an ectopic expression in immortalized fibroblast cell lines resulting in cell transformation (Bischoff et al. 1998, Zhou et al. 1998). Aurora A mutants with defective kinase activity do not induce cell transformation, indicating that the active kinase is oncogenic.

Genetic variants of the aurora kinase A gene have more recently been implicated in cancer risk, including breast cancer (Lo et al. 2005, Cox et al. 2006). One of these genetic variants has been shown to be more effective in transforming cells to a more malignant phenotype (Ewart-Toland et al. 2003). The prevalence of the homozygous state of this allele is higher in Asian populations than Caucasians (Lo et al. 2005). It has been shown that the genetic variants are associated with breast cancer in both populations (Cox et al. 2006).

Several small molecule inhibitors have been designed from the aurora crystal structure (Harrington et al. 2004). Protein kinase inhibitors are among the top new mechanisms for cancer therapy development that are under investigation, with significant progress.

Cell Cycle Checkpoint Proteins

One of the most fundamental events in the G1-S cell cycle checkpoint is the stabilization and activation of p53. TP53 is somatically mutated in about 25% of breast tumors, and germline mutations have been described in the Li-Fraumeni Syndrome, where one of the increased susceptibility disease phenotypes is breast cancer (Malkin et al. 1990; Srivastava et al. 1990). P53 is a rather well defined transcription factor, and its role in cell-cycle checkpoint is generally accepted. In the case of DNA aberrations or other defined stress on the cell, the increased amount of p53 due to stabilization of this otherwise unstable protein is responsible for blocking the cell cycle and inducing apoptosis. Several molecular mechanisms have been described, including the promoter-directed elevated expression of p21, a protein that can block the cyclin-dependent kinase/cyclin function, resulting in halting of the cell cycle at the G1 checkpoint. P53 plays also a central role in the decision of a cell to undergo apoptosis after exposure to diverse stresses, including DNA damage. Interaction of p53 with Brca1 and other proteins important for DNA repair has been reported, but functional evidence for the role of p53 in DNA repair is still limited (Zhang 1998). A feasible model is that p53 is important for blocking the cell from entering the S-phase of the cell cycle upon cell damage, and induces apoptosis if the damage is overwhelming. With failure of p53 normal function due to mutation, there is a risk of accumulation of genomic instability and mutations in additional genes.

The majority of TP53 mutations are missense, in contrast to mutations in several other tumor suppressor genes, where the majority of mutations result in a truncated protein. Some of the TP53 mutations are dominant negative, presumably due to incompetent transcription factor, if one or more mutant copies of the protein are included in the p53 tetrameric form. The germline mutation spectrum is slightly different from the somatic pattern, in line with endogenous mutagenic processes (Olivier 2001). A high frequency of codon 163 mutation of the TP53 is detected in breast tumors, particularly in a BRCA1 mutational background (Crook et al. 1997, 1998; Greenblatt et al. 2001). The mutation spectrum of TP53 in BRCA1 and BRCA2 carriers is different from that of sporadic tumors, which is consistent with a repair function of Brca1 and Brca2 (Greenblatt et al. 2001). The p53 mutants are presumably selected during the malignant progression in the genetic background of BRCA1 and BRCA2 associated tumors.

Somatic and germline mutations in the CHK2 gene have been described in relation to breast cancer, suggesting that loss of Chk2 is functionally equivalent to TP53 mutations, while mutation frequency is lower in CHK2 than in TP53 (Bell et al. 1999; Ingvarsson et al. 2002; Sullivan et al. 2002). Germline mutations of CHK2 have been found in Li-Fraumeni and Li-Fraumeni-like families, and by population screening of breast cancer patients (Bell et al. 1999; Ingvarsson et al. 2002; Sullivan et al. 2002). The germline variants of CHK2 analyzed so far by population screening seem to be low penetrance alleles conferring susceptibility to breast cancer (Ingvarsson et al. 2002; Meijers-Heijboer et al. 2002). Population-based analysis of a mutation that abolishes kinase activity indicated a 5% frequency in individuals with breast cancer, and a twofold and tenfold increased risk of breast cancer in females and males respectively (Meijers-Heijboer et al. 2002). Tumors in BRCA1 carriers have a relatively high frequency of somatic CHK2 mutations, as do tumors in patients with medullary carcinoma (Sullivan et al. 2002). This is of particular interest, since TP53 somatic mutations are also found at a high level in BRCA1 tumors (Crook et al. 1997, 1998; Greenblatt et al. 2001). These findings of somatic mutations in cell-cycle checkpoint genes such as TP53 and CHK2 are in line with the theory that they increase the rate of tumorigenesis in BRCA1 associated tumors.

As p53 is a cell-cycle checkpoint protein in DNA-damaged cells, it is not surprising that cells that lack functional p53 accumulate genomic defects, even though all target genes of this transcription factor and protein networks are not fully characterized. Tp53 mutations have been implicated as a cause for CIN in breast cancer in some studies, but not all (Sigurdsson et al. 2000, Lingle et al. 2002).

Mouse knockout experiments support the association of dysfunctional p53 and genomic instability (Fukasawa et al. 1996, 1997). Homozygous p53 knockout mouse embryo fibroblasts undergo centrosome amplification (Fukasawa et al. 1996). Further experiments suggested that p53 inactivation induces CIN through centrosome amplification, and a putative mechanism is through loss of transcriptional activation of p21, and subsequent activation of cyclin-dependent kinase 2/cyclin E complexes controlling the centrosome duplication cycle (Mussman et al. 2000). Of interest is the finding that p53 loss induces centrosome amplification and CIN in human cells, in concert with cyclin E overexpression (Kawamura et al. 2004). This may explain some of the discrepancies between different studies, but needs further analysis in breast cancer. Centrosome amplification in p53 negative cells does not necessarily imply a role for p53 in the regulation of centrosome duplication, but instead may reflect the involvement of a p53-dependent checkpoint in the elimination of cells that emerge from aborted divisions. The mechanism for centrosome amplification associated with loss of p53 is poorly understood, but some additional clues come from an experimental system, in which centrosomes undergo multiple rounds of duplication in rodent cells during S-phase (Tarapore et al. 2001). This occurs only if p53 is mutated or lost, and in the presence of wild-type p53 the centrosome re-duplication is blocked. Increased levels of p21 block the initiation of centrosome duplication via inhibition of cyclin-dependent kinase 2/cyclin E. In hydroxyurea-treated cells with mutant p53 there is an abnormal centrosome accumulation, whereas cells with wild-type p53 arrest centrosome duplication under these conditions (Dassoro et al. 2004).

Human and mouse heterozygous ATM mutation carriers are at increased risk for tumors, including breast cancer (Shiloh et al. 2003, Spring et al. 2002). Atm is a key player in the cellular response to DNA damage. It is a phosphadidyl inositol 3-kinase which phosphorylates substrates in response to DNA damage. This includes p53 and results in stabilization and activation of it since it loses the inhibitory interaction of the Mdm2 ubiquitin ligase complex. Brca1 presumably serves as a scaffold for Atm to pass on its phosphorylation to downstream targets required for apoptosis and checkpoint activation. Also, the Chk2 kinase is phosphorylated by Atm.

DNA Repair, BRCA1 and BRCA2

BRCA1 is a familial breast and ovarian cancer susceptibility gene (Miki et al. 1994). Brca1 is involved in diverse cellular events and functions, including homologous recombination DNA repair, transcriptional regulation, chromatin remodeling, cell- cycle checkpoint control and ubiquitin ligation (Moyhanan et al. 1999, Welcsh et al. 2002, Bochar et al. 2000, Baer et al. 2002). BRCA2 is also a familial breast cancer susceptibility gene that is structurally unrelated to BRCA1, but its protein product plays a partial role in the same pathways (Wooster et al. 1995). The main function of Brca2 is in homologous recombination DNA repair. Both Brca1 and Brca2 bind to Rad51, a protein implicated in recombination and double stranded DNA repair (Ingvarsson 1999). The Brca1 and Brca2 proteins participate in the BASC (Brca1 associated genome surveillance complex). They are multifunctional proteins involved in complex protein-protein interactions. The factors binding to Brca1 are both specific transcription factors and factors involved in chromatin remodeling. Brca2 is involved in loading of Rad51 to damaged DNA. Mainly active in S and G2 phases of the cell cycle, Brca1 and Brca2 are essential for preserving chromosome structure, suggesting that, in their role as tumor suppressors, they behave as caretakers, suppressing genomic instability. While the role of Brca1 and Brca2 in homologous recombination repair of double-strand DNA breaks is well established, more data are needed to clarify how they act as regulators of cell-cycle events independent of their role in DNA repair.

Even though BRCA1 and BRCA2 are the major genes involved in hereditary breast cancer, they explain only less than 10% of breast cancers. The majority of breast cancers are believed to be sporadic, where somatic mutations have a major role, or are due to the combined effects of low-penetrance sequence variants and genetic background. The mechanism of BRCA1 or BRCA2 inactivation in tumors is believed to be a double hit, a germline mutation and a somatic deletion (Smith et al. 1992; Gudmundsson et al. 1995). However, experimental data are lacking to clarify whether losses of the wild-type chromosomes are a prerequisite for non- or abnormal function of the proteins, or whether dominant negative or haplo-insufficient mechanisms can explain the original pathogenesis (Fan et al. 2001). Since germline mutations of BRCA1 and BRCA2 are relatively frequent in relation to familial breast cancer, the rarity of somatic mutations has been regarded as surprising (Khoo et al. 1998; Signori et al. 2001). This situation is different from the TP53 mutation story, where somatic mutations are relatively common and germline mutations are rare. It is not clear whether some prevention of the molecular mechanism leads to somatic mutations of BRCA1 and BRCA2, or whether the mutations do not give growth advantage for the cells. There could be a particular time frame in normal tissue maturation, after which somatic BRCA1 and BRCA2 mutations are not selected during sporadic breast tumor development, although gene silencing mechanisms and large rearrangements and deletions can influence tumor progression. Even though somatic mutations are rare in BRCA1, it is frequently deleted and expression is decreased in breast tumors, although not always by a known mechanism (Thompson et al. 1995; Wilson et al. 1999). Hypermethylations at the promoter region may partly explain the BRCA1 downregulation in sporadic breast tumors (Catteau et al. 1999; Niwa et al. 2000, Rice et al. 1999).

Molecular and pathological data suggest not only a difference between BRCA1 and BRCA2 associated tumors, but also between them and sporadic tumors. BRCA1 and BRCA2 tumors are more aggressive than sporadic tumors, as indicated by S-phase, mitosis, aneuploidy, genomic instability and pathological appearance (Breast cancer linkage consortium 1997). Other characteristics of BRCA1 tumors are low ER content, elevated lymphocyte infiltration and appearance of medullary phenotype (Marcus et al. 1996; Johannsson et al. 1997). The gross genomic instability detected in BRCA1 and BRCA2 tumors fits well with their documented function in DNA repair (Ingvarsson et al. 1998; Tirkkonen et al. 1997). Moreover, the chromosome aberration profiles of BRCA1 and BRCA2 tumors differ from each other and from other breast cancers, suggesting that specific genetic pathways operate in the progression of genomic instability in these inherited tumors (Ingvarsson et al. 1998; Tirkkonen et al. 1997). Functional support for the discrimination between BRCA1, BRCA2 and sporadic breast tumors is also evident from genome-wide gene expression profiles (Hedenfalk et al. 2002).

It can be hypothesized that in the early stage of BRCA1 and BRCA2 pathogenesis, cells progress through a preliminary crisis phase with massive apoptosis due to accumulation of genetic changes. Further gene alterations, for instance in TP53 or CHK2, rescue the cell from this senescence phase, and progression is towards reduced apoptosis, enhanced cell growth and a fully malignant phenotype (Crook et al. 1997; Greenblatt et al. 2001; Sullivan et al. 2002). Even though TP53 mutations are not as frequent in BRCA2 as in BRCA1 associated tumors, overexpression of p53 is detected, suggesting that in BRCA2 mutation carriers the p53 pathway is deregulated by some other mechanisms in addition to mutation (Crook et al. 1998; Eiriksdottir et al. 1998; Greenblatt et al. 2001; Gretarsdottir et al. 1998). Mouse knockout experiments support the hypothesis of a preliminary crisis phase, and it has been shown that inactivation of p53, or other checkpoint proteins like Bub1 and Mad3L, is of importance in tumor progression in mouse cells lacking Brca (Lee et al. 1999).

In addition to the role of Brca1 and Brca2 in DNA repair, these proteins have multiple functions, one of which seems to be regulation of centrosome number. Brca1 can bind the γ-tubulin which is one of the major centrosomal proteins (Hsu et al. 2001). It has been shown that embryonic fibroblasts derived from mice deficient for a full-length wild-type BRCA1 contain amplified centrosomes (Xu et al. 1999). Similarly, loss of BRCA2 results in centrosome amplification (Tutt et al. 1999). The Brca1 and Brca2 proteins are participants in large protein complexes and, as described earlier, one of the proteins that is considered to be of major importance is Rad51. This refers both to the DNA repair function and to centrosome amplification. The functional inhibition of Rad51 by expression of dominant negative Rad51, or conditional repression of Rad51, results in centrosome amplification (Bertrand et al. 2003, Dodson et al. 2004). This may imply a link between DNA repair and numeral homeostasis of centrosomes. In support of this, centrosome amplification is induced by irradiation, which is otherwise a well-known inducer of DNA breaks (Sato et al. 2000). There seems to be a link between the Brca1 and aurora A kinase, since the former is phosphorylated by the latter, an event that is considered to be important for the regulation of the G2-M transition in the cell cycle (Ouchi et al. 2004). A recent report has suggested that Brca1-dependent ubiquitination activity in concert with Bard1 marks the centrosomes, and inhibits their reduplication (Ko et al. 2006, Starita et al. 2004). Mutations of BARD1 are found at low frequency in breast cancer (Thai et al. 1998, Ghimenti et al. 2002). The role of Bard1 in the Brca1 and Brca2 pathways and genomic stability is further established in knockout mouse experiments (McCarthy et al. 2003).

Fanconi anemia is a rare genetic cancer susceptibility syndrome. In addition to abnormalities in skeleton and skin pigmentation and bone marrow failure, it is characterized by CIN in the form of rearrangements between non-homologous chromosomes, and sensitivity to DNA cross-linking agents (D'Andrea and Grompe 2003). Fanconi anemia patients are also predisposed to developing cancer of several types (Rosenberg et al. 2003). Eight Fanconi anemia genes have been cloned and one of them appears to be BRCA2. The situation is different from typical breast cancer predisposition where one allele is mutated in germline, since Fanconi anemia patients express biallelic BRCA2 mutations (Howlett et al. 2002).

MYC and Telomerase

Another pathway of CIN induction in breast tumors involves telomere maintenance and release of cell senescence, presumably due to elevated expression of the enzyme telomerase. Telomere shortening is a natural consequence of somatic cell proliferation. Loss of telomeres leads to apoptosis unless an event is activating telomerase, leading to maintenance of telomeres and a situation where cells accumulating genomic changes become more viable. Telomerase maintains cell viability and maintenance of telomeres through the addition of repeats to chromosome ends. The reactivation of telomerase through the upregulation of TERT, the telomerase protein subunit, is an important step during cancer development, yet TERT protein function and regulation remain incompletely understood. Telomerase is of importance for cell immortalization and it can establish genomic instability that favors growth advantage of tumor cells. Telomerase overexpression is detected in the majority of breast cancers (Artandi et al. 2003). In mouse models where telomerase is lacking in a p53 heterozygous background, end-joining and unequal translocations between chromosomes are frequent, but these are not detected in mice with long telomeres (Artandi et al. 2000). Analysis of the genome in mouse tumors lacking telomerase shows that uneven translocations lead to a high number of aberrations on chromosome regions, which are not seen in tumors with normal telomeres (O'Hagen et al. 2002).

The well defined oncoprotein Myc has elevated expression in a subset of breast cancer cells. It is a transcription factor involved in cell growth and cell turnover control. Myc seems to affect tumor pathogenesis in several ways, including increased proliferation and immortalization of the cancer cells and induction of CIN. Myc overexpression in breast cancer can partially be explained by gene amplification. Myc amplifications are detected in early stage breast cancer, especially in younger patients, but also occur later in tumor development and appear to be associated with disease progression (Aulmann et al. 2006). The effects of Myc on increased CIN in breast cancer have been documented (Rummikainen et al. 2001). Myc can bind to the promoter of the TERT gene and activate transcriptional expression, resulting in elevated telomerase (Wu et al. 1999). It is also of interest that the aurora kinase A upregulates Myc and then indirectly telomerase expression (Yang et al. 2004). This provides further support for the postulated cross-regulation between different pathways leading to genomic instability.

Epigenetics

An epigenetic mechanism may also be of importance for the development of genomic instability in breast cancer progression. It is generally accepted that global DNA hypomethylation leads to genomic instability and increased tumor progression, but there has been little study of the role of epigenetics in genomic instability of breast tumor cells (Feinberg 2006). Evidence for the involvement of hypomethylation in genomic instability comes from an animal model, as global reduction in methylation was shown to increase chromosomal instability in DNA methyltransferase knockout mice (Chen et al. 1998). Also, chromosomal instability events correlate with the extent of global hypomethylation and expression of MBD2/demethylase in breast cancer cell lines (Vilain et al. 1999). Is it possible to restore genomic stability by affecting global DNA methylation? Further studies will doubtless elucidate the role of global DNA methylation in genomic instability of breast cancer progression, and possibly give some clues on therapeutic intervention.

Therapeutic Intervention

Genomic instability is believed to play a role in the mechanism of action of chemotherapy and possibly radiotherapy. In a background of genomic instability, there is an increased rate of acquiring mutations which facilitate tumor progression, but can also accelerate pathways induced by cancer drugs, leading to reduced viability of the cancer cell. The majority of chemotherapeutic agents interfere with DNA metabolism and are mutagens. In a genetically unstable cancer cell, a further increase in mutagenesis due to chemotherapy could lead to accumulation of mutation and extinction of the cell. An obvious side effect of chemotherapy and of radiotherapy is induction of secondary malignancies, and the state of the genome probably affects this progression. In individuals with breast cancer due to predisposition genes such as ATM , BRCA1, BRCA2 and TP53, it is debatable whether radiation should be used, but this will hopefully be clarified through additional follow-up studies. Ionising radiation has a central role, not only in the treatment of breast cancer, but also in diagnosis and surveillance. Valid questions may be asked, about whether defects in the genes that cause inherited predisposition to breast cancer may also affect radiosensitivity, entailing a predisposition to altered radiation-induced effects in tumor tissue, healthy tissue, or both.

Recent developments in understanding of molecular networks involved in genomic instability are already providing some clues in therapy strategies. Can the function of a tumor suppressor protein be restored, as has been suggested for p53, by blocking degradation pathways or using small molecules that reactivate the protein (Issaeva et al. 2003)? To restore Brca1 or Brca2 activity seems more complicated; it may be more relevant to induce further genomic damage in order to make cells less viable, as has been suggested using PARP inhibitors (Farmer et al. 2005). Emerging data on the role of aurora kinases in genomic instability and breast cancer pathogenesis are opportune, and could give some clues on novel kinase inhibitor treatment.

Instability of the genome may also play a role in resistance to cancer therapy. In a background of genomic instability, there might not only be accelerated rate of mutations that are required for tumor progression but it could also in parallel generate an even larger number of mutations that would render cells resistant to chemotherapeutic agents. Within a tumor there may be multiple cells that contain mutations in genes or regulatory sequences that render those cells resistant to specific chemotherapies. In the presence of chemotherapy, the mutant cells would have a growth advantage. Accordingly, treatment with chemotherapy selects resistant mutants, and genomic instability exacerbates this problem.

Conclusion

There is strong evidence that genomic instability has a role in breast cancer pathogenesis, as well as a possible role in sensitivity and resistance to therapy. CIN is frequent in breast tumor cells, and some chromosome regions are more unstable than others, particularly in hereditary breast cancer. Why would a cell with elevated CIN be viable? This must be due to selective pressure of genes involved in cell turnover such as cell proliferation, cell-cycle checkpoints, apoptosis etc. Indeed some experimental data support this hypothesis for breast cancer: both information from human tumors and from mouse models, such as knockout mice. An example of such an explanation derives from the work on Brca1 and Brca2. As genomic instability can result in an increased number of gene abnormalities by growth selection, some of these gene abnormalities can induce development of further genomic instability. Perhaps an autonomous loop of events is induced in breast cancer, as well as in some other cancer types, where gene abnormalities induce CIN, and the induced instability gives rise to further gene abnormalities. There must be some equilibrium in the amount and speed of such events to favor appropriate growth selection for the cancer cell; too much instability could result in poor cell survival. Clearer understanding is being achieved on the networks involved in genomic instability in breast tumors, but molecular pathways need to be studied further. Presumably there is some sort of synergism between the progression of genomic instability and tumor suppressor dysfunction/oncoprotein activation, to facilitate breast tumor development. Genomic instability is probably one of the most common causes of tumor cell evasion of therapy. Hence a complete understanding of the biological basis of genomic instability is essential for effective diagnostic and prognostic evaluation and therapeutic intervention in breast cancer.

References

Artandi SE. (2003). Complex roles for telomeres and telomerase in breast carcinogenesis. *Breast Cancer Res.* 5, 37-41.

Artandi SE, Chang S, Lee SL, Alson S, Gottlieb GJ, Chin L, DePinho RA. (2000) Telomere dysfunction promotes non-reciprocal translocations and epithelial cancers in mice. *Nature* 406, 641-645.

Aulmann S, Adler N, Rom J, Helmchen B, Schirmacher P, Sinn HP (2006) C-myc amplifications in primary breast carcinomas and their local recurrences. *J. Clin. Pathol.* 59, 424-428.

Baer R and Ludwig T. (2002) The BRCA1/BARD1 heterodimer, a tumor suppressor complex with ubiquitin E3 ligase activity. *Curr. Opin. Genet Dev.* 12, 86-91.

Bell DW, Varley JM, Szydlo TE, Kang DH, Wahrer DC, Shannon KE, Lubratovich M, Verselis SJ, Isselbacher KJ, Fraumeni JF, Birch JM, Li FP, Garber JE, Haber DA. (1999) Heterozygous germ line hCHK2 mutations in Li-Fraumeni syndrome. *Science* 286, 2528-2531.

Bertrand P, Lambert S, Joubert C, Lopez BS. (2003) Overexpression of mammalian Rad51 does not stimulate tumorigenesis while a dominant-negative Rad51 affects centrosome fragmentation, ploidy and stimulates tumorigenesis, in p53-defective CHO cells. *Oncogene* 22, 7587-7592.

Bischoff JR, Anderson L, Zhu Y, Mossie K, Ng L, Souza B, Schryver B, Flanagan P, Clairvoyant F, Ginther C, Chan CS, Novotny M, Slamon DJ, Plowman GD. (1998) A homologue of Drosophila aurora kinase is oncogenic and amplified in human colorectal cancers. *EMBO J.* 17, 3052-3065.

Bochar DA, Wang L, Beniya H, Kinev A, Xue Y, Lane W, Wang W, Kashanchi F, Shiekhattar R. (2000) BRCA1 is associated with a human SWI/SNF-related complex: linking chromatin remodeling to breast cancer. *Cell* 102, 257-265.

Boveri T. (1914) *Zur Frage der Entsehung Maligner Tumoren*. Fisher, Jena.

Bragadottir G, Eiriksdottir G, Sigurdsson A, Barkardottir RB, Gudmundsson J, Jonasson JG, Ingvarsson S. (1995) Loss of heterozygosity at chromosome 6q correlates with tumor progression and patient survival. *Int. J. Oncol.* 7, 871-876.

Breast Cancer Linkage Consortium. (1997) Pathology of familial breast cancer: differences between breast cancers in carriers of BRCA1 or BRCA2 mutations and sporadic cases. *Lancet* 349, 1505-1510.

Cahill DP, Kinzler KW, Vogelstein B, Lengauer C. (1999) *Genetic instability and darwinian selection of tumours.* TCB 9, TIBS 24, TIG 15, M57-M60.

Catteau A, Harris WH, Xu CF, Solomon E. (1999) Methylation of the BRCA1 promoter region in sporadic breast and ovarian cancer: correlation with disease characteristics. *Oncogene* 18, 1957-1965.

Chen RZ, Pettersson U, Beard C, Jackson-Grusby L, Jaenisch R. (1998) DNA hypomethylation leads to elevated mutation rates. *Nature* 395, 89–93.

Courjal F, Cuny M, Rodriguez C, Louason G, Speiser P, Katsaros D, Tanner MM, Zeillinger R, Theillet C. (1996) DNA amplifications at 20q13 and MDM2 define distinct subsets of evolved breast and ovarian tumours. *Br. J. Cancer* 74, 1984-1989.

Cox DG, Hankinson SE, Hunter DJ. (2006) Polymorphisms of the AURKA (STK15/Aurora kinase) gene and breast cancer risk. *Cancer Caus. Contr.* 17, 81-83.

Crook T, Crossland S, Crompton MR, Osin P, Gusterson BA. (1997) p53 mutations in BRCA1-associated familial breast cancer. *Lancet* 350, 638-639.

Crook T, Brooks LA, Crossland S, Osin P, Barker KT, Waller J, Philp E, Smith PD, Yulug I, Peto J, Parker G, Allday MJ, Crompton MR, Gusterson BA. (1998) p53 mutation with frequent novel codons but not a mutator phenotype in BRCA1- and BRCA2-associated breast tumours. *Oncogene* 17, 1681-1689.

D'Andrea AD, Grompe M. (2003). The Fanconi anemia/BRCA pathway. *Nat. Rev. Cancer* 3, 23-334.

D'Assoro AB, Barrett SL, Folk C, Negron VC, Boeneman K, Busby R, Whitehead C, Stivala F, Lingle WL, Salisbury JL. (2002) Amplified centrosomes in breast cancer: A potential indicator of tumor aggressiveness. *Breast Cancer Res. Treat* 75, 25-34.

D'Assoro AB, Busby R, Suino K, Delva E, Almodovar-Mercado GJ, Johnson H, Folk C, Farrugia DJ, Vasile V, Stivala F, Salisbury JL. (2004) Genotoxic stress leads to centrosome amplification in breast cancer cell lines that have an inactive G1/S cell cycle checkpoint. *Oncogene* 23, 4068-4075.

Dodson H, Bourke E, Jeffers LJ, Vagnarelli P, Sonoda E, Takeda S, Earnshaw WC, Merdes A, Morrison C. (2004) Centrosome amplification induced by DNA damage occurs during a prolonged G2 phase and involves ATM. *EMBO J.* 23, 3864-3873.

Eiriksdottir G, Bergthorsson JT, Sigurdsson H, Gudmundsson J, Skirnisdottir S, Egilsson V, Barkardottir RB, Ingvarsson S. (1995) Mapping of chromosome 3 alterations in human breast cancer using microsatellite PCR markers: correlation with clinical variables. *Int. J. Oncol.* 6, 369-375.

Eiriksdottir G, Barkardottir RB, Agnarsson BA, Johannesdottir G, Olafsdottir K, Egilsson V, Ingvarsson S. (1998) High incidence of loss of heterozygosity at chromosome 17p13 in breast tumours from BRCA2 mutation carriers. *Oncogene* 16, 21-26.

Ewart-Toland A, Briassouli P, de Koning JP, Mao JH, Yuan JW, Chan F, MacCarthy-Morrogh L, Ponder BAJ, Nagase H, Burn J, Ball S, Almeida M, Linardopoulos S, Balmain A (2003) Identification of Stk6/STK15 as a candidate low-penetrance tumor-susceptibility gene in mouse and human. *Nat. Genet.* 34, 403-412.

Fan SJ, Yuan RQ, Ma YX, Meng QH, Goldberg ID, Rosen EM. (2001) Mutant BRCA1 genes antagonize phenotype of wild-type BRCA1. *Oncogene* 20, 8215-8235.

Farmer H, McCabe N, Lord CJ, Tutt ANJ, Johnson DA, Richardson TB, Santarosa M, Dillon KJ, Hickson I, Knights C, Martin NMB, Jackson SP, Smith GCM, Ashworth A. (2005) Targeting the DNA repair defect in BRCA mutant cells as a therapeutic strategy. *Nature* 434, 917-921.

Feinberg AP, Ohlsson R, Henikoff S. (2006) The epigenetic progenitor origin of human cancer. *Nat. Rev. Genet* 7, 21-33.

Fukasawa K, Choi T, Kuriyama R, Rulong S, Woude G. (1996) Abnormal centrosome amplification in the absence of p53. *Science* 271, 1744-1747.

Fukasawa K, Wiener F, VandeWoude GF, Mai SB. (1997) Genomic instability and apoptosis are frequent in p53 deficient young mice. *Oncogene* 15, 1295-1302.

Ghimenti C, Sensi E, Presciuttini S, Brunetti IM, Conte P, Bevilacqua G, Caligo MA. (2002) Germline mutations of the BRCA1-associated ring domain (BARD1) gene in breast and breast/ovarian families negative for BRCA1 and BRCA2 alterations. *Genes Chrom.* Cancer 33, 235-242.

Glover DM, Leibowitz MH, Mclean DA, Parry H. (1995) Mutations in aurora prevent centrosome separation leading to the formation of monopolar spindles. *Cell* 81, 95-105.

Greenblatt MS, Chappuis PO, Bond JP, Hamel N, Foulkes WD. (2001) TP53 mutations in breast cancer associated with BRCA1 or BRCA2 germ-line mutations. *Cancer Res.* 61, 4092-4097.

Gretarsdottir S, Thorlacius S, Valgardsdottir R, Gudlaugsdottir S, Sigurdsson S, Steinarsdottir M, Jonasson JG, Anamthawat-Jonsson K, Eyfjord JE. (1998) BRCA2 and p53 mutations in primary breast cancer in relation to genetic instability. *Cancer Res.* 58, 859-862.

Gudmundsson J, Johannesdottir G, Bergthorsson JT, Arason A, Ingvarsson S, Egilsson V, Barkardottir RB. (1995) Different tumor types from BRCA2 carriers show wild-type chromosome deletions on 13q12-q13. *Cancer Res.* 55, 4830-4832.

Hanahan D, Weinberg RA. (2000) The hallmarks of cancer. *Cell* 100, 57-70.

Hansen LL, Yilmaz M, Overgaard J, Andersen J, Kruse TA. (1998) Allelic loss of 16q23.2-24.2 is an independent marker of good prognosis in primary breast cancer. *Cancer Res.* 58, 2166-2169.

Harrington EA, Bebbington D, Moore J, Rasmussen RK, Ajose-Adeogun AO, Nakayama T, Graham JA, Demur C, Hercend T, Diu-Hercend A, Su M, Golec JMC, Miller KM. (2004) VX-680, a potent and selective small-molecule inhibitor of the Aurora kinases, suppresses tumor growth in vivo. *Nat. Med.* 10, 262-267.

Hedenfalk I, Duggan D, Chen Y. (2002) Gene-expression profiles in hereditary breast cancer. *Adv. Anat. Pathol.* 9, 1-4.

Howlett NG, Taniguchi T, Olson S, Cox B, Waisfisz Q, de Die-Smulders C, Persky N, Grompe M, Joenje H, Pals G, Ikeda H, Fox EA, D'Andrea AD. (2002). Biallelic inactivation of BRCA2 in Fanconi anemia. *Science* 297, 606-609.

Hsu LC, Doan TP, White RL. (2001) Identification of a gamma-tubulin-binding domain in BRCA1. *Cancer Res.* 61, 7713-7718.

Hu BC, Wang HY, Wang X, Lu HR, Huang CF, Powell SN, Huebner K, Wang Y. (2005) Fhit and CHK1 have opposing effects on homologous recombination repair. *Cancer Res.* 65, 8613-8616.

Huebner K. (2001) Tumor suppressors on 3p: A neoclassic quartet. Proc Natl Acad Sci USA 98, 14763-14765.

Huiping C, Johannsdottir JT, Arason A, Olafsdottir GH, Eiriksdottir G, Egilsson V, Ingvarsson S. (1999a) Replication error in human breast cancer: Comparison with clinical variables and family history of cancer. *Oncol. Rep.* 6, 117-122.

Huiping C, Sigurgeirsdottir JR, Jonasson JG, Eiriksdottir G, Johannesdottir JT, Egilsson V, Ingvarsson S. (1999b) Chromosome alterations and E-cadherin gene mutations in human lobular breast cancer. *Br. J. Cancer* 81, 1103-1110.

Ingvarsson S, Geirsdottir EK, Johannesdottir G, Sigbjörnsdóttir BI, Eiriksdottir G, Ragnarsson G, Agnarsson BA, Gudmundsson J, Jonasson JG, Sigurdsson A, Egilsson V, Barkardottir RB. (1998) High incidence of loss of heterozygosity in breast tumors from carriers of the 999del5 BRCA2 mutation. *Cancer Res.* 58, 4421-4425, 1998.

Ingvarsson S, Agnarsson BA, Sigbjornsdottir BI, Kononen J, Kallioniemi OP, Barkardottir RB, Kovatich A, Schwarting R, Hauck WW, Huebner K, McCue PA. (1999a) Reduced Fhit expression in sporadic and BRCA2-linked breast carcinomas. *Cancer Res.* 59, 2682-2689.

Ingvarsson S. (1999b) The Brca1 and Brca2 proteins and tumor pathogenesis. *Anticancer Res.* 19, 2853-2862.

Ingvarsson S. (2001) FHIT alterations in breast cancer. *Sem. Cancer Biol.* 11, 361-366, 2001.

Ingvarsson S, Sigbjornsdottir BI, Huiping C, Hafsteinsdottir SH, Ragnarsson G, Barkardottir RB, Arason A, Egilsson V, Bergthorsson JT. (2002) Mutation analysis of the CHK2 gene in breast carcinoma and other cancers. *Breast Cancer Res.* 4: R4.

Ingvarsson S. (2004) Genetics of breast cancer. *Drugs Today* 40, 991-1002.

Ingvarsson S. (2005) Tumor suppressor genes on human chromosome 3 and cancer pathogenesis. *Cancer Gen. Prot.* 2, 247-254.

Issaeva N, Friedler A, Bozko P, Wiman KG, Fersht AR, Selivanova G. (2003) Rescue of mutants of the tumor suppressor p53 in cancer cells by a designed peptide. *Proc. Natl. Acad. Sci. USA* 100, 13303-13307.

Jeng YM, Peng SY, Lin CY, Hsu HC. (2004) Overexpression and amplification of Aurora-A in hepatocellular carcinoma. *Clin. Cancer Res.* 10, 2065-2071.

Johannsdottir JT, Jonasson JG, Bergthorsson JT, Amundadottir L, Olafsdottir GH, Magnusson J, Egilsson V, Ingvarsson S. (2000) The effect of mismatch repair deficiency on tumorigenesis; Microsatellite instability affecting genes containing short repeated sequences. *Int. J. Oncol.* 16, 133-139.

Johannsson OT, Idvall I, Anderson C, Borg A, Barkardottir RB, Egilsson V, Olsson H. (1997) Tumor biological features of BRCA1-induced breast and ovarian cancer. *Eur. J. Cancer* 33, 362-371.

Kawamura K, Izumi H, Ma Z, Ikeda R, Moriyama M, Tanaka T, Nojima T, Levin LS, Fujikawa-Yamamoto K, Suzuki K, Fukasawa K. (2004) Induction of centrosome amplification and chromosome instability in human bladder cancer cells by p53 mutation and cyclin E overexpression. *Cancer Res.* 64, 4800-4808.

Kimura M, Kotani S, Hattori T, Sumi N, Yoshioka T, Todokoro K, Okano Y. (1997) Cell cycle-dependent expression and spindle pole localization of a novel human protein kinase, Aik, related to Aurora of Drosophila and yeast Ipl1. *J. Biol. Chem.* 272, 13766-13771.

Khoo US, Ozcelik H, Cheung ANY, Chow LWC, Ngan HYS, Done SJ, Liang ACT, Chan VWY, Au GKH, Ng WF, Poon CSP, Leung YF, Loong F, Ip P, Chan GSW, Andrulis IL, Lu J, Ho FCS. (1999) Somatic mutations in the BRCA1 gene in Chinese sporadic breast and ovarian cancer. *Oncogene* 18: 4643-4646.

Ko MJ, Murata K, Hwang DS, Parvin JD. (2006) Inhibition of BRCA1 in breast cell lines causes the centrosome duplication cycle to be disconnected from the cell cycle. *Oncogene* 25, 298-303.

Koff A, Giordano A, Desai D, Yamashita K, Harper JW, Elledge S, Nishimoto T, Morgan DO, Franza BR, Roberts JM. (1992) Formation and activation of a cyclin E-CDK2 complex during the G(1)-phase of the human cell-cycle. Science 257, 1689-1694.

Lee SB, Kim SH, Bell DW, Wahrer DC, Schiripo TA, Jorczak MM, Sgroi DC, Garber JE, Li FP, Nichols KE, Varley JM, Godwin AK, Shannon KM, Harlow E, Haber DA. (1999) Destabilization of CHK2 by a missense mutation associated with Li-Fraumeni Syndrome. *Cancer Res.* 15, 8062-8067.

Lingle WL, Barrett SL, Negron VC, D'Assoro AB, Boeneman K, Liu WG, Whitehead CM, Reynolds C, Salisbury JL. (2002) Centrosome amplification drives chromosomal instability in breast tumor development. *Proc. Natl. Acad. Sci. USA* 99, 1978-1983.

Lo YL, Yu JC, Chen ST, Yang HC, Farm CSJ, Mau YC, Shen CY. (2005) Breast cancer risk associated with genotypic polymorphism of the mitosis-regulating gene Aurora-A/STK15/BTAK. *Int. J. Cancer* 115, 276-283.

Loeb LA. A mutator phenotype in cancer. (2001) *Cancer Res.* 61: 3230-3239.

Malkin D, Li FP, Strong LC, Fraumeni JF Jr, Nelson CE, Kim DH, Kassel J, Gryka MA, Bischoff FZ, Tainsky MA, Friend SH. (1990) Germ line p53 mutations in a familial syndrome of breast cancer, sarcomas, and other neoplasms. *Science* 250, 1233-1238.

Marcus JN, Watson P, Page DL, Narod SA, Lenoir GM, Tonin P, Linder-Stephenson L, Salerno G, Conway TA, Lynch HT. (1996) Hereditary breast cancer: pathobiology, prognosis, and BRCA1 and BRCA2 gene linkage. *Cancer* 77, 697-709.

McCarthy EE, Celebi JT, Baer R, Ludwig T. (2003) Loss of Bard1, the heterodimeric partner of the Brca1 tumor suppressor, results in early embryonic lethality and chromosomal instability. *Mol. Cell Biol.* 23, 5056–5063.

Meijers-Heijboer H, Van Den Ouweland A, Klijn J, Wasielewski M, De Snoo A, Oldenburg R, Hollestelle A, Houben M, Crepin E, Van Veghel-Plandsoen M, Elstrodt F, Van Duijn C, Bartels C, Meijers C, Schutte M, McGuffog L, Thompson D, Easton DF, Sodha N, Seal S, Barfoot R, Mangion J, Chang-Claude J, Eccles D, Eeles R, Evans DG, Houlston R, Murday V, Narod S, Peretz T, Peto J, Phelan C, Zhang HX, Szabo C, Devilee P, Goldgar D, Futreal PA, Nathanson KL, Weber BL, Rahman N, Stratton MR (2002). Low-penetrance susceptibility to breast cancer due to CHEK2(*)1100delC in noncarriers of BRCA1 or BRCA2 mutations. *Nature Genet.* 31, 55-59.

Miki Y, Swensen J, Shattuck-Eidens D, Futreal PA, Harshman K, Tavtigian S, Liu Q, Cochran C, Bennett LM, Ding W, Bell R, Rosenthal J, Hussey C, Tran T, Mcclure M, Frye C, Hattier T, Phelps R, Haugenstrano A, Katcher H, Yakumo K, Gholami Z, Shaffer D, Stone S, Bayer S, Wray C, Bogden R, Dayananth P, Ward J, Tonin P, Narod S, Bristow PK, Norris FH, Helvering L, Morrison P, Rosteck P, Lai M, Barrett JC, Lewis C, Neuhausen S, Cannonalbright L, Goldgar D, Wiseman R, Kamb A, Skolnick MH. (1994) A strong candidate for the breast and ovarian cancer susceptibility gene BRCA1. *Science* 266, 66-71.

Moynahan ME, Chiu JW, Koller BH, Jasin M. (1999) Brca1 controls homology-directed DNA repair. *Mol. Cell* 4, 511-518.

Mussman JG, Horn HF, Carroll PE, Okuda M, Tarapore P, Donehower LA, Fukasawa K. (2000) Synergistic induction of centrosome hyperamplification by loss of p53 and cyclin E overexpression. *Oncogene* 19, 1635-1646.

Niwa Y, Oyama T, Nakajima T. (2000). BRCA1 expression statis in relation to DNA methylation of the BRCA1 promoter region in sporadic breast cancers. *Jpn. J. Cancer Res.* 91, 519-526.

O'Hagan RC, Chang S, Maser RS, Mohan R, Artandi SE, DePinho RA. (2002) Telomere dysfunction provokes regional amplification and deletion in cancer genomes. *Cancer Cell* 2, 149-155.

Olivier M and Hainaut P. (2001) TP53 mutation pattern in breast cancers: searching for clues of environmental carcinogenesis. *Sem. Cancer Biol.* 11, 353-360.

Ouchi M, Fujiuchi N, Sasai K, Katayama H, Minamishima YA, Ongusaha PP Deng CX, Sen S, Lee SW, Ouchi T. (2004) BRCA1 phosphorylation by Aurora-A in the regulation of G(2) to M transition. *J. Biol. Chem.* 279, 19643-19648.

Percy M, Myrie EA, Neeley CK, Azim JN, Ethier SP, Petty EM. (2000) Expression and mutational analyses of the human MAD2L1 gene in breast cancer cells. *Genes Chrom. Cancer* 29, 356-362.

Pihan GA, Wallace J, Zou YN, Doxsey SJ. (2003) Centrosome abnormalities and chromosome instability occur together in pre-invasive carcinomas. *Cancer Res.* 63, 1398-1404.

Rice JC, Ozcerlik H, Maxeiner P, Andrulis I, Futscher BW. (1999) Methylation of the BRCA1 promoter is associated with decreased BRCA1 mRNA levels in clinical breast cancer specimens. *Carcinogenesis* 21, 1761-1765.

Rosenberg PS, Greene MH, Alter BP. (2003) Cancer incidence in persons with Fanconi anemia. *Blood* 101, 822-826.

Rummukainen JK, Salminen T, Lundin J, Joensuu H, Isola J. (2001) Amplification of c-myc oncogene by chromogenic and fluorescence in situ hybridization in archival breast cancer tissue array samples. *Lab. Invest.* 81: 1545-1551.

Sato N, Mizumoto K, Nakamura M , Tanaka M. (2000) Radiation-induced centrosome overduplication and multiple mitotic spindles in human tumor cells. *Exp. Cell Res.* 255, 321-326.

Sen S, Zhou HY, White RA. (1997) A putative serine/threonine kinase encoding gene BTAK on chromosome 20q13 is amplified and overexpressed in human breast cancer cell lines. *Oncogene* 14, 2195-2200.

Shiloh Y. (2003) ATM and related protein kinases: safeguarding genome integrity. *Nt. Rev. Cancer* 3, 155-168.

Sigbjörnsdottir BI, Ragnarsson G, Agnarsson BA, Huiping C, Barkardottir RB, Egilsson V, Ingvarsson S. (2000) Chromosome 8p alterations in sporadic and BRCA2 999del5 linked breast cancer. *J. Med. Genet.* 37, 342-347.

Signori E, Bagni C, Papa S, Primerano B, Rinaldi M, Amaldi F, Fazio VM.(2001) A somatic mutation in the 5 ' UTR of BRCA1 gene in sporadic breast cancer causes down-modulation of translation efficiency. *Oncogene* 20, 4596-4600.

Sigurdsson S, Bodvarsdottir SK, Anamthawat-Jonsson K, Steinarsdottir M, Jonasson JG, Ogmundsdottir HM, Eyfjord JE. (2000) p53 abnormality and chromosomal instability in the same breast tumor cells. *Cancer Genet. Cytogenet.* 121, 150-155.

Skirnisdottir S, Eiriksdottir G, Baldursson T, Barkardottir RB, Egilsson V, Ingvarsson S. (1995) High frequency of allelic imbalance at chromosome region 16q22-q23 in human breast cancer: correlation with high PgR and low S-phase. *Int. J. Cancer* 64, 112-116.

Smith SA, Easton DF, Evans DG, Ponder BA. (1992) Allele losses in the region 17q12-21 in familial breast and ovarian cancer involve the wild-type chromosome. *Nature Genet.* 2, 128-131.

Spring K, Ahangari F, Scott SP, Waring P, Purdie DM, Chen PC, Hourigan K, Ramsay J, McKinnon PJ, Swift M, Lavin MF (2002) Mice heterozygous for mutation in Atm, the gene involved in ataxia-telangiectasia, have heightened susceptibility to cancer. *Nat. Genet* 32, 185-190.

Srivastava S, Zhou ZQ, Pirollo K, Blattner W, Chang EH. (1990) Germ-line transmission of a mutated p53 gene in a cancer-prone family with Li-Fraumeni syndrome. *Nature* 348, 747-749.

Starita LM, Machida Y, Sankaran S, Elias JE, Griffin K, Schlegel BP, Gygi SP, Parvin JD. (2004) BRCA1-dependent ubiquitination of gamma-tubulin regulates centrosome number. *Mol. Cell Biol.* 24, 8457-8466.

Suizu F, Ryo A, Wulf G, Lim J, Lu KP. (2006) Pin1 regulates centrosome duplication, and its overexpression induces centrosome amplification, chromosome instability, and oncogenesis. *Mol. Cell Biol.* 26, 1463-1479.

Sullivan A, Yuille M, Repellin C, Reddy A, Reelfs O, Bell A, Dunne B, Gusterson BA, Osin P, Farrell PJ, Yulug I, Evans A, Ozcelik T, Gasco M, Crook T. (2002) Concomitant inactivation of p53 and Chk2 in breast cancer. *Oncogene* 21, 1316-1324.

Tarapore P, Horn HF, Tokuyama Y, Fukasawa K. (2001) Direct regulation of the centrosome duplication cycle by the p53-p21Wafl/Cip1 pathway. *Oncogene* 20, 3173-3184.

Thai TH, Du F, Tsan JT, Jin Y, Phung A, Spillman MA, Massa HF, Muller CY, Ashfaq R, Mathis JM, Miller DS, Trask BJ, Baer R, Bowcock AM. (1998) Mutations in the BRCA1-associated RING domain (BARD1) gene in primary breast, ovarian and uterine cancers. *Hum. Mol. Genet.* 7, 195-202.

Thompson ME, Jensen RA, Obermiller PS, Page DL, Holt JT. (1995) Decreased expression of BRCA1 accelerates growth and is often present during sporadic breast-cancer progression. *Nature Genet.* 9, 444-450.

Tirkkonen M, Johannsson O, Agnarsson BA, Olsson H, Ingvarsson S, Karhu R, Tanner M, Isola J, Barkardottir RB, Borg A, Kallioniemi OP. (1997) Distinct somatic genetic changes associated with tumor progression in carriers of BRCA1 and BRCA2 germ-line mutations. *Cancer Res.* 57, 1222-1227.

Tsukasaki K, Miller CW, Greenspun E, Eshaghian S, Kawabata H, Fujimoto T, Tomonaga M, Sawyers C, Said JW and Koeffler HP. Mutation in the mitotic checkpoint gene, MAD1L1, in human cancers. *Oncogene* 20, 3301-3305, 2001.

Tutt A, Gabriel A, Bertwistle, Connor F, Paterson H, Peacock J, Ross G, Ashworth A. (1999) Absence of Brca2 causes genomic instability by chromosome breakage and loss associated with centrosome amplification. *Curr. Biol.* 9, 1107-1110.

Vilain A, Vogt N, Dutrillaux B, Malfoy B. (1999) DNA methylation and chromosome instability in breast cancer cell lines. *FEBS Let.* 460, 231-234.

Welcsh PL, Lee MK, Gonzalez-Hernandez RM, Black DJ, Mahadevappa M, Swisher EM, Warrington JA, King MC. (2002) BRCA1 transcriptionally regulates genes involved in breast tumorigenesis. *Proc. Natl. Acad. Sci. USA* 99, 7560-7565.

Wilson CA, Ramos L, Villasenor MR, Anders KH, Press MF, Clarke K, Karlan B, Chen JJ, Scully R, Livingston D, Zuch RH, Kanter MH, Cohen S, Calzone FJ and Slamon DJ. (1999) Localization of human BRCA1 and its loss in high-grade, non-inherited breast carcinomas. *Nature Genet.* 21, 236-240.

Wooster R, Bignell G, Lancaster J, Swift S, Seal S, Mangion J, Collins N, Gregory S, Gumbs C, Micklem G, Barfoot R, Hamoudi R, Patel S, Rice C, Biggs P, Hashim Y, Smith A, Connor F, Arason A, Gudmundsson J, Ficenec D, Kelsell D, Ford D, Tonin P, Bishop DT, Spurr NK, Ponder BAJ, Eeles R, Peto J, Devilee P, Cornelisse C, Lynch H, Narod S, Lenoir G, Egilsson V, Barkardottir RB, Easton DF, Bentley DR, Futreal PA, Ashworth A, Stratton MR. (1995) Identification of the breast cancer susceptibility gene BRCA2. *Nature* 378, 789-792.

Wu KJ, Grandori C, Amacker M, Simon-Vermot N, Polack A, Lingner J, Dalla-Favera R. (1999) Direct activation of TERT transcription by c-Myc. *Nature Genet.* 21: 220-224.

Xu XL, Weaver Z, Linke SP, Li CL, Gotay J, Wang XW, Harris CC, Ried T, Deng CX. (1999) Centrosome amplification and a defective G2-M cell cycle checkpoint induce genetic instability in BRCA1 exon 11 isoform-deficient cells. *Mol. Cell* 3, 389-395, 1999.

Yang H, Ou CC, Feldman RI, Nicosia SV, Kruk PA, Cheng JQ (2004) Aurora A kinase regulates telomerase activity through c-Myc in human ovarian and breast epithelial cells. *Cancer Res*. 64, 463-467.

Zhang HB, Somasundaram K, Peng Y, Tian H, Zhang HX, Bi DK, Weber BL, El-Deiry WS. (1998) BRCA1 physically associates with p53 and stimulates its transcriptional activity. *Oncogene* 16, 1713-1721.

Zhou HY, Kuang J, Zhong L, Kuo WL, Gray JW, Sahin A, Brinkley BR, Sen S (1998). Tumour amplified kinase STK15/BTAK induces centrosome amplification, aneuploidy and transformation. *Nat. Genet.* 20, 189-193.

In: Frontiers in Breast Cancer Research
Editor: Louis P. Fortugno, pp. 141-156
ISBN: 978-1-60021-671-8

Chapter VI

The Pathology of Male Breast Cancer

J. Chakrabarti[1], R. S. Rampaul[1], C. Guevara[2], S. E. Pinder[2], I. O. Ellis[2] and J. F. Robretson[1]*

[1]Professorial Unit of Breast Surgery, Nottingham City Hospital, Hucknall Road, Nottingham NG5 1PB

[2]Department of Pathology, Nottingham City Hospital, Nottingham

Abstract

The incidence of male breast cancer is rising, but it is still an uncommon condition. There are a limited number of large studies in male breast cancer, and most of the treatments are extrapolated from female breast cancer. This review aims to summarize the pathological similarities and differences between male and female breast cancer, with a specific emphasis on the genetic aspects, and molecular markers.

Introduction

Male breast cancer is a rare disease, accounting for less than one percent of all breast cancers. Approximately 1600 new cases were diagnosed in the US in 2004, compared with 200,000 new cases in women [1]. In the U.K, there are approximately 200-300 cases per year [2].

Recently the reported incidence has risen significantly from 0.86 to 1.08 per 100,000 population in the US, and has also been reflected in other nations [3].

The precise cause for male breast cancer is unknown and is still under investigation. Cases have shown that changes in hormonal balance between androgens and estrogens may be implicated.

---

*Correspondence: RS Rampaul MRCS, Specialist Registrar in Surgery, University of Nottingham, Tel: 0115 9691169. Fax: 0115 8402618, Email: ajendra.rampaul@nottingham.ac.uk

Men who are on oestrogen, oestrogen-like compounds or anti-androgens, for example in the treatment of prostate cancer, are at an increased risk.[4] In breasts of male to female transsexuals, where progestative chemical castration is combined with feminising estrogen therapy, full acini and lobules form. Metaplasia has been reported, but only four cases of breast carcinoma have been reported to date, and it has been suggested that if treated with oestrogens, they have the same annual risk of breast malignancy as do genetic females.[5] Androgen deficiency also increases the risk of developing breast cancer such as in males with testicular atrophy from mumps, orchitis, injury or undescended testes [6].

Kleinfelters disease, caused by chromosome aneuploidy, characteristically presents with small testes, gynaecomastia, hypogonadism and high levels of FSH. Most studies in these patients show that there is a slightly increased risk of approximately 3% of developing breast carcinoma [7]. Hultborn et al found the risk was as high as 50%, [8] but certain environmental factors have also been implicated, such as men working in steel mills, blast furnaces and rolling mills. This has been suggested to be due to chronic heat exposure, which can suppress testicular function [9].

Pathologically, there are similarities and also distinct differences between male and female breast cancer. This review aims to summarise the difference, and describe recently reported genetic aspects of male breast cancer.

Pathology

Grossly and microscopically carcinomas of the male breast are remarkably similar to those seen in females and exhibit the same range of morphological diversity of grade and type. As a consequence the histological classification and grading of male and female invasive breast carcinoma use identical criteria.

Male breast cancers are predominantly invasive carcinomas of no special type, comprising about 80% of cases. Medullary, tubular, papillary, small cell and mucinous carcinoma have also been noted in men, but are seen in less than 15% of cases [10, 11].

About 10% of all breast tumours in men are non-invasive. Virtually all of these are ductal carcinoma in situ [12]. The histological features are in general similar to those in the female breast but two major studies have found that the most frequent architectural pattern is papillary [13]. The in situ carcinomas are generally of the non-necrotic cribriform or papillary types. Though necrosis develops in some cases composed of either micropapillary or the cribriform types, true comedo DCIS is rare [14].

Due to the absence of lobules and acini in the male breast, lobular cancer is extremely rare in men, and to our knowledge only 20-30 cases have been reported in the literature. Lobular carcinoma in situ has only been reported in conjunction with invasive lobular carcinoma [15, 16]. This does not usually occur in men even in those exposed to endogenous or exogenous hormone stimulation and should only be diagnosed if E-Cadherin expression is absent [17, 18].

Despite these broad similarities in the morphological features of breast cancer in male and female patients some differences, particularly related to frequency of occurrence, have been identified. Male patients' tumours are more likely to be of poorer prognostic type or have adverse prognostic characteristics such as higher frequency of grade 3 morphology, cerb-B2 positivity and p53 positivity [19]. In contrast male breast cancers are more likely to be ER and PGR positive [19]. Male breast cancers have a somewhat higher frequency of ER positivity in 60-95% range while PR positivity occurs in 45-85% of cases [14].

DCIS in Males

DCIS in the male breast is rare; in one series comprised about 7% of all male breast cancer [20]. Differences between male and female subtypes of DCIS have been noted. Macroscopically, pure DCIS lesions in men tend to be well circumscribed and retroareolar. Hittmair et al found that the commonest architectural growth patterns of DCIS were papillary, cribriform and solid. Within papillary DCIS, most frequently observed were solid and cribriform patterns supported by fibrovascular cores.

The papillary architecture was seen in larger ducts whereas cribriform, solid, and micropapillary patterns were seen in more frequently in smaller and peripheral ducts.

The majority of pure DCIS in the series by Hittmair et al. was low grade with occasional cases displaying necrosis. High grade DCIS appears to be rare in the male breast [13].

Unlike in males, the majority of breast carcinoma in females arises within the terminal duct lobular units (TDLU). The female breast generally shows greater development of the more central portion of the duct system than in males. The periphery of the organ differentiates only under the physiologic influence of estrogens. Therefore, DCIS patterns observed within the male breast are similar to those also present in the more central ducts of the female breast [13].

Another difference described is that low grade forms are generally found more often in males, for example in the series described by Hittmair et al. which showed that only 7 of 114 DCIS cases were high grade [13]. The site of derivation of high grade DCIS compared to low grade disease which may develop from larger ducts develops only in conditions of relative or absolute hyperestrogenism, for example in Kleinfelters syndrome [21].

Genetics of Male Breast Cancer

Around 15-20 % of male breast cancer is associated with a positive family history. Women with BRCA1 or BRCA2 mutations have a cumulative lifetime risk of 55-85% of developing breast cancer whereas men have only a 6.3% risk [22, 23] (Table 1).

In women, a germ line genetic mutation in either BRCA1 or BRCA2 gives rise to an increased risk of breast cancer. However, in men a mutation in BRCA2 has been shown to be a risk factor.

Tumours associated with BRCA1 mutations in men are more frequently of a higher pathological grade, show high proliferation rates, aneuploidy and lack ER which are all factors associated with a poorer prognosis. Male BRCA2 associated tumours similarly are often of a higher grade, more frequently lobular and show less tubule formation than sporadic male breast cancer cases. They also present at an earlier age and are associated with a shorter survival rate [24] (Table 1).

Table 1. BRCA 1 and 2 Mutations in Male Breast Cancer

Year	Institution	Author and Reference	Total no of patients tested	No. with BRCA2 mutations	%	No. with BRCA1 mutations	%
1996	Pennsylvania	Couch FJ et al [77]	50	7	14	0	0
1997	California	Friedman LS et al. [78]	54	2	3.7	0	0
1997	Leeds	Mavraki E et al. [79]	28	3	10.7	0	0
1998	Sweden	Haraldsson K et al. [80]	34	7	20.6	0	0
	Hungary	Csokay et al [81]	18	6	33.3	0	0
2000	Israel	Sverdlov RS et al.[82]	31	1	3.2	1	3.2
2001	Poland	Kwiatkowska E [83]					
2002	Poland	Kwiatkowska E et al. [84]	27	8	29.6	0	0
2000	Canada	Wolpert N et al. [85]	14	2	14.3	0	0
	U.K	Basham VM et al. [86]	94	5	5.3	0	0
	Italy	Ottini L et al. [87]	25	3	12	1	4
1999	Finland	Tirkkonen M et al. [88]	26	5	19.2	0	0

Molecular Markers in Male Breast Cancer

Expression of molecular markers such as HER-2/neu, p53, Bcl-2, cyclin D1 and Epidermal growth factor receptor (EGFR) have been extensively studied in female breast cancer. However, few studies have evaluated their role in male breast cancer.

HER-2/neu

HER-2/neu is a proto-oncogene, whose product is a transmembrane receptor protein with tyrosine kinase activity which is related to the EGF receptor. In females, Her-2/neu gene expression is found in 20-30% of breast cancers [25].

Slamon et al. showed that Her-2/neu amplification independently predicted overall survival (OS) and disease free survival (DFS) in node positive patients, by multivariate analysis [26]. There is however less agreement about the importance of HER-2 overexpression in node negative patients and regarding associations with other prognostic factors such as increasing tumour size, grade and hormone receptor status. Due to the rarity of male breast cancer and low numbers of patients the significance of HER-2/neu expression in these carcinomas is not well defined.

There has been little work on whether it is the protein expression or gene amplification that occurs in these patients. As a result of differing scoring systems, cut off values and methods of assessment there is conflicting evidence. Pooled data shows that 0-95% of tumours overexpress HER-2/neu as detected by IHC. However, many investigators have been unable to demonstrate HER-2/ neu gene overexpression in male breast carcinoma. Recently, Rudlowski et al. examined expression of Her-2 in 99 male patients with primary breast cancer with 60% diagnosed with T2-T4 disease and ER positivity of 90%. Eleven percent of cases had HER-2/neu FISH amplification [27]. Examination of any potential association between HER-2/neu protein and prognosis in male breast cancer also shows conflicting results. Some studies have shown no correlation, [28-31] whereas others show an association [32-34] although it is not apparent whether this was with multivariate or univariate analysis.

Pich et al showed in a series of 50 patients, that immunopositivity for Her-2 protein was strongly correlated with poor patient survival and was the most significant independent prognostic variable in multivariate analysis ($p<0.01$). Simultaneous expression of p53 and her-2/neu proteins had an additive negative impact on survival. When patients were grouped by Her-2 and p53 immunoreactivity, all patients, with tumors which did not express Her-2 and p53 were alive after 58 months whereas none of the 14 patients with tumour expressing both proteins survived at 61 months [35].

In comparison with several female breast cancer studies, it has been reported that there is no association between Her-2 expression and histological grade, tumour size, or hormone receptor status [25].

p53

Approximately 30% of female breast cancers have been found to have a p53 mutation [29-31]. This has been shown to be associated with a poorer prognosis [32, 33]. In males, there have been mixed results. Immunohistochemical detection of mutated p53 protein has been reported ranges between 0-54% of cases but when measured with PCR the detection rate is higher [35, 93.] Other reasons for the discrepancy between results could potentially be due to lack of sensitivity as certain point mutations give rise to overexpression whilst frame shifts may not. There is also a lack of consensus on what constitutes a significant accumulation and when p53 assesment by immunohistochemistry should be considered as positive; some investigators regarding any nuclear reactivity for p53 as positive and others requiring at least 5-10% of the cells to be positive.

Therefore, not only expression,but also prognostic significance of p53 in male breast cancer is difficult to assess. Pich et al.'s series (n=50) showed that p53 immunoreactivity was associated with poor survival with a median survival of 99 months for p53 negative tumours vs. 33 months for p53 positive tumors, and p53 retained independent prognostic significance in multivariate analysis. ($p=0.001$) A cut-off value of 10% nuclear staining was used.

These authors also found that MIB-1 scores were higher in p53 positive tumours compared to negative ones, and postulated that the prognostic relevance of p53 overexpression mainly depends on the association between protein overexpression and cell proliferative activity [35]. Rayson et al. examined p53 expression in male breast cancer, and using a cut-off of 20%, found no prognostic significance of this molecular marker [28].

Bcl-2

Bcl-2 is a proto-oncogene, which has a role in the inhibition of apoptosis and subsequently promotes cell growth [36]. In female breast cancer, bcl-2 expression has been found in 48-90% of cases [37]. High expression has been associated with low grade, small, node positive tumours and in oestrogen and progesterone positive tumours. Conversely, low bcl-2 expression has been found in concordance with p53 positive tumours, and highly proliferating tumours. Some studies have shown a longer disease free survival and overall survival particularly in node-positive cases [38-40]. Thus the prognostic significance of bcl-2 expression in female breast cancer is unclear.

In male breast cancer the rate of expression appears to be higher than in female cancers, with expression rates varying between 57-94% [28, 41-44] in the few studies examining this marker. These conflicting results may again be due to differences in scoring procedures. Rayson et al postulated that the high frequency of bcl-2 expression in male breast cancer involves antiapoptotic mechanisms [28].

Bcl-2 expression in males is less likely to be acting through an oestrogen dependent transcription pathway, or to be regulated by oestrogen.

Idelevich et al showed in 30 patients that the 5-year survival rate was marginally better for those patients with tumours staining positively for bcl-2 ($p = 0.05$). [41] No other studies report any correlation between bcl-2 and patient survival.

Cyclin D1

Cyclin D1 is a product of the CCND1 gene and has been implicated as playing a role in cell cycle progression in breast cancer. The gene is found on chromosome 11q13 and is amplified in approximately 15% of female breast cancers. The protein is expressed in 30-60% of female breast cancers [45].

Barnes et al, and Gillett et al recently showed that over-expression of cyclin D1 is aassociated with good outcome, both in terms of prognosis and response to endocrine treatment [46].

In male breast cancer cyclin D1 protein overexpression is seen in 41-63% of cases [28, 47, 48] with 12% of cases showing amplification of the CCND1 gene. The latter was also associated with positive ER expression. ($p<0.0001$) In a single study of 73 patients by Rayson et al, Cyclin D1 negativity was associated with a significantly decreased DFS ($p= 0.009$). This may be due to interactions between cyclin D1 and pRb mutations or inactivation of pRB which leads to down regulation of cyclin D1.

AR (Androgen Receptor)

Few studies have evaluated the role of androgen receptor (AR) in either male or female breast cancer and most have included relatively small numbers of patients.

Teller et al showed that androgens cause regression of DMBA-induced breast cancers in rats and suppress growth in human breast cancers [49, 50]. AR has been reported to be expressed in 31-91% of cases.

No association with tumor size, lymph node stage, or tumour stage of female breast cancer has been reported [51-53]. Nomura found a higher response in AR positive tumours with hormone therapy and some studies have shown a longer disease free survival or overall survival [54-57]. However, in larger series, AR has not been shown to provide significant prognostic information.

AR positivity has been found in 34- 91% of cases of male breast cancer [58-64] However, some investigators have performed AR assay from cytosol preparation [58-60] whilst others have used immunohistochemistry [63]. To our knowledge, there has been no reported association between AR status and survival and no correlation has been found with other prognostic features such as tumour size, stage or lymph node status.

Pich et al. [63] and Pachecho et al. [60] have reported a relationship between AR and ER (p=0.0001) Pich also showed a weak but significant association between AR and cell proliferative activity.

ER (Oestrogen Receptor)

Approximately 64-91% of male breast cancers have been found to express ER [28]. This is greater than that found in many series of female breast cancer. The reason for this may be likened to that of the disease process in post menopausal women. Hormone–receptor positive cancers are believed to occur as a result of abnormal steroid receptor up-regualation in the estrogen starved post-menopausal setting. Tumours overexpressing the steroid receptor may then have constitutive activation of downstream targets. The observation that most cancers arising in male breasts are ER positive could thus be due to the lack of circulating oestrogen, as in post menopausal women [42].

It is not clear whether there is any association between ER positivity and prognosis in male breast cancer. Munoz de Toro showed no correlation between ER status and prognosis. [65] Stalsberg et al., in a series of 282 men found a marginally significant trend for patients with ER positive tumours to present with higher stage disease although no data on DFS or OS was presented [66]. Rayson et al. in a study of 76 patients found that 91% were ER positive by immunohistochemistry but due to the high degree of positivity, were unable to assess whether there was an association with DFS and OS. [28] However, in a series of 77 patients Donegan et al. reported that the survival of patients with ER positive tumours was significantly superior to those with ER negative tumours (p=0.0001). A similar association was found with PR positive patients (p=0.0012) [67].

Table 2. Expression of Molecular Markers in male breast cancer (all markers were assessed by immunohistochemistry unless otherwise stated)

Marker	no. studies	total pts	total +ve by IHC	% +ve	total + by fish	Refs.
HER-2	14	547	164	30	11/99 (11%)	[19, 27-29,31, 33, 34, 41, 42, 44, 89, 90-92]
p-53	13	507	111	22		[19, 28, 31, 33, 34, 41, 42, 44, 89-91, 93,104]
bcl-2	5	218	178	82		[28, 41-44]
cyclin D1	3	249	144	58	15 /128 (12%)	[28, 47, 48]
EGFR	3	33	17	52		[19,94,95]
ER	20	1254	1028	82		[12, 19, 28, 31, 34, 44, 65, 67, 75, 90, 94-103]
PR	14	1074	835	78		[12, 19, 28, 34, 44, 65, 67, 96-102]
AR	3	75	34	45		[63, 65, 102]

Treatment and Prognosis

The prognostic factors in male breast cancer are similar to those in females. Willcher et al. showed that grade and lymph node status were the strongest parameters influencing survival. The risk of death was three fold greater for patients with nodal metastases and high grade tumours ($p<0.01$) [68, 69].

A multi-institutional study in Portland, USA showed that overall disease free survival was 100% and 71% for early stage (0-2A), but 71% and 20% for advanced disease. Only the AJCC stage and its components (tumor size, nodal status, and metastases) correlated with survival by multivariate analysis; other factors such as age, family history and presenting symptoms/signs did not [70]. Rudan et al. showed that for TNM stages III and IV, male patients had a significantly worse five-year overall survival than females. Three predictors that explained most of the survival variance in males were TNM-stage, number of affected lymph nodes and delay in treatment [71].

The low incidence of male breast cancer prevents therapeutic questions from being addressed in single institution prospective randomised trials. To date, treatment algorithms have generally been extrapolated from those used in female breast cancer. The currently recommended surgical therapy for male patients is a modified radical mastectomy along with axillary lymph node dissection. Due to the morbidity associated with axillary dissection, sentinel node biopsy is becoming common practice in female breast cancer and sentinel node biopsy has also now been reported to have accurately predicted lymph node status in male breast cancer patients [72].

As in female breast cancer patients, in a small number of male patients, the addition of radiation decreased the incidence of local recurrence, but there was no difference in patient survival [73].

As in women, tamoxifen therapy for male breast cancer has shown a benefit of increasing disease free and overall survival. Riberio noted an increase in 5 year disease free survival from 28-55% in patients who received adjuvant tamoxifen for a year compared with controls [74].

In a study by Vinod et al, 67 % of patients who received tamoxifen remained free of relapse [75]. Studies have also showed that chemotherapy is beneficial. Bagley found 24 patients treated with CMF chemotherapy had a projected 5 year survival of greater than 80% [76].

There is conflicting data from studies of survival rates of male breast cancer patients. Data from the National Cancer Data Base reported that the survival rates are equivalent for stage 1 and 2 disease, but a trend for poorer survival for men with stage 3 and 4 disease has been noted. Overall survival rates for men with breast carcinoma stratified by stage of disease have been recorded to be lower than for women with breast carcinoma, but these differences may be due to older age distribution of male patients [3].

Conclusion

Male breast cancer remains a rare disease but its incidence has risen recently. There are many similarities between male and female breast cancer and most of the present management strategies have been extrapolated from studies involving female breast cancer.

More multi institutional studies need to be undertaken to advance our understanding of the risk factors, disease biology, prognostic factors, prognosis and optimal treatments.

References

[1] Perkins, H; Middleton, LP. Breast cancer in men. *BMJ* 2003; 327: 239-240.

[2] Iredale, R; Williams, B; Brain K. Breast Cancer in men: Group is exploring issues for men in the United Kingdom. *BMJ* 2003 327: 930-931.

[3] Giordano, SH; Cohen, DS; Buzdar, AU. et al. Breast Carcinoma in Men: *Cancer* 2004; 101:51-7.

[4] Giordano, SH; Buzdar, AU; Hortobagyi, GN. Breast Cancer in Men: *Ann. Int. Med.*; 2002;137:678-687.

[5] Kanhai; Robert, CJ; Hage, J et al. Short term and Long Term Histologic Effects of Castration and Estrogen Treatment on Breast Tissue of 14 Male to female Transsexuals in Comparison with Two Chemically Castrated Men. *The American Journal of Surgical Pathology*. 2000(24)1.

[6] Ravandi-Kashani, F; Hayes, TG Male Breast Cancer: A Review of the Literature. *European Journal of Cancer*. 1998 34(9) 1341-1347.

[7] Lanfranco, F; Kamischke, A; Zitzmann, M; Nieschlag, E. Klinefelter's syndrome. *Lancet*. 2004 Jul 17; 364(9430):273-83.

[8] Hultborn, R; Hanson, C; Kopf, I. Prevalence of Klinefelter's syndrome in male breast cancer patients: *Anticancer Res*. 1997 Nov-Dec; 17(6D):4293-7.

[9] Cocco, P; Figgs, L; Dosemeci, M et al. Case-control study of occupational exposures and male breast cancer. *Occupational and Environmental Medicine*. 1998(55) 599-604.

[10] Erlichman, C; Murphy, KC; Elhakim, T. Male breast cancer: A 13-year review of 89 patients. *J Clin Oncol* 1984 (2) 903-9.

[11] Borgen, PI; Wong, GY; Vlamis, V et al. Current management of male breast cancer: a review of 104 cases. *Ann. Surg.* 1992 (215) 451-9.

[12] Stalsberg, H; Thomas, DB; Rosenblatt, KA; Jimenez, LM; McTiernan, A; Stemhagen, A; Thompson, WD; Curnen, MG; Satariano, W; Austin DF. Histologic types and hormone receptors in breast cancer in men: a population-based study in 282 United States men. *Cancer Causes Control*. 1993 Mar;4(2):143-51.

[13] Hittmair, AP; Lininger, RA; Tavassoli, FA. Ductal Carcinoma in the Male Breast. *Cancer* 1998 Nov 83(10): 2139-49.

[14] Tumours of the male breast (1) 110-112 in Tavassoli, FA; Devilee P.(2003) WHO Classification of Tumours. Pathology and Genetics. *Tumours of the Breast and the Female Organs.*

[15] Sanchez, AG; Villaneuva, AG; Redondo, C. Lobular carcinoma of the breast in a patient with Kleinfelter's syndrome. A case with bilateral, synchronous, histologically different breast tumors. *Cancer* 1986: 57:1181-3.

[16] Schiedbach, H; Dworak, O; Schmucker, B et al. Lobular carcinoma of the breast in an 85-year-old man. *European Journal of Surgical Oncology* 1999.

[17] Michaels, BM; Nunn, CR; Roses, DF Lobular *Carcinoma of the male breast Surgery* 115:402-405.

[18] Acs, G; Lawton, TJ; Rebbeck, TR; LiVolsi, VA; Zhang, PJ. Differential expression of E-cadherin in lobular and ductal neoplasms of the breast and its biologic and diagnostic implications. *Am. J. Clin. Pathol.* 115:85-98.

[19] Willsher, PC; Leach, IH; Ellis, IO; Bell, JA; Elston, CW; Bourke, JB; Blamey RW, Robertson, JFR. Male Breast Cancer: Pathological and Immunohistochemical Features. *Anticancer Research* 17:2335-2338.

[20] Cutuli, B; Dilhuydy, JM; de la Fontan, B; Berlie, J; Lacroze, M; Lesaunier, F; Graic, Y; Tortochaux, J; Resbaut, M; Lesimple, T; Gamelin, E; Campana F, Reme-Saumon, M; Moncho-Bernier, V; Cuilliere, JC; Marchal, C; De Gislain, G; Nguyen TD, Teissier E, Velten M(1997). Ductal carcinoma in situ of the male breast. Analysis of 31 cases. *Eur. J. Cancer* 33:35-38.

[21] Evans, DB; Chichlow, RW. Carcinoma of the male breast and Kleinfelters syndrome: is there an association? CA: *A Cancer Journal For Clinicians* 1987 37(4); 246-251.

[22] Antoniou, P. D. P; Pharoah, S; Narod, H. Average Risks of Breast and Ovarian Cancer Associated with *BRCA1* or *BRCA2* Mutations Detected in Case Series Unselected for Family History: A Combined Analysis of 22 Studies. *The American Journal of Human Genetics*, volume 72 (2003), page 1117.

[23] Easton, DF; Steele, L; Fields, P; Ormiston, W; Averill, D et al. Cancer risks in two large breast cancer families linked to BRCA2 on chromosome 13q12-13 *Am. J. Hum. Genet* 1997; 61: 120-8.

[24] Kwiatkowska, E; Teresiak, M; Filas, V; Karczewska, A; Breborowicz, D; Mackiewicz A. BRCA2 mutations and androgen receptor expression as independent predictors of outcome of male breast cancer patients. *Clin. Cancer Res.* 2003 Oct 1; 9(12):4452-9.

[25] Rampaul, RS; Pinder, SE; Gullick, WJ et al. HER-2 in breast cancer-methods of detection, clinical significance and future prospects for treatment. *Critical reviews in Oncology/Haematology* 43 (2002) 231-244.

[26] Slamon, DJ; Clark, GM; Wong, SG; Levin, WJ; Ulrich, A; McGuire, WL Human breast cancer: correlation of relapse and survival with amplification of the HER-2/neu oncogene. *Science* 1987;235:177-82.

[27] Rudlowski, C; Friedrichs, N; Faridi, A; Fuzesi, L; Moll, R; Bastert, G; Rathg Buttner R. HER-2/neu gene amplification and protein expression in primary male breast cancer. *Breast Cancer Research and Treatment* 84: 215-233, 2004.

[28] Rayson, D; Erlichman, C; Suman, VJ. Molecular markers in male breast carcinoma. *Cancer.* 1998 Nov 1;83(9):1947-55.

[29] Blin, N; Kardas, I; Welter, C et al: Expression of the c-erbB-2 proto-oncogene in male breast carcinomas: lack of prognostic significance. *Oncology* 50:408–411, 1993.

[30] Payne, S; Bruce, DM; Heys, SD et al: Prognostic parameters in male breast cancer. *J. Pathol.* 175s:143, 1994 (abstr).

[31] Bruce, DM; Heys, SD; Payne, S et al: Male breast cancer: Clinico-pathological features, immunocytochemical characteristics and prognosis. *Eur. J. Surg. Cancer* 22:42–46, 1996.

[32] Wang-Rodriguez, J; Cross, K; Gallagher, S; Djahanban, M; Armstrong, JM; Wiedner, N; Shapiro, DH. Male breast carcinoma: correlation of ER, PR, Ki-67, Her2-Neu, and p53 with treatment and survival, a study of 65 cases. *Mod. Pathol.* 2002 Aug;15(8):853-61.

[33] Mourao Netto, M; Logullo, AF; Nonogaki, S; Brentani, RR; Brentani, MM.Expression of c-erbB-2, p53 and c-myc proteins in male breast carcinoma: Comparison with traditional prognostic factors and survival. *Braz. J. Med. Biol. Res.* 2001 Jul; 34(7):887-94.

[34] Joshi, MG; Lee, AK; Loda, M; Camus, MG; Pedersen, C; Heatley, GJ; Hughes, KS. Male breast carcinoma: an evaluation of prognostic factors contributing to a poorer outcome. *Cancer.* 1996 Feb 1;77(3):490-8.

[35] Pich, A; Margaria, E; Chiusa, L. Oncogenes and male breast carcinoma: c-erbB-2 and p53 coexpression predicts a poor survival. *J. Clin. Oncol.* 2000 Aug;18(16):2948-56.

[36] Hockenbery, D; Nunez, G; Milliman, C; Schreiber, RD; Korsmeyer, SJ. Bcl-2 is an inner mitochondrial membrane protein that blocks programmed cell death. *Nature.* 1990 Nov 22;348(6299):334-6.

[37] Alsabeh, R; Wilson, CS; Ahn, CW; Vasef, MA; Battifora, H. Expression of bcl-2 by breast cancer: a possible diagnostic application. *Mod. Pathol.* 1996 Apr;9(4):439-44.

[38] Bargmann, CI; Hung, M-C; Weinberg, RA: The neu oncogene encodes an epidermal growth factor receptor-related protein. *Nature* 319: 226-230.

[39] Bhargava, V; Thor, A; Deng, G et al: The association of p53 immunopositivity with tumour proliferation and other indicators in breast cancer. *Modern Pathol.* 7: 361-368, 1994 (Abstract).

[40] Locker, AP; Dowle, CS; Ellis, IO et al: c-myc oncogene product expression and prognosis in operable breast cancer. *Br. J. Cancer* 60:669-672, 1989.
[41] Idelevich, E Mozes, M; Ben-Baruch, N; Huszar, M; Kruglikova, A; Katsnelson, R; Shani A. Oncogenes in male breast cancer. *Am. J. Clin. Oncol.* 2003 Jun;26(3):259-61.
[42] Muir, D; Kanthan, R; Kanthan, SC. Male versus female breast cancers. A population-based comparative immunohistochemical analysis. *Arch. Pathol. Lab. Med.* 2003 Jan;127(1):36-41.
[43] Pich, A; Margaria, E; Chiusa, L. Bcl-2 expression in male breast carcinoma. *Virchows Arch.* 1998 Sep;433(3):229-35.
[44] Temmim, L; Luqmani, YA; Jarallah, M; Juma, I; Mathew, M. Evaluation of prognostic factors in male breast cancer. *Breast*. 2001 Apr;10(2):166-75.
[45] Sutherland, RL; Musgrove, EA. Cyclins and breast cancer. *J. Mammary Gland. Biol. Neoplasia*. 2004 Jan;9(1):95-104.
[46] Barnes, DM; Gillett, CE. Cyclin D1 in breast cancer. *Breast Cancer Res Treat.* 1998;52(1-3):1-15.
[47] Barlund, M; Kuukasjarvi, T; Syrjakoski, K; Auvinen, A; Kallioniemi A. Frequent amplification and overexpression of CCND1 in male breast cancer. *Int. J. Cancer.* 2004 Oct 10; 111(6):968-71.
[48] Arber, N; Hibshoosh, H; Zhang, Y; Han, E; Sgambato, A; Weinstein I. Overexpression of cyclin D1 in both female and male breast cancers [Abstract]. *Proc. Annu. Meet Am. Assoc. Cancer Res.* 1995;36:1350-1350.
[49] Teller, MN; Stock, CC; Stohr, G; Merker, PC; Kaufman, RJ; Escher, GC; Bowie, M. Biologic characteristics and chemotherapy of 7,12-dimethylbenz[a]anthracene-induced tumors in rats. *Cancer Res*. 1966 Feb;26(2):245-52.
[50] Poulin, R; Baker, D; Labrie F. Androgens inhibit basal and estrogen-induced cell proliferation in the ZR-75-1 human breast cancer cell line. *Breast Cancer Res. Treat.* 1988 Oct;12(2):213-25.
[51] Allegra, JC; Lippman, ME; Thompson, EB; Simon, R; Barlock, A; Green, L; Huff, KK; Do, HM; Aitken, SC. Distribution, frequency, and quantitative analysis of estrogen, progesterone, androgen, and glucocorticoid receptors in human breast cancer. *Cancer Res.* 1979 May;39(5):1447-54.
[52] Langer, M; Kubista, E; Schemper, M; Spona J. Androgen receptors, serum androgen levels and survival of breast cancer patients. *Arch. Gynecol. Obstet*. 1990;247(4):203-9.
[53] Miller, WR; Telford, J; Dixon, JM; Hawkins, RA. Androgen receptor activity in human breast cancer and its relationship with oestrogen and progestogen receptor activity. *Eur J. Cancer Clin. Oncol.* 1985 Apr;21(4):539-42.
[54] Bryan, RM; Mercer, RJ; Bennett, RC; Rennie, GC; Lie, TH; Morgan, F Androgen receptors in breast cancer. *Cancer.* 1984 Dec 1;54(11):2436-40.
[55] Birrell, SN; Roder, DM; Horsfall, DJ; Bentel, JM; Tilley WD. Medroxyprogesterone acetate therapy in advanced breast cancer: the predictive value of androgen receptor expression. *J. Clin. Oncol.* 1995 Jul;13(7):1572-7.
[56] Kuenen-Boumeester, V; Van der Kwast, TH; Claassen, CC; Look, MP; Liem, GS; Klijn, JG; Henzen-Logmans, SC. The clinical significance of androgen receptors in

breast cancer and their relation to histological and cell biological parameters. *Eur. J. Cancer.* 1996 Aug;32A(9):1560-5.

[57] Nomura, Y; Yamagata, J; Takenaka, K; Tashiro, H. Steroid hormone receptors nd clinical usefulness in human breast cancer. *Cancer*. 1980 Dec 15;46(12 Suppl):2880-3.

[58] Calandra, RS; Charreau, EH; Royer de Giaroli, M; Baldi, A. Incidence of estrogen, progesterone and prolactin receptors in human breast cancer. *Prog. Clin. Biol. Res.* 1984;142:97-108.

[59] Mercer, RJ; Bryan, RM; Bennett, RC. Hormone receptors in male breast cancer. *Aust. NZ J. Surg*. 1984 Jun;54(3):215-8.

[60] Pacheco, MM; Oshima, CF; Lopes, MP; Widman, A; Franco, EL; Brentani, MM. Steroid hormone receptors in male breast diseases. *Anticancer Res*. 1986 Sep-Oct;6(5):1013-7.

[61] Sasano, H; Kimura, M; Shizawa, S; Kimura, N; Nagura, H. Aromatase and steroid receptors in gynecomastia and male breast carcinoma: an immunohistochemical study. *J. Clin. Endocrinol. Metab*. 1996 Aug;81(8):3063-7.

[62] Soreide, JA; Lea, OA; Varhaug, JE; Skarstein, A; Kvinnsland, S. Androgen receptors in operable breast cancer: relation to other steroid hormone receptors, correlations to prognostic factors and predictive value for effect of adjuvant tamoxifen treatment. *Eur. J. Surg. Oncol.* 1992 Apr;18(2):112-8.

[63] Pich, A; Margaria, E; Chiusa, L; Candelaresi, G; Dal Canton, O. Androgen receptor expression in male breast carcinoma: lack of clinicopathological association. *Br. J. Cancer*. 1999 Feb;79(5-6):959-64.

[64] Kidwai, N; Gong, Y; Sun, X; Deshpande, CG; Yeldandi, AV; Rao, MS; Badve S. Expression of androgen receptor and prostate-specific antigen in male breast carcinoma. *Breast Cancer Res*. 2004;6(1):R18-23. Epub 2003 Nov. 07.

[65] Munoz de Toro, MM; Maffini, MV; Kass, L; Luque, EH. Proliferative activity and steroid hormone receptor status in male breast carcinoma. *J. Steroid. Biochem. Mol. Biol.* 1998 Nov;67(4):333-9.

[66] Stalsberg, H; Thomas, DB; Rosenblatt, KA; Jimenez, LM; McTiernan, A; Stemhagen, A; Thompson, WD; Curnen, MG; Satariano, W; Austin, DF. Histologic types and hormone receptors in breast cancer in men: a population-based study in 282 United States men. *Cancer Causes Control*. 1993 Mar;4(2):143-51.

[67] Donegan, WL; Redlich, PN; Lang, PJ; Gall, MT. Carcinoma of the breast in males: A multiinstitutional survey. *Cancer*. 1998 Aug 1;83(3):498-509.

[68] Willsher, PC; Leach, IH; Ellis, IO; Bourke, JB; Blamey, RW; Robertson, JFR. A comparison outcome of male breast cancer with female breast cancer. *Am. J. Surg.* 1997 Mar;173(3):185-8.

[69] Herman, K; Lobaziewicz, W; Skotnicki, P; Fortuna, J; Kusy, T; Lesniak. Male Breast cancer. Does the prognosis differ compared to female? *Neoplasma*. 2000;47(3):191-5.

[70] Vetto, J; Jun, SY; Paduch, D; Eppich, H; Shih, R. Stages at presentation, prognostic factors, and outcome of breast cancer in males. *Am. J. Surg*. 1999 May; 177(5):379-83.

[71] Rudan, I; Rudan, N; Basic, N; Basic, V; Rudan, D; Jambrisak, Z. Differences between male and female breast cancer. III. Prognostic features. *Acta Med. Croatica.* 1997;51(3):135-41.

[72] Goyal, A; Horgan, K; Kissin, M; Yiangou, C; Sibbering, M; Lansdown, M; Newcombe, RG; Mansel, RE; Chetty, U; Ell, P; Fallowfield, L. Sentinel lymph node biopsy in male breast cancer patients. *Eur. J. Surg. Oncol.* 2004 Jun;30(5):480-3.

[73] Erlichman, C; Murphy, KC; Elhakim, T. Male breast cancer: A 13 year reviw of 89 patients. *J. Clinical Oncol.* 1984;(2): 903-9.

[74] Ribeiro, G; Swindell, R. Adjuvant tamoxifen for male breast cancer (MBC). *Br. J. Cancer*. 1992;(65):252-4.

[75] Vinod, SK; Pendlebury, SC. Carcinoma of the male breast: A review of adjuvant therapy. *Australas Radiol.* 1999 Feb;43(1):69-72.

[76] Bagley, CS; Wesley, MN; Young, RC; Lippman ME. Adjuvant chemotherapy in males with cancer of the breast. *Am. J. Clin. Oncol.* 1987 Feb;10(1):55-60.

[77] Couch, FJ; Farid, LM; DeShano, ML; Tavtigian, SV; Calzone, K; Campeau, L; Peng, Y; Bogden, B; Chen, Q; Neuhausen, S; Shattuck-Eidens, D; Godwin AK; Daly, M; Radford, DM; Sedlacek, S; Rommens, J; Simard, J; Garber, J; Merajver, S; Weber, BL. BRCA2 germline mutations in male breast cancer cases and breast cancer families. *Nat. Genet.* 1996 May;13(1):123-5.

[78] Friedman, LS; Gayther, SA; Kurosaki, T; Gordon, D; Noble, B; Casey, G; Ponder, BA; Anton-Culver, H. Mutation analysis of BRCA1 and BRCA2 in a male breast cancer population. *Am. J. Hum. Genet.* 1997 Feb;60(2):313-9.

[79] Mavraki, E; Gray, IC; Bishop, DT; Spurr, NK. BRCA2 germline mutations in male breast cancer cases and breast cancer families. *Br. J. Cancer.*1997;76(11):1428-31.

[80] Haraldsson, K; Loman, N; Zhang, QX; Johannsson, O; Olsson, H; Borg, A. BRCA2 germ-line mutations are frequent in male breast cancer patients without a family history of the disease. *Cancer Res.* 1998 Apr 1;58(7):1367-71.

[81] Csokay, B; Udvarhelyi, N; Sulyok, Z; Besznyak, I; Ramus, S; Ponder, B; Olah, E. High frequency of germ-line BRCA2 mutations among Hungarian male breast cancer patients without family history. *Cancer Res.* 1999 Mar 1;59(5):995-8.

[82] Sverdlov, RS; Barshack, I; Bar Sade, RB; Baruch, RG; Hirsh-Yehezkel, G; Dagan, E; Feinmesser, M; Figer, A; Friedman, E. Genetic analyses of male breast cancer in Israel. *Genet Test.* 2000;4(3):313-7.

[83] Kwiatkowska, E; Teresiak, M; Lamperska, KM; Karczewska, A; Breborowicz, D; Stawicka, M; Godlewski, D; Krzyzosiak, WJ; Mackiewicz, A. BRCA2 germline mutations in male breast cancer patients in the Polish population. *Hum. Mutat.* 2001;17(1):73.

[84] Kwiatkowska, E; Teresiak, M; Breborowicz, D; Mackiewicz, A. Somatic mutations in the BRCA2 gene and high frequency of allelic loss of BRCA2 in sporadic male breast cancer. *Int. J. Cancer*. 2002 Apr 20;98(6):943-5.

[85] Wolpert, N; Warner, E; Seminsky, MF; Futreal, A; Narod, SA. Prevalence of BRCA1 and BRCA2 mutations in male breast cancer patients in Canada. *Clin. Breast Cancer.* 2000 Apr;1(1):57-63; discussion 64-5.

[86] Basham, VM; Lipscombe, JM; Ward, JM; Gayther, SA; Ponder, BA; Easton, DF; Pharoah, PD. BRCA1 and BRCA2 mutations in a population-based study of male breast cancer. *Breast Cancer Res.* 2002;4(1):R2. Epub 2001 Nov 21.

[87] Ottini, L; Masala, G; D'Amico, C; Mancini, B; Saieva, C; Aceto, G; Gestri, D; Vezzosi, V; Falchetti, M; De Marco, M; Paglierani, M; Cama, A; Bianchi, S; Mariani-Costantini, R; Palli, D. BRCA1 and BRCA2 mutation status and tumor characteristics in male breast cancer: a population-based study in Italy. *Cancer Res.* 2003 Jan 15;63(2):342-7.

[88] Tirkkonen, M; Kainu, T; Loman, N; Johannsson, OT; Olsson, H; Barkardottir, RB; Kallioniemi, OP; Borg, A. Somatic genetic alterations in BRCA2-associated and sporadic male breast cancer. *Genes Chromosomes Cancer.* 1999 Jan;24(1):56-61.

[89] Andre, S; Fonseca, I; Pinto, AE et al. Male Breast Cancer- A reappraisal of clinical and biologic indicators of prognosis. *Acta Oncol.* 2001; 40(4):472-8.

[90] Shiptz, B; Bomstein, Y; Sternberg, A et al. Angiogenesis, p53, and c-erbB-2 immunoreactivity and clinicopathological features in male breast cancer. *J. Surg. Oncol.* 2000 Dec; 75(4):252-7.

[91] Clark, JL; Nguygen, PL; Jaszcz, WB, et al. Prognostic Variables in male breast cancer. *Am. Surg.* 2000 May; 66(5):502-11.

[92] Bloom, KJ; Govil, H; Gatusso, P et al. Status of HER-2 in male and female breast carcinoma. *Am. J. Surg.* 2001 Oct;182(4):389-92.

[93] Anelli, A; Anelli, TFM, Youngson, B; Rosen, PP; Borgen, PI. Mutations of the p53 gene in male breast cancer. *Cancer* 1995; 75: 2233-8.

[94] Fox, SB; Rogers, S; Day, CA; Underwood, JC. Oestrogen receptor and epidermal growth factor receptor expression in male breast carcinoma. *Journal of Pathology* 1992 Jan;166(1):13-8.

[95] Chung, HC; Kim, DL; Koh, EH; Kim, JH; Roh, JK; Min, JS; Lee, KS; Yang, WI; Kim, BS; Lee, KB. Expression of prognostic factors (EGFR, ER) by immunohistochemical staining method in male breast cancer. *Yonsei Med. J.* 1991 Jun; 32(2):126-30.

[96] Takeuchi, H; Shirasaka, C; Tsuji, K; Ueo, H. Clinicopathological study of Japanese male breast carcinoma. *Breast Cancer.* 2003; 10(3):249-53.

[97] Williams, WL Jr; Powers, M; Wagman, LD. Cancer of the male breast: a review. *J. Natl. Med. Assoc.* 1996 Jul; 88(7):439-43.

[98] Cutuli, B; Lacroze, M; Dilhuydy, JM et al. Male breast cancer: results of the treatments and prognostic factors in 397 cases. *Eur. J. Cancer.* 1995 Nov; 31A (12):1960-4.

[99] Morimoto, T; Komaki, K; Yamakawa, T; Tanaka, T; Oomine, Y; Konishi, Y; Mori, T; Monden, Y. Cancer of the male breast. *J. Surg. Oncol.* 1990 Jul; 44(3):180-4.

[100] Goss, PE; Reid, C; Pintilie, M; Lim, R; Miller, N. Male breast carcinoma: a review of 229 patients who presented to the Princess Margaret Hospital during 40 years: 1955-1996. *Cancer.* 1999 Feb 1; 85(3):629-39.

[101] Tan, PH; Sng, IT. Male breast cancer: a retrospective study with immunohistochemical analysis of hormone receptor expression. *Pathology.* 1997 Feb; 29(1):2-6.

[102] Sasano, H; Kimura, M; Shizawa, S; Kimura, N; Nagura, H. Aromatase and steroid receptors in gynecomastia and male breast carcinoma: an immunohistochemical study. *J. Clin. Endocrinol. Metab.*1996 Aug;81(8):3063-7.

[103] Borgen, PI; Senie, RT; McKinnon, WM; Rosen, PP. Carcinoma of the malebreast: analysis of prognosis compared with matched female patients. *Ann. Surg. Oncol.* 1997 Jul-Aug; 4(5):385-8.

[104] Dawson, PJ; Schroer, KR; Wolman, SR. ras and p53 genes in male breast cancer. *Mod. Pathol.* 1996 Apr;9(4):367-70.

In: Frontiers in Breast Cancer Research
Editor: Louis P. Fortugno, pp. 157-173

ISBN: 978-1-60021-671-8

Chapter VII

Detection of HER-2/Neu Status by Immunohistochemistry and Fluorescence *In Situ* Hybridization in Breast Cancer

A. Skalova[1, 3,*], T. Vanecek[2], Z. Kinkor[3] and M. Michal[1]

[1]Department of Pathology, Medical Faculty, Charles University, Plzen, Czech Republic
[2]Molecular and Genetic Laboratory, Department of Pathology, Medical Faculty Hospital, Plzen, Czech Republic
[3]Private Histopathology and Cytology Laboratory, Plzen, Czech Republic

Abstract

Introduction: HER-2/neu protein is overexpressed in 15-20% of invasive breast carcinomas and has been reported to be an independently adverse prognostic and predictive factor in patients with breast cancer. Recently, HER-2/neu overexpression has gained therapeutic implications, because the use of trastuzumab/Herceptin™, recombinant humanized monoclonal antibody directed against extracellular domain of HER-2/neu molecule, has been shown to result in clinical response in patients with breast cancer overexpressing HER-2/neu.

Aims: As a result of these developments, there has been increasing demand for pathologists to perform exact evaluation of HER-2/neu in breast cancer specimens.

Methods and Results: In our series of 449 cases of breast cancer we have examined HER-2/neu protein and gene by means of immunohistochemistry and fluorescence in situ hybridization, respectively. The results of HER-2/neu study were compared with hormonal status, cancer grade and proliferative activity as assessed using immunohistochemistry with MIB1 antibody. Of these 449 cases 18 randomly chosen samples were examined for HER2/neu gene status. All 7 cases of breast cancer with

* Correspondence concerning this article should be addressed to Dr. Alena Skálová, Šikl's Department of Pathology, Medical Faculty Hospital, dr. E. Beneše 13, 305 99 Plzeň, Czech Republic. Fax: +420-37-7421561; Tel: +420-37-7402545; e-mail: skalova@fnplzen.cz.

strong overexpression of HER-2/neu (score 3+) revealed an amplification of the gene. In contrast, among 11 cases of breast cancers with mild HER-2/neu overexpression (score 2+), the gene amplification was demonstrated in 5 cases (45%).

Conclusions: Good concordance was achieved between immunohistochmistry in negative and strongly positive cases (score 3+). Immunohistochemical assessment and fluorescence in situ hybridization (FISH) are complementary methods for detection of HER-2/neu status in breast cancer. While immunohistochemistry is excellent screening method, FISH should be used for confirmation of positive result of HER-2/neu status analysis before Herceptin treatment.

Keywords: *breast cancer, HER-2/neu gene, oncoprotein cerbB2, immunohistochemistry, FISH.*

Introduction

Breast cancer is the most common type of cancer in women. As in other human tumors, multiple genetic changes have been identified in breast carcinomas that might be involved in uncontrolled tumor cell growth [1-2]. Among other genes, the human epidermal growth factor receptor-2 (also known as the HER-2/neu or c-erbB-2 gene) is one of the genes involved in human breast cancer [3].

The human HER-2/neu gene, present on chromosome 17q11, encodes a 185-kDa transmembrane glycoprotein with tyrosine kinase activity closely related to epidermal growth factor receptor [4]. The HER-2/neu protein is expressed normally at low levels in a variety of epithelial cells including breast duct epithelium, and has an importat role in normal cellular proliferation [5]. HER-2/neu protein overexpression most commonly results from gene amplification [6].

HER-2/neu gene amplification is seen in about 15 to 20% of invasive breast carcinomas [6]. HER-2/neu expression has gained increasing importance as an independent adverse prognostic indicator in clinical management of patients with breast cancer. Most studies indicated that HER-2/neu gene amplification and protein overexpression are associated with aggressive clinical course of breast cancer [7]. Recent clinical studies have also implicated HER-2/neu overexpression as a predictive marker of resistance to chemotherapy [8]. Breast carcinomas that overexpress HER-2/neu protein have been found to show resistance to drugs, such as cyclophosphamide, methotrexate, and tamoxifen and increased sensitivity to others, such as doxorubicin and paclitaxel [9-10].

The advent of Trastuzumab (Herceptin™, Genentech, San Francisco, CA, USA) treatment for invasive ductal breast cancer has increased interest in assessment of HER-2 status. Trastuzumab, a humanized monoclonal antibody to HER-2 protein, binds directly to the extracellular domain of the HER-2/neu protein preventing interaction of the receptor with growth-stimulatory signals [11-12]. This therapy specifically targets HER-2 over-expressing tumor cells. As immunohistochemistry (IHC) assesses the level HER-2/neu protein over-expression, it is expected to represent the best method of determination of HER-2/neu status in this setting. However, IHC for HER-2/neu analysis has been criticized because of lack of standardization and poor reproducibility in interpretation of the results as numerous immunohistochemical methods with different antibodies to HER-2/neu molecule are used. HercepTest was proposed as a standardized IHC method, approved by Food and Drug Administration (FDA), capable of overcoming these problems. However, several recent studies have demonstrated the excessive sensitivity of this kit [13-15].

Recently, HER-2-FISH status was found to be more predictive of clinical response to trastuzumab than IHC alone and was therefore proposed as the best method to select the patients that would benefit from Herceptin therapy [13,16-17], even though gene amplification is not a direct target of anti-HER-2 therapy. However, FISH is more expensive and more time consuming than IHC. This sophisticated procedure also requires highly trained laboratory personnel, and moreover not all problems regarding FISH standardization and interpretation were solved [18].

For this purpose, we examined in our series of 449 cases of breast cancer HER-2/neu protein over-expression and gene amplification by means of immunohistochemistry and fluorescence in situ hybridization, respectively. The results of HER-2/neu study were compared with hormonal status, cancer grade and proliferative activity as assessed using immunohistochemistry with MIB1 antibody.

Materials and Methods

Patients

A total of 449 patients diagnosed with breast cancer who underwent diagnostic curative surgery within six months period (January-June 2001) were included in the study. For all patients, information was recorded at diagnosis about family history of breast cancer, age, menopausal status, histologic type of tumor, tumor size, nodal status, tumor grade, disease stage, proliferative activity, and estrogen/progesterone receptor levels.

The mean age of patients at diagnosis was 63 (range 32 to 89 years). All patients were women, 20 % were premenopausal. Histologically, most tumors, 370 cases (82%) were infiltrating ductal carcinomas, 37 cases (8%) were infiltrating lobular carcinomas, the remaining cases included 6 cases (2%) of ductal in situ carcinoma,14 cases (3%) of medullary carcinoma, 9 cases of mucinous carcinoma (2%). The remaining 9 cases (2%) represent rare variants (see Table 1).

Immunohistochemistry, Including HER-2/neu Protein Expression

The formalin-fixed, paraffin-embedded tissues were processed routinely and stained with hematoxylin and eosin. For immunohistochemical studies, 4-μm-thick sections were cut from paraffin blocks, mounted on slides coated with 3-aminopropyltriethoxy-silane (Sigma, St. Louis, MO), deparaffinized in xylene, and rehydrated in descending grades (100% to 70%) of ethanol. Sections were then subjected to heat-induced epitope retrieval by immersion in a 0.01 mol/l concentration of citrate buffer (pH 6.0) in microwave oven Micromed TTmega for

40 minutes. Endogenous peroxidase was blocked by a 5-minute treatment with 3% hydrogen peroxidase in absolute methanol. The slides were incubated in an autostainer LabVision for 60 minutes at room temperature with primary antibodies (Table 2).

Table 1. Characteristics of Tumors in the Study

Histological Type	Grade	Number of Cases	%
Ductal infiltrating	Grade 1	149	33
	Grade 2	164	36
	Grade 3	57	13
	TOTAL	370	82
Tubular		4	1
Lobular infiltrating		37	8
Medullary		14	3
Mucinous		9	2
Ductal carcinoma in situ (DCIS)	Grade 1	3	1
	Grade 2	0	
	Grade 3	3	1
Others***		9	2
TOTAL		449	100

*** non-invasive papillary carcinoma (2 cases), invasive papillary carcinoma (2 cases), myoepithelial, metaplastic, Paget carcinoma of the nipple associated with DCIS grade 3, mucoepidermoid carcinoma, solid noninvasive papillary carcinoma (one case each).

Table 2. Antibodies Used for Immunohistochemistry

Antibody	Clone	Dilution	Source
HercepTest			DakoCytomation A/S, Glostrup, Denmark
Ki67	MIB1	1:500	DakoCytomation, A/S, Glostrup
anti-HER-2/neu Ab17	clone e2-4001 and 3B5	1:2000	NeoMarker(BioTech), Fremont, Ca
anti-HER-2/neu NCL-HER-356	clone 10 A7	1:150	Novocastra, Newcastle/Tyne, Great Britain

The bound antibodies were visualized using the supersensitive streptavidin-biotin-peroxidase complex (Novocastra, Newcastle upon Tyne, UK) and 3-3´-diaminobenzidine (Sigma) as chromogen. The slides were counterstained with Mayer´s hematoxylin.

Similar sections were stained for HER-2/neu according to instructions of the manufacturer using the reagents included in the HercepTest kit. The primary antibody included in the kit was polyclonal, raised in rabbits, and provided in a prediluted form. For each run, a composite slide of 3 formalin-fixed human breast carcinoma cell lines representing different HER-2/neu protein expression levels (MDA-231 for score 0, MDA-175 for score 1+, and SKBR3 for score 3+) were used as controls. In addition, for each case, one slide was incubated with normal rabbit serum instead of the primary antibody and used as negative control. An EnVision™ system included in the HercepTest was used to detect positive immunoreaction.

IHC Interpretation

The immunohistochemical preparations were interpreted following the criteria recommended by DAKO for the HercepTest (Table 3.). Overexpression of HER-2/neu was defined as positive membrane staining in more than 10% of the neoplastic cells. Partial or incomplete, weak to moderate, and moderate to strong membrane staining in more than 10% of the tumor cells was scored as 1+ (negative), 2+ (weakly positive), and 3+ (strongly positive), respectively.

Table 3. Scoring System for Assessment of Immunohistochemical Overexpression of HER-2/neu Protein

Colour Reaction	Score	HER-2/neu Protein Overexpression Assessment
No staining is observed, or membrane staining in less than 10% of the tumor cells	0	Negative
A faint/barely perceptible membrane staining is detected in more than 10% of the tumor cells The cells are only stained in part of the membrane	1+	Negative
A weak to moderate complete membrane staining is observed in more than 10% of the tumor cells	2+	Weakly positive
A strong complete membrane staining is observed in more than 10% of the tumor cells	3+	Strongly positive

FISH for HER-2/neu Gene Amplification

FISH analysis of HER-2/neu gene was performed using the PathVysion™ HER-2/neu DNA probe kit (VYSIS/Abbott, IL, USA) or the Oncor/Ventana INFORM® HER-2/neu Gene Detection System S8000-KIT (Ventana Medical Systems, Frankfurt, Germany).

Slide Preparation and Pretreatment

An appropriate formalin fixed paraffin embedded tissue block was selected in each case by pathologist, cut into 4 μm thick section, and placed on silanized or positively charged slide (Menzel-Glaser, Braunschweig, Germany). The slide was baked overnight at 65 ^{0}C. After that, routine deparaffinization was carried out, and slide was treated by 30% sodium bisulphite for 30 minutes at 42^{0}C followed by digestion in 2x Sodium Salt Citrate (2xSSC)/proteinase K (0.25 mg/ml) solution for 45 to 60 minutes at 42^{0}C. Then, the slide was immersed in H_2O and in 2xSSC each for 2 minutes at room temperature. Finally, slide was dehydrated in 70%, 85% and 100% ethanol series, each for 2 minutes at room temperature and air dryed.

FISH Using PathVysion™ HER-2/neu DNA Probe Kit

An amount of 4-15 μl of directly labelled LSI HER-2/neu SpectrumOrange™/CEP 17 SpectrumGreen™ probe mix was applied on specimens, covered with the coverslip, sealed and co-denatured simultaneously for 8 minutes at 75^{0}C. After the hybridization overnight in a humidified chamber at 37^{0}C, the coverslip was carefully removed and slide was washed for two minutes in Post-Hybridization Wash Buffer (2xSSC/0.3% NP-40 (pH 7.0 – 7.5)) at 72^{0}C. The slide was then air-dried in the dark, counterstained with DAPI in an antifade medium, and either immediately examined or kept at -20^{0}C in the dark before examination.

FISH Interpretation

The sections were examined with an Olympus BX60 fluorescence microscope using a 100x objective and filter sets DAPI and Triple Band Pass (DAPI/FITC/Texas Red). Scoring of amplification was performed by counting the ratio between the number of both fluorescent signals (HER-2/neu:CEP17) in 60 randomly selected non-overlapping cancer nuclei. Each slide was independently enumerated by two observers (AS and TV). Tumors with a ratio of signals < 2 as a mean per nucleus were interpreted as non-amplified, whereas cases exhibiting a ratio of signals ≥ 2 as a mean were classified as amplified ones. The samples with ratio 1.8 - 2.0 were considered as suspicious for amplification and were interpreted with care.

FISH Using INFORM® HER-2/neu Gene Detection System

Dryed slide was denatured in 70 % formamide/2xSSC (pH 7.0) for 8 minutes at 75 ^{0}C and dehydrated in ice cold 70%, 85% and 100% ethanol series each for 2 minutes. After the air drying, 4-10μl of biotinylated HER-2/neu probe prewarmed at 37^{0}C for 5 minutes was applied on specimen, covered with coverslip, sealed and hybridized overnight in humidified chamber at 37 ^{0}C. Then, the slide was immersed twice for 2 minutes in 2xSSC and washed in Post-Hybridization Wash Solution (50% formamide/2xSSC (pH 7.0)) at 43^{0}C for 15 minutes followed by incubation in 2xSSC at 43^{0}C for 10 minutes. After that, the HER-2/neu probe was visualised by fluorescein-labeled avidin solution, and the signal was amplified by successive incubations with anti-avidin antibody. The slide was counterstained with DAPI in an antifade medium, and was immediately examined or kept at -20^{0}C in the dark before examination.

FISH Interpretation

The sections were examined with Olympus BX60 fluorescence microscope using filter sets DAPI and Triple Band Pass (DAPI/FITC/Texas Red). Scoring was performed by counting the number of fluorescent signals twice in 60 randomly selected non-overlapping cancer cell nuclei. A technologist (TV) and pathologist (AS) independently enumerated each case. Tumours with ≤ 4 mean signals per nucleus were interpreted as nonamplified, whereas cases exhibiting >4 signals as a mean were classified as amplified ones.

Results

Tables 4 and 5 summarize the immunohistochemical results of HER-2/neu over-expression grouped by tumor type, grade and hormonal status, respectively. Seventy-six (17%) of the cases showed strong overexpression (score 3+) of HER-2/neu protein by immunohistochemistry (Figure 1). Thirty-six (8%) of the cases were mildly positive (score 2+), and no significant staining for HER-2/neu was seen in 337 cases (75%).

Table 4. HER-2/neu Overexpression in Different Types of Breast Carcinoma

Histologic type	Grade	HER-2/neu Positive 3+	HER-2/neu Positive 2+	HER-2/neu Negative 0/1+	Total
Ductal infiltrating	Grade 1	13	10	126	149
	Grade 2	36	18	110	164
	Grade 3	18	6	33	57
Total		67	34	269	370
Tubular		1	0	3	4
Lobular infiltrative		3	1	33	37
Medullary		0	0	14	14
Mucinous		1	0	8	9
Ductal in situ DCIS	Grade 1	0	0	3	3
	Grade 2	0	0	0	0
	Grade 3	3	0	0	3
Total		3	0	3	6
Others***		1	1	7	9
Total		76	36	337	449

*** non-invasive papillary carcinoma (2 cases), invasive papillary carcinoma (2 cases), myoepithelial, metaplastic, Paget carcinoma of the nipple associated with DCIS grade 3, mucoepidermoid carcinoma, solid noninvasive papillary carcinoma (one case each).

In the group of ductal invasive carcinomas, the total number of which were 370 cases, there were 101 patients (27%) with HER-2/neu overexpression (score 3+ or 2+). The highest percentage of HER-2/neu positive cases was among poorly differentiated ductal invasive carcinomas (grade 3). Within the group of grade 3 ductal invasive carcinomas, the HER-2/neu positive cases (score 2+ and 3+) represent 42%. In contrast, only 15% of well differentiated ductal invasive carcinomas (grade 1) over-expressed the HER-2/neu protein (see Table 4).

There were 37 cases of lobular invasive carcinoma in our series, among them 3 cases displayed immunohistochemically strong overexpression of HER-2/neu with score 3+. In one such case, the tumor represented a combined ductal/lobular invasive carcinoma, and in two cases the tumors were diagnosed as pleomorphic variant of invasive lobular carcinoma. Still other poorly differentiated clear cell lobular invasive carcinoma demonstrated mild overexpression of HER-2/neu (score 2+). The remaining thirty three cases of lobular invasive carcinoma were negative for HER-2/neu. All fourteen cases of medullary carcinoma of the breast were consistently ngative for HER-2/neu.

Table 5. Comparison of HER-2/neu Overexpression and Hormonal Status in Breast Carcinoma

Hormonal status	HER-2/neu positive 3+		HER-2/neu positive 2+		HER-2/neu Negative 0/1+	
	Number of cases	%	Number of cases	%	Number of cases	%
ER+/PR+	32	42	22	61	242	72
ER+/PR-	10	13	5	14	28	8
ER-/PR+	4	5	0	0	7	2
ER-/PR-	30	40	9	25	60	18
Total	76	100	36	100	337	100

ER – estrogen receptor.
PR – progesterone receptor.

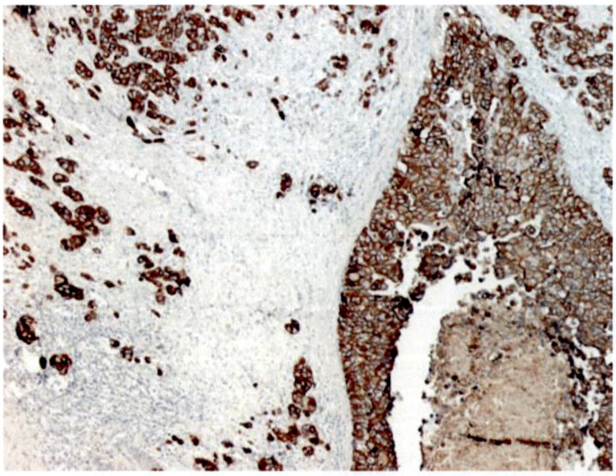

Figure 1. Immunohistochemical analysis of HER-2/neu protein in invasive ductal carcinoma: strong membrane staining showing overexpression (score 3+).

Histologically, six tumors were pure ductal non-invasive carcinomas (in situ) (Table 4). Three tumors revealed well-differentiated features as monomorphic tumor cells with uniform size nuclei, fine chromatin, and marked cell polarization. No necrosis was found in these well differentiated tumors. None of them showed HER-2/neu immunoreactivity. Three ductal in situ carcinomas had poor differentiation features as pleomorphic nuclei, irregular nuclear membrane, coarse chromatin, prominent nucleoli, and mitotic figures. Necrosis and comedo features were also present in these tumors. All these three poorly differentiated in situ ductal carcinomas displayed a strong membrane over-expression of HER-2/neu (Figure 2.).

In the group of invasive ductal carcinomas, there were 13 cases with prominent poorly differentiated high grade in situ component (grade 3). Eleven of them (85%) demonstrated strong over-expression of HER-2/neu. Ten cases of ductal invasive carcinomas were associated with prominent well differentiated (grade 1) and intermediate differentiated (grade 2) in situ component. Among these ten tumors, only one (10%) in situ carcinoma showed a HER-2/neu immunoreactivity. The cells of Paget carcinoma of the nipple revealed a strong membrane overexpression of HER-2/neu (Figure 3.).

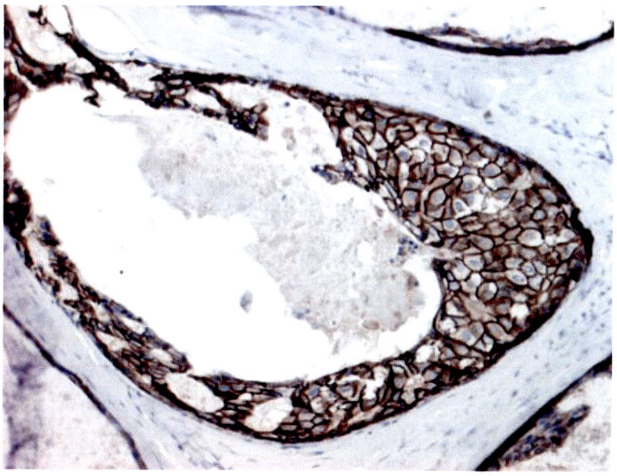

Figure 2. Immunohistochemical analysis of HER-2/neu protein in poorly differentiated in situ ductal carcinomas (grade 3): the cells display strong membrane overexpression.

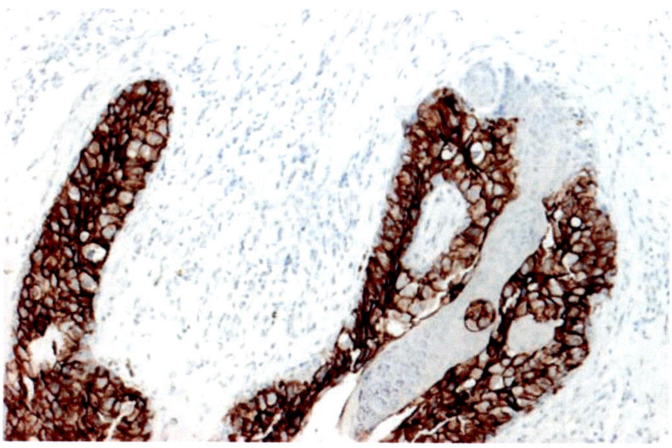

Figure 3. Immunohistochemical analysis of HER-2/neu protein: cells of Paget carcinoma of the nipple reveal strong membrane overexpression of HER-2/neu.

If we compare hormonal status and HER-2/neu overexpression, high percentage of hormone negative cases (both estrogen and progesterone negative) among HER-2/neu positive tumors is apparent. As shown in Table 5, thirty of total number of 76 tumors (40%) with strong HER-2/neu overexpression (score 3+) were completely negative for estrogen and progesterone receptors (ER-/PR-). In contrast, in the group of HER-2/neu negative tumors, only 60 cases of total number of 337 (18%) were estrogen and progesterone negative (ER-/PR-). There is also a considerable difference in hormonal status between HER-2/neu positive and negative groups, if absence of one hormone receptor is taken into account (see Table 5). As shown in the Table 5, only 42% of patients reveales immunoreactivity for both hormon receptors (ER+/PR+) in HER-2/neu positive group compared to 72% of patients in HER-2/neu negative group.

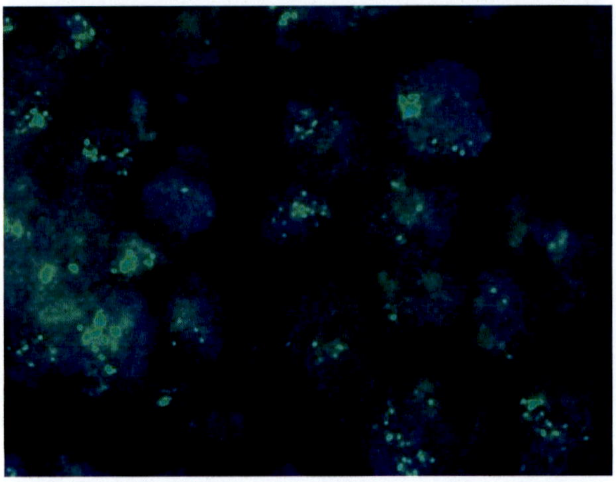

Figure 4. FISH analysis of HER-2/neu gene using the Oncor/Ventana INFORM® HER-2/neu Gene Detection System S8000-KIT: strong amplification (specimen # 3).

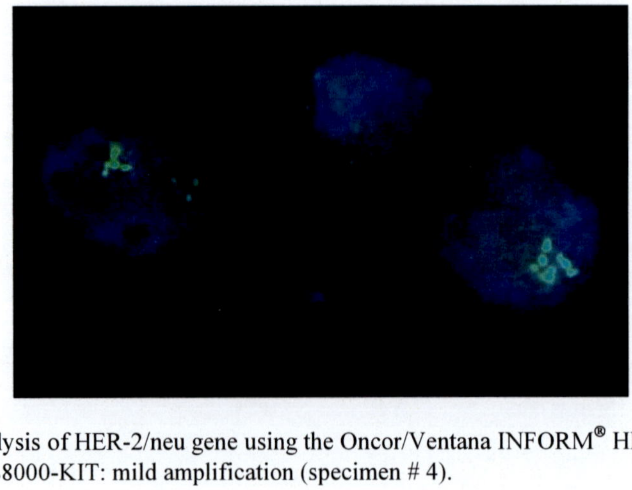

Figure 5. FISH analysis of HER-2/neu gene using the Oncor/Ventana INFORM® HER-2/neu Gene Detection System S8000-KIT: mild amplification (specimen # 4).

The results of fluorescence in situ hybridization (FISH) of HER-2/neu gene amplification in eighteen patients with HER 2/neu positive tumors are shown in Table 6. All seven tumor with strong membrane HER-2/neu immunoreactivity (score 3+) displayed HER-2/neu amplification (Figures 4, 5 and 6) or were suspicious for amplification (case # 14). In contrast, the group of eleven tumors with mild or intermediate expression of HER-2/neu by immunohistochemistry (score 1+/2+ or 2+/2+) was heterogeneous. In this particular group, FISH analysis demonstrated gene amplification in 5 carcinomas (45%), four carcinomas (36%) were not amplified and in two remaining cases, the results were interpreted as borderline (see Table 6).

Table 6. Results of HER-2/neu Immunohistochemistry in Comparison with Fluorescence in Situ Hybridization (FISH) in Breast Carcinoma

Case	ER/PR	MIB1 Index %	IHC expression of HER-2/neu protein		FISH analysis of HER-2/neu gene		Histologic Type Grade
			NeoMarker	Novocastra	Ventana*	Vysis**	
1	+/-	25	2+	2+		(1.1) NEG	IDC 3
2	+/+	20	2+	1+		(1.8)SUSP	IDC1
3	+/+	60	2+	2+	(>10)+	(>10)+	IDC 2
4	-/-	60	3+	3+	(5.3)+		IDC 3
5	-/-	10	2+	2+	(>10)+		IDC 3
6	-/-	10	2+	1+	NEG		IDC 1
7	+/+	40	2+	2+	(5.2)+		IDC 2
8	+/+	35	2+	2+	(2.5)NEG		IDC 2
9	-/+	50	2+	0		(2.1)+	IDC 3
10	+/+	15	2+	1+		(1.6)SUSP	IDC 1
11	-/-	17	3+	3+		(2.5)+	IDC 2
12	-/+	25	3+	3+		(2.4)+	IDC 2
13	+/+	20	3+	3+		(2.2)+	IDC 3
14	+/-	15	3+	3+		(1.8)+	IDC 3
15	+/+	35	1+	2+		(1.2)NEG	IDC 2
16	-/-	29	3+	3+		(2.2)+	DCIS 3
17	+/+	20	3+	3+		(2.1)+	IDC 2
18	-/-	25	2+	2+	(5.7)+		IDC 2/DCIS 3

*number in ( ) means average number of HER-2/neu gene copies per nucleus. ** -ratio of both fluorescent signals HER-2/neu:CEP17. NEG – negative, SUSP – borderline value, ER – estrogen receptor, PR – progesterone receptor, MIB1- antibody against Ki-67, MIB1 index – percentage of proliferating cells. IDC –infiltrating ductal carcinoma, DCIS – ductal in situ carcinoma.

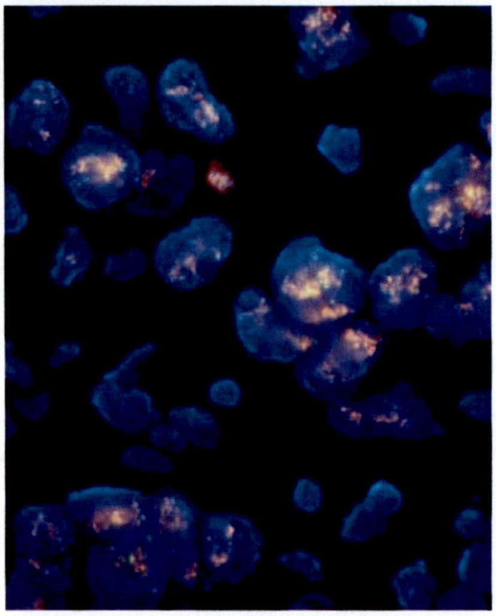

Figure 6. FISH analysis of HER-2/neu gene using the PathVysionTM HER-2/neu DNA probe kit : strong amplification (specimen # 3).

Discussion

The most frequently implicated receptors and growth factors in human breast carcinoma are members of the epidermal growth factor receptor family with tyrosine kinase activity. Type 1 protein tyrosine kinases consist of four transmembranous growth factor receptors, i.e. EGFR (epidermal growth factor receptor), c-erbB-2, c-erbB-3, and c-erbB-4 [19-21]. These receptors share a common molecular architecture, they all possess a large glycosylated extracellular ligand-binding domain, a single hydrophobic transmembrane domain, and cytoplasmic tyrosine kinase domain. HER-2/neu (also known as c-erbB-2 or neu) is a proto-oncogene localized to chromosome 17q and it encodes a 185-kDa tyrosine kinase glycoprotein. Amplification of HER-2/neu gene plays an important role in pathogenesis of breast cancer [6,22]. Little is known about starting point of amplification of HER-2/neu and how it is involved in the progression of breast malignant disease. Xu et al [23] addressed these questions by evaluating amplification of HER-2/neu in benign, premalignant and malignant breast lesion using FISH. Their study indicated that amplification of HER-2/neu appears de novo at any stage of the disease process, from atypical ductal hyperplasia to metastatic breast cancer, but most often is emerges in atypical ductal hyperplasia and carcinoma in situ. The degree of HER-2/neu amplification increases with progression to invasive carcinoma, with no further increase in metastases. These data suggest that amplification of HER-2/neu appears to be mainly involved in the initiation of breast oncogenesis, and that its role in progression of breast cancer is uncertain.

It is well known that estrogen (ER) and progesterone receptor (PR) expression is inversely related to tumor histologic grade and prognosis [24-26]. It means that ER/PR positive tumors are associated with a lower histologic grade and better prognosis than ER/PR negative tumors. As in our study, HER-2/neu positive carcinomas have been shown to be associated more often with ER/PR negativity than HER-2/neu negative tumors [27-28]. Moreover, patients with ER/PR positive-HER-2/neu negative tumors have better disease-free interval and overall survival than patients with ER/PR positive- HER-2/neu positive tumors [27,29], suggesting that HER-2/neu overexpression may be a better predictor of response to tamoxifen therapy than ER status alone [27,29].

Previous studies have suggested that HER-2/neu protein overexpression may predict responsiveness to anthracycline-based therapy. Preliminary results of clinical trials using Herceptin therapy were promising, showing that women with HER-2/neu-overexpressing tumors resistant to multiple previous therapies, showed objective response when Herceptin was used in combination with doxorubicyn-Cytoxan or paclitaxel [11]. Herceptin has also achieved an excellent overall response rate when administrated as a single agent in metastatic breast cancer [30].

One of the main reasons for the clinical utility of the assessment of HER-2/neu is for selection of patients with invasive breast cancer for trastuzumab monoclonal antibody therapy (Herceptin™, Genentech, San Francisco, CA, USA). Appropriate HER-2/neu testing has been discussed over past several years, but controversy remains. Various techniques are available for the assessment of HER-2/neu gene amplification and HER-2/neu protein overexpression, such as fluorescence in situ hybridization FISH and immunohistochemistry, respectively. Substantial variability among different methods and laboratories has been reported [31]. Immunohistochemical methods for HER-2/neu analysis have been criticized because of lack of standardization and poor reproducibility as plentiful immunohistochemical methods with different antibodies against HER-2/neu molecule are used. Previous studies have shown that sensitivity and specificity of immunohistochemical methods to detect HER-2/neu overexpression in formalin-fixed paraffin-embedded material varied according to the fixative, performance of antigen epitope retrieval and primary antibody [32-33]. HercepTest was proposed as a standardized immunohistochemical method, approved by Food and Drug Administration (FDA), capable of overcoming these problems [34]. As in our recent study [35], several others have also demonstrated the excessive sensitivity of this kit [13-15,36]. Several subsequent studies comparing HercepTest and FISH analysis demonstrated a low specificity of this technique, with a substantial number of HercepTest positive / HER-2-FISH negative cases [37-9].

Recently, HER-2/neu-FISH status was found to be more predictive of clinical response to trastuzumab than immunohistochemistry alone, and was therefore proposed as the best method for selection of patients for Herceptin therapy [13,16-17]. However, FISH is more expensive and more time consuming than immunohistochemistry. Moreover not all problems regarding FISH standardization and interpretation were solved. Thus, there is still debate about the best method for measuring the marker to select patients for therapy. Lack of standardization of immunohistochemistry (IHC) has been considered responsible for discrepancies between HER-2/neu status detected by IHC and FISH [40-41]. In our study, all tumors with strong overexpression of HER-2/neu detected by immunohistochemistry (score 3+) were amplified by FISH, while the tumors non-reactive for HER-2/neu using immunohistochemistry (score 0/1+) were non-amplified by FISH. In contrast, among 11 tumors that were 2+ according to the HercepTest scoring system, seven tumors (64 %) revealed an amplification of HER-2/neu gene by FISH, while four (35 %) were non-amplified.

In this study, we have achieved a fairly good accuracy and concordance between immunohistochemistry (IHC) using the HercepTest scoring system and FISH in strongly positive cases (score 3+) and in negative cases. However, a substantial proportion of IHC-HER-2/neu 2+ positive cases are not HER-2/neu amplified by FISH. This happened in 45% in the present series and in 64-83% in other studies [42-43]. The overall rate of cancer response with trastuzumab used as single chemotherapy for metastatic breast cancer was 9.3 % and 20.2 % for 2+ and 3+ tumours, respectively [17]. These figures suggest that selection of the patients for Herceptin (trastuzumab) therapy should be restricted to those tumors with high levels of overexpression and amplification [40].

In conclusion, we have shown that immunohistochemistry is an accurate method for detection of tumors with high levels of overexpression of HER-2/neu (3+). In our opinion, there is no universal immunohistochemical method for demonstration of HER-2/neu, and different antibodies directed against different epitopes can be used, provided that critical steps in the IHC procedure, such as dilution of primary antibody and heat-induced epitope retrieval are taken into consideration. Immunohistochemical assessment and fluorescence in situ hybridization (FISH) are complementary methods for detection of HER-2/neu status in breast cancer. While immunohistochemistry is excellent screening method, FISH should be used for confirmation of 2+ IHC -positive cases before Herceptin (trastuzumab) treatment.

References

[1] van de Vijver MJ. Molecular genetic changes in human breast cancer. *Adv. Cancer Res.* 1993: 61:25-56.

[2] Bieche I, Lindereau R. Genetic alterations in breast cancer. *Genes Chromosomes Cancer* 1995:14:227-251.

[3] De Potter CR. The neu-Oncogene: more than a prognostic indicator? *Hum. Pathol.* 1994: 25:1264-68.

[4] Akiyama T, Sudo C, Ogawara H, et al. The product of the human c-erbB-2 gene: a 185-kilodalton glycoprotein with tyrosine kinase activity. *Science* 1986:232:1644-1646.

[5] Popescu NC, King CR, Kraus MH. Localization of the human erbB-2 gene on normal and rearranged chromosomes 17 to bands q12-21.32. *Genomics* 1989:4:362-366.

[6] Slamon DJ, Godolphin W, Jones LA, Holt JA, Wong SG, Keith DE, et al. Studies of the HER-2/neu proto-oncogene in human breast and ovarian cancer. *Science* 1989:244:707-12.

[7] Ross JS, Fletcher JA. The HER-2/neu oncogene in breast cancer: prognostic factor, predictive factor, and target for therapy. *Stem Cells* 1998:16:413-28.

[8] Vargas-Roig LM, Gago FE, Tello O, De Civetta MTM, Ciocca DR. C-erbB-2(HER-2/neu) protein and drug resistance in breast cancer patients treated with induction chemotherapy. *Int. J. Cancer (Pred Oncol)* 1999: 84:129-134.

[9] Stal O, Sullivan S, Wingren S, et al. C-erbB-2 expression and benefit from adjuvant chemotherapy and radiotherapy of breast cancer. *Eur J Cancer* 1995:31A:2185-2190.

[10] Tetu B, Brisson J, Plante V, et al. P53 and c-erbB-2 as markers of resistance to adjuvant chemotherapy in breast cancer. *Mod. Pathol.* 1998:11:823-830.

[11] Ross JS, Fletcher JA. HER-2/neu (c-erb-B2) gene and protein in breast cancer. *Am. J. Clin. Pathol.* 1999:112 (Suppl 1): S 53-67.

[12] Pegram MD Lipton A, Ayes DF, et al. Phase II study of receptor-enhanced chemosensitivity using recombinant humanized anti-p185$^{HER-2/neu}$ monoclonal antibody plus cisplatin in patients with HER-2/neu –overexpressing metastatic breast cancer refractory to chemotherapy treatment. *J. Clin. Pathol.* 1998: 16:2659-2671.

[13] Bánkfalvi A, Brandt RS, Burger H, Vollmer I, Dockharn-Dworniczak B, Lellé R-J, Boecker W. Comparative methodological analysis of erbB-2/HER-2 gene dosage, chromosomal copy number and protein overexpression in breast carcinoma tissues for diagnostic use. *Histopathology* 2000:37:411-419.

[14] Jacobs TW, Gown AM, Yaziji H, Barnes MJ, Schnitt SJ. Specificity of HercepTest in determining HER-2/neu status of breast cancers using the United States Food and Drug Administration-approved scoring system. *J. Clin. Oncol.* 1999:17:1983-7.

[15] Roche P, Ingle JN. Increased HER 2 with Food and Drug Administration-approved antibody. *J. Clin. Oncol.* 1999: 17:434.

[16] Hoang MP, Sahin AA, Ordonez NG, et al. HER-2/neu gene amplification compared with HER-2/neu protein overexpression and interobserver reproducibility in invasive breast carcinoma. *Am. J. Clin. Pathol*, 113, 2000, s.852-859.

[17] Mass RD, Sanders C, Charlene K. The concordance between the clinical trials assay (CTA) and fluorescence in situ hybridization (FISH) in the Herceptin pivotal trials. In *Oncol. PASC* ed. ASCO 2000.

[18] Taucher S, Rudas M, Mader RM, Gnant M, et al: Do we need HER-2/neu testing for all patients with primary breast carcinoma? *Cancer* 2003:98:2547-53.

[19] Gullick WJ, Srinivasan R. The type 1 growth factor receptor family: new ligands and receptors and their role in breast cancer. *Breast Cancer Res. Treat* 1998:52:43-53.

[20] Klapper LN, Kirschbaum MH, Sela M, Yarden Y. Biochemical and clinical implications of the ErbB/HER signaling network of growth factor receptors. *Adv. Cancer Res.* 2000:77:25-79.

[21] Bacus SS, Gudkov AV, Esteva FJ, Yarden Y. Expression of erbB recptors and their ligands in breast cancer: implications to biological behavior and therapeutic response. *Breast Dis.* 2000:11:63-75.

[22] Di Fiore PP, Pierce JH, Kraus MH, Segatto O, King CR, Aaronson SA. ErbB-2 is a potent oncogene when overexpressed in NIH/3T3 cells. *Science* 1987: 237:178-182.

[23] Xu R, Perle MA, Inghirami G, et al. Amplification of HER-2/neu gene in HER-2/neu-overexpressing and-nonexpressing breast carcinomas and their synchronous benign, premalignant, and metastatic lesions detected by FISH in arcival material. *Mod. Pathol.* 2002:15:116-124.

[24] Moriki T, Takahashi T, Hoiroi M, et al. Histological grade in invasive ductal carcinoma of the breast correlates with proliferative activity evaluated by BrdU: an immunohistochemical study including correlations with p53, c-erbB-2 and estrogen recptor status. *Pathol. Intern.* 1996: 46:417-25.

[25] Joonjic N, Mustac E, Krstulja M, et al. Nuclear grade in invasive ductal breast carcinoma: comparative study on nuclear grade and morphometric parameters,

hormonal receptor status, flow cytometric analysis and lectin histochemistry. *Gen. Diagn Pathol.* 1996:142:83-88.
[26] Ruibal A, Arias JI, Del Rion MC, et al. The correlations of clinicopathologic features, hormon receptor level with prognosis of breast cancer: report of 308 cases in elderly women. *Clin. Med. Sci. J.* 1997:12:60-62.
[27] Pinto AE, Andre S, Nobrega S, et al. C-erbB-2 oncoprotein overexpression identifies a subgroup of estrogen receptor positive (ER+) breast cancer patients with poor prognosis. *Ann Oncol* 2001:12:525-33.
[28] Anderson JM, Ariga R, Govil H, Bloom KJ, Francescatti D, Reddy VB, Gould VE, Gattuso P. Assessment of HER-2/neu status by immunohistochemistry and fluorescence in situ hybridization in mammary Paget disease and underlying carcinoma. Appl Immunohistoch *Mol. Morphol.* 2003:11:120-124.
[29] Ferrero-Pous M, Hacene K, Bouchet C, et al. Relationship between C-erbB-2 and other tumor characteristics in breast cancer prognosis. *Clin. Cancer Res.* 2000:6:4745-54.
[30] Cobleigh MA, Vogel CL, Tripathy NJ, et al Efficacy and safety of Herceptin as a single agent in 222 women with HER2 overexpression who relapsed following chemotherapy for metastatic breast cancer (abstract). *Proceedings of the American Society of Clinical Oncology,* vol 17. Alexandria, VA: American Society of Clinical Oncology, 1998:97.
[31] Tubbs R, Skacel M, Pettay J, et al. Interobserver interpretative reproducibility of GOLGFISH, a first generation gold-faciliated autometallographic bright field in situ hybridization assay for HER-2/neu amplification in invasive mammary carcinoma. *Am J. Surg. Pathol.* 2002:26:908-913.
[32] Press M, Hung C, Godolphin W, et al. Sensitivity of HER-2/neu antibodies in archival tissue samples: potential source error in immunohistochemical studies of oncogene expression. *Cancer Res.* 1994: 54:2771-2777.
[33] Penault-Llorca F, Adelaide J, Houvenaeghel G et al. Optimization of immunohistochemical detection of ERBB2 in breast cancer: impact of fixation. *J. Pathol.* 1994:173:65-75.
[34] Espinoza F. HercepTest assay. Another perspective. *J. Clin. Oncol.*, 17, 1999, s.2293-4.
[35] Skálová A, Vaněček T, Lošan F, Papatsidesová L, Fínek J. Detection of HER-2/neu in breast carcinoma. *Čas. Lék. Čs.* 2003:142 (2): 93-98 (in Czech).
[36] O´Malley FP, Parkes R, Latta E, Tjan S, Zadro T, Mueller R, Arneson N, Blacksein M, Andrulis I. Comparison of HER2/neu status assessed by quantitative polymerase chain reaction and immunohistochemistry. *Am. J. Clin. Pathol.* 2001:115: 504-511.
[37] Lebeau A, Deimling D, Kaltz C, et al. HER-2/neu analysis in archival tissue samples of human breast cancer: comparison of immunohistochemistry and fluorescence in situ hybridization. *J. Clin. Oncol.* 2001: 19:354-363.
[38] Pauletti G, Dandekar S, Rong HM, et al. assessment of methods tissue-based detection of the HER-2/neu alteration in breast cancer: a direct comparison of fluorescence in situ hybridisation and immunohistochemistry. *J. Clin. Oncol.* 2000: 18: 3651-3664.
[39] Roche P, Ingle JN. Increased HER2 with U.S. Food and Drug Adminitration approved antibody. *J. Clin. Oncol.* 1999:17:434.

[40] Vincent-Salomon A, MacGrogan G, Couturier J, et al. Calibration of immunohistochemistry for assessment of HER2 in breast cancer: results of French Multicentre GEFPICS Study. *Histopathology* 2003:42:337-347.

[41] Hammond ME, Barker P, Taube S, Gutman S. Standard reference material for HER2 testing. *Appl. Immunohistochem. Mol. Morphol.* 2003:11:103-106.

[42] Ridolfi R, Mehdi R, Jamehdor MD, et al. HER-2/neu testing in breast carcinoma: a combined immunohistochemical and fluorescence in situ hybridisation approach. *Mod. Pathol.* 2000: 13:886-873.

[43] Tubbs RR, Pettay JD, Roche PC et al. Discrepancies in clinical laboratory testing of eligibility for Trastuzumab therapy: apparent immunohistochemical false-positives do not get the message. *J. Clin. Oncol.* 2001: 19:2714-2721.

In: Frontiers in Breast Cancer Research
Editor: Louis P. Fortugno, pp. 175-186
ISBN: 978-1-60021-671-8

Chapter VIII

Fruit Intake and Risk of Breast Cancer: A Case-Control Study

Alvaro L. Ronco[1,*], Eduardo De Stéfani[2] and Hugo Deneo-Pellegrini[3]
[1]Oncology Unit, Pereira Rossell Women's Hospital, Ministry of Public Health, Montevideo, Uruguay
[2]Unit of Epidemiology, Department of Pathology, School of Medicine, State University, Montevideo, Uruguay
[3]Department of Pathology, National Institute of Oncology, Ministry of Public Health, Montevideo, Uruguay

Abstract

In order to know possible associations of fruit consumption and the risk of breast cancer (BC) in Montevideo, the authors carried out a case-control study in the period 1999-2001. A total number of 333 women were interviewed with a specific questionnaire, 111 of which were certified cases of BC and 222 were frequency-matched healthy women, with a recent normal mammography (Birads 1). The questionnaire included a detailed 120-item food frequency section, as well as sociodemographic, reproductive, familial, medical and lifestyle variables. There was particular emphasis set on types of fruits. After controlling for age, age at menarche, menopausal status, duration of menses, energy, family history of BC, smoking, total vegetables, total meat, dairy, frequency of exercise and number of live births, a multivariate analysis found that high intakes of orange (OR=0.51), orange juice (OR=0.26), citrus fruits (OR=0.27) and total fruits (OR=0.44) were associated with significant reduced risk of BC. The inclusion of dietary ascorbic acid in the regression models made even stronger the decrease of risk for orange (OR= 0.22) and citrus fruits (OR=0.13), suggesting that this constituent of fruits might be co-responsible for the results.

* Correspondence concerning this article should be addressed to Dr. Alvaro L. Ronco, Laureles 923, 11900 Montevideo Uruguay. Tel/fax: (+598 2) 304 3678; E-mail address: alronco@redfacil.com.uy; alronco@gmail.com.

Keywords: *breast cancer, citrus, diet, epidemiology, fruits, risk factors.*

Introduction

Breast cancer (BC) is the leading malignancy among Uruguayan women, with an age-adjusted incidence rate of 114 per 100.000 (Parkin et al, 2002) for women living in the capital city, Montevideo. In international comparisons, Uruguayan rate of female BC is the highest among South American registries (Parkin et al, 2002). Theoretically, this could be the result of an unusually high prevalence of risk factors or of a low prevalence of protective factors.

Although the etiology of human BC remains unknown, risk factors associated with the disease can be grouped into three broad determinants (DeBruin and Josephy 2002): family history (hereditary) factors, hormonal and reproductive factors, and environmental (including lifestyle) factors. A recent epidemiologic analysis concluded that 73% of breast cancers are attributable to environmental factors (Lichtenstein P et al 2000). From these latter, diet appears as the most relevant factor and the relationship between vegetables fruits and breast cancer has been examined in at least three prospective and nine teen case-control studies (World Cancer Research Fund, 1997). According to an international panel, diets high in vegetables and fruits probably decrease the risk of breast cancer (World Cancer Research Fund, 1997). Diets with five or more daily servings of fruits and vegetables have been recognized to be a potential protective against breast cancer (*Snyderwine 1998*), but a later study did not support a protective role for dietary fruits and vegetables in adulthood (*Smith-Warner 2001*).

Plant foods are a rich source of nutrients and non-nutritive substances which are, probably, anticarcinogens (Steinmetz and Potter 1991a; Steinmetz and Potter, 1991b, Steinmetz and Potter, 1996; La Vecchia and Tavani, 1998). Among these, carotenoids, vitamin C, vitamin E, and flavonoids have been associated with reduced risks in several cancer sites (World Cancer Research Fund, 1997). Nevertheless, the interaction among phytochemicals, micro- and macronutrient components of whole foods features the challenge of quantifiying phytochemical intakes, which were not yet determined for most foods (Greenwald et al, 2001).

Previous epidemiological studies conducted in Uruguay analyzed the relationship between diet and the risk of BC among women admitted at public hospitals (Ronco et al, 1996; De Stéfani et al, 1997a,b; De Stéfani et al, 1998; Ronco and De Stéfani, 1999) and, more recently, also in women belonging to the pre-paid healthcare system (Ronco et al 2002, Ronco et al 2003). In one of these previous studies (De Stefani et al , 1997b), a reduced risk of BC was associated with high dietary fiber intake. In particular, diets high in fiber and quercetin and fiber and lutein were associated with a substantial protective effect (De Stefani et al, 1997b). Besides, we should remark that only some vegetables but no fruits were part of the discriminant models for low- and high-risk BC populations (restricted only to women belonging to the public hospitals healthcare system) we had found some years ago through the application of artificial neural networks (Ronco 1999, Ronco and De Stéfani 1999).

Uruguayan population is particularly difficult for studying the relationship between plant foods and BC, since its diet is rich in meat and low in vegetable and fruit consumption. More specifically, Uruguayan diet is relatively poor in vegetables and fruits, being tomato, lettuce, onion, spinach, orange, apple, and banana the most frequently consumed food items (Comision Honoraria de Lucha Contra el Cancer, 1993). In this sense, the study of a populational subset who has higher socioeconomic and cultural levels and also higher incidence rates of breast cancer, appears as advantageous in order to explore possible associations of certain food items with the risk of this disease.

After some initial exploratory analyses, whose findings were no relevant concerning the role of vegetable consumption, we decided to conduct a case-control study exclusively based on fruit intake and the risk of BC in Uruguay.

Subjects and Methods

A case-control study designed to study the relationship among environmental factors and BC within the Uruguayan private health system was conducted between October 1999 and July 2001 in Montevideo, the capital city of Uruguay where around 45% of the Uruguayan inhabitants live. The research was performed exclusively in IMPASA (Instituto Médico de Previsión, Asistencia y Servicios Afines), an Institution which is well-representative of the pre-paid system in the country.

During the study period, 111 cases of breast cancer were collected. Cases were women with incident (i.e. diagnosed within two years before the interview) and mainly histologically verified carcinomas (103 cases in 111, 92.8%). One control and two cases rejected the interview and other three cases (0.9%) died during the study period, leading to a final response rate of 99.6% for controls and 95.7 % for cases.

In the same time period 222 healthy women with a normal control mammography (BIRADS 1) (Feig, 1999) performed no longer than one year before the interview, were selected as controls (2 controls per case). They were frequency-matched by age (± 5 years) and residence (Montevideo and its neighbourhood), being mandatory requirements for the controls not to be hospitalized at the moment of the interview and not being afflicted by a cancer.

All interviews were conducted in the hospital and performed face-to-face by a trained nurse, who was blinded concerning major risk factors. The questionnaire included the following sections: (1) sociodemographic variables; (2) a section on occupation based on job titles and the duration of each activity; (3) history of cancer in first and second degree relatives; (4) self-reported height and weight 5 years before the interview, at 18 years old and the most frequent weight during the adulthood; (5) a tobacco smoking section; (6) a history on alcohol drinking (including type of beverage, age at start, age of quit, and average amount of alcohol drinked per day); (7) a history of "mate" drinking ("mate" is the folk name of a local infusion, which is highly prevalent in the Uruguayan population; (8) menstrual and reproductive events; and (9) a detailed food-frequency questionnaire (FFQ) on 120 items representative of the diet of the Uruguayan population. The current FFQ was not validated, but was tested for reproducibility with reasonably good results. It is a modification of a previous one, having added some details concerning selected items. Furthermore, it allowed to estimate the total energy intake of each subject.

Data Analysis

The following fruits were analyzed: (sum of all individual variables). Other groups were also created: all vegetables, all fruits, red meat, white meat, grain and desserts. Food groups and food items were adjusted for total energy intake, using the residuals method (Willett and Stampfer, 1986). Each food group was categorized in tertiles according to the controls distribution. Intake of foods was recorded as servings per year. Odds Ratios (OR)s and 95% Confidence Intervals (CI)s were calculated by unconditional logistic regression (Breslow and Day, 1980). Potential confounders were included in the multivariate analysis. All equations included terms for age, age at menarche, menopausal status, duration of menses, energy, family history of BC, smoking status, total vegetables, total meat, dairy, frequency of exercise and number of live births. All variables were entered in the models as continuous ones. All the calculations were performed with the software STATA (STATA, 1999).

Results

Table 1 show selected variables featuring the studied population, which exhibited a marked homogeneity, regarding sociodemographic, menstrual and reproductive variables. Dietary energy (kcalories) ($p<0.001$) and family history of BC ($p=0.016$) were the only variables with statistically significant differences between cases and controls.

In Table 2 are indicated the OR's calculated for different fruits, even crude as well as adjusted. Although total fruit intake was negatively and significantly associated with the risk of BC (OR= 0.44), there are few items which displayed an association in the same sense: oranges (OR= 0.51), orange juice (OR= 0.26) and citrus fruits, which include tangerines (OR= 0.27).

Table 3 compares the adjusted OR's for the highest tertiles with and without including Vitamin C (ascorbic acid) in the regression model. A general reduction trend is observed, even stronger, as a consequence of the quoted inclusion.

Table 4 shows adjusted OR's for fruits, stratified by levels of vegetable intake, according to the median level of consumption (low <=1104 servings/year, high >=1105 servings/year). Even with low vegetable intakes, orange juice and citrus fruits showed strong inverse associations, in a protective sense. One of the grape types (moscatel) tended to show an increase of risk for low vegetable consumers (OR=4.02 and OR=1.72). On the other hand, red apple consumption tended to be positively associated with BC for high vegetable consumers (OR=3.58 significant).

The adjusted OR's calculated according to BMI are presented in Table 5. Categories of BMI were dichotomized according to Normal weight (<=24.99 kg/m2) and Overweight-Obesity (>=25 kg/m2). Significant negative associations were found for the highest tertiles of orange juice (OR=0.22), citrus fruits (OR=0.19) and total fruit consumption (OR=0.34) among normal-weight women. Also a significant protective association was found among overweight-obese women in orange juice (OR=0.09), plum (OR=0.17) and citrus fruits (OR=0.25), but only in the medium tertile of consumption.

Finally, Table 6 displays the calculated OR's for fruits according to smoking status, dichotomized into never and ever (current + former) smokers. Significant negative associations were found almost only among non smokers: orange (OR=0.47), orange juice (OR=0.20) and citrus fruits (OR=0.21), in all cases related to high consumers of fruits.

Table 1. Distribution of cases and controls by selected variables

	Controls		Cases		Significance
Variable	n	%	n	%	
Age, yrs					
<=49	31	14.0	15	13.5	
50-59	74	33.3	29	26.1	
60-69	77	34.7	41	36.9	
>=70	40	18.0	26	23.4	p=0.48
Urban status, yrs					
<=54	76	34.2	35	31.5	
55-65	79	35.6	33	29.7	
>=66	67	30.2	43	38.7	p=0.28
Education, yrs					
<=10	81	36.5	40	36.0	
11-14	68	30.6	25	22.5	
>=15	73	32.9	46	41.4	p=0.20
Body Mass Index (kg/m2)					
<=22.51	69	31.1	41	36.9	
22.52-25.39	77	34.7	32	28.8	
>=25.40	76	34.2	38	34.2	p=0.46
Menopausal status					
Pre	24	10.8	11	9.9	
Post	198	89.2	100	90.1	p=0.80
Menarche, yrs					
<=11	76	34.2	29	26.1	
12	71	32.0	35	31.5	
>=13	75	33.8	47	42.3	p=0.22
No. of living births					
Nulliparous	23	10.4	12	10.8	
1	47	21.2	23	20.7	
2	99	44.6	45	40.5	
>=3	53	23.9	31	27.9	p=0.85
Energy, kcal					
<=1761	73	32.9	15	13.5	
1762-2064	74	33.3	46	41.4	
>=2065	75	33.8	50	45.0	p=0.00076
Family history of BC					
No	180	81.1	77	69.4	
Yes	42	18.9	34	30.6	p=0.016
Total number of subjects	222	100.0	111	100.0	

Table 2. Distribution of cases and controls according to variables of interest. Crude and adjusted odds ratios of breast cancer for each analyzed variable

Variable		Controls	Cases	p- value for trend	Crude	Adjusted **
Tertils Intake*		n %	n %		*OR* (95% CI)	*OR* (95% CI)
Orange						
Low	0-52	73 32.9	46 41.4		1.00 -	1.00 -
Mid	53-364	74 33.3	44 39.6		0.94 (0.56-1.59)	0.62 (0.33-1.16)
High	>=365	75 33.8	21 18.9	0.012	0.44 (0.24-0.82)	0.51 (0.26-0.98)
Orange juice						
Low	0-156	73 32.9	77 69.4		1.00 -	1.00 -
Mid	157-364	74 33.3	18 16.2		0.23 (0.13-0.42)	0.16 (0.08-0.3
High	>=365	75 33.8	16 14.4	<0.0001	0.20 (0.11-0.38)	0.26 (0.13-0.54)
Tangerine						
Low	0	73 32.9	28 25.2		1.00 -	1.00 -
Mid	1-52	74 33.3	46 41.4		1.62 (0.92-2.87)	1.03 (0.54-1.99)
High	>=53	75 33.8	37 33.3	0.439	1.28 (0.71-2.31)	1.20 (0.64-2.26)
Red apple						
Low	0-104	73 32.9	39 35.1		1.00 -	1.00 -
Mid	105-260	74 33.3	33 29.7		0.83 (0.47-1.47)	0.92 (0.49-1.73)
High	>=261	75 33.8	39 35.1	0.925	0.97 (0.56-1.68)	1.31 (0.71-2.43)
Green apple						
Low	0-104	73 32.9	52 46.8		1.00 -	1.00 -
Mid	105-208	74 33.3	30 27.0		0.57 (0.33-0.99)	0.66 (0.36-1.21)
High	>=209	75 33.8	29 26.1	0.025	0.54 (0.31-0.95)	0.55 (0.31-1.01)
Grapes – Moscatel type						
Low	0	73 32.9	23 20.7		1.00 -	1.00 -
Mid	1-52	74 33.3	67 60.4		2.87 (1.62-5.10)	2.61 (1.37-4.98)
High	>=53	75 33.8	21 18.9	0.760	0.89 (0.45-1.74)	0.96 (0.46-1.99)
Grapes – common type						
Low 0		73 32.9	42 37.8		1.00 -	1.00 -
Mid	1-12	74 33.3	21 18.9		0.49 (0.27-0.91)	0.93 (0.45-1.94)
High	>=13	75 33.8	48 43.2	0.647	1.11 (0.66-1.88)	1.48 (0.82-2.65)
Banana						
Low	0-104	73 32.9	45 40.5		1.00 -	1.00 -
Mid	105-156	75 33.8	19 17.1		0.41 (0.22-0.77)	0.44 (0.23-0.87)
High	>=157	74 33.3	47 42.3	0.891	1.03 (0.61-1.74)	1.14 (0.64-2.03)
Plum						
Low	0-12	74 33.3	50 45.0		1.00 -	1.00 -
Mid 13-24		74 33.3	21 18.9		0.42 (0.23-0.77)	0.59 (0.30-1.15)
High	>=25	74 33.3	40 36.0	0.360	0.80 (0.47-1.35)	0.62 (0.34-1.11)
Peach						
Low	0-24	73 32.9	30 27.0		1.00 -	1.00 -
Mid	25-48	75 33.8	38 34.2		1.23 (0.69-2.19)	1.56 (0.82-2.96)
High	>=49	74 33.3	43 38.7	0.233	1.41 (0.80-2.49)	1.29 (0.68-2.43)
Watermelon						
Low	0	73 32.9	47 42.3		1.00 -	1.00 -
Mid	1-12	74 33.3	24 21.6		0.50 (0.28-0.91)	0.98 (0.48-2.00)
High	>=13	75 33.8	40 36.0	0.461	0.83 (0.49-1.41)	0.79 (0.45-1.40)

Variable		Controls	Cases	p- value for trend	Crude	Adjusted **
Tertils Intake*		n %	n %		*OR* (95% CI)	*OR* (95% CI)
Pear						
Low	0-5	73 32.9	29 26.1		1.00 -	1.00 -
Mid	6-24	74 33.3	31 27.9		1.05 (0.58-1.92)	0.65 (0.33-1.27)
High	>=25	75 33.8	51 45.9	0.049	1.71 (0.98-2.99)	1.35 (0.72-2.54)
Tertils Intake*		n %	n %		*OR* (95% CI)	*OR* (95% CI)
Fruit cocktail						
Low	0	73 32.9	34 30.6		1.00 -	1.00 -
Mid	1-24	74 33.3	49 44.1		1.42 (0.83-2.45)	0.99 (0.54-1.82)
High	>=25	75 33.8	28 25.2	0.495	0.80 (0.44-1.45)	0.86 (0.45-1.64)
Citrus fruits						
Low	0-348	73 32.9	71 64.0		1.00 -	1.00 -
Mid	349-663	74 33.3	25 22.5		0.35 (0.20-0.61)	0.32 (0.18-0.60)
High	>=664	75 33.8	15 13.5	<0.0001	0.21 (0.11-0.39)	0.27 (0.13-0.55)
Non-citrus fruits						
Low 0-554		74 33.3	33 29.7		1.00 -	1.00 -
Mid	555-867	73 32.9	35 31.5		1.08 (0.60-1.91)	0.99 (0.53-1.87)
High	>=868	75 33.8	43 38.7	0.371	1.29 (0.74-2.24)	1.07 (0.58-1.97)
Total fruits						
Low	<=1019	74 33.3	46 41.4		1.00 -	1.00 -
Mid	1020-1436	73 32.9	40 36.0		0.88 (0.52-1.50)	0.86 (0.48-1.55)
High	>=1437	75 33.8	25 22.5	0.040	0.54 (0.30-0.96)	0.44 (0.23-0.86)

* Intake is expressed in number of servings per year.

** Logistic regression model adjusted for: age, age at menarche, menopausal status, duration of menses, energy, family history of BC, smoking, total vegetables, total mea, dairy, frequency of exercise and number of live births.

Table 3. Odds Ratios estimated after inclusion of vitamin C as a term of adjustment for selected fruits

Variable	Adjusted OR Without Vitamin C	Adjusted OR Including Vitamin C	
		Tertile II	Tertile III
Orange	0.51 (0.26 – 0.98)	0.44 (0.19 – 1.03)	0.22 (0.08 – 0.64)
Orange juice	0.26 (0.13 – 0.54)	0.16 (0.08 – 0.31)	0.23 (0.11 – 0.48)
Citrus	0.27 (0.13 – 0.55)	0.23 (0.11 – 0.46)	0.13 (0.05 – 0.33)
Total fruits	0.44 (0.23 – 0.86)	0.81 (0.43 – 1.55)	0.35 (0.16 – 0.76)

Discussion

Our study found an inverse association between high intakes of some fruits (citrical, in particular) and the risk of BC. On one hand, an explanation arises from the contribution of fibre, ascorbic acid, and some bioactive substances like bioflavonoids. The antioxidant capability of substances like glutathion, especially present in these fruits like orange, together with the improvement of immune system provided by vitamin C, result in a plausible explanation for our findings. Since flavonoid is mostly concentrated in the orange pulp and not in juice, it seems logic the outcome concerning to the inclusion of this item in multivariate analysis, being even more negative in the association with orange (OR decreases from 0.51 to 0.22) than with orange juice, which was slightly modified (OR=0.26 to

OR=0.23). Furthermore, the risk of citrus fruits was reduced up to a half (from 0.27 to 0.13), probably due to an effect of the same factors.

Table 4. Odds ratios of breast cancer for each fruit according to level of vegetable intake

	Low intake of vegetables (<=1104 servings/year) Tertiles of fruit intake			High intake of vegetables (>=1105 servings/year) Tertiles of fruit intake		
Variable	I	II	III	I	II	III
Orange	1.00	0.46	0.63	1.00	0.71	0.53
Orange juice	1.00	0.13*	0.16*	1.00	0.17*	0.42
Tangerine	1.00	0.83	0.67	1.00	1.18	1.80
Red apple	1.00	0.74	0.77	1.00	1.49	3.58*
Green apple	1.00	0.83	0.97	1.00	0.66	0.42
Moscatel grape	1.00	4.02*	1.72	1.00	1.53	0.50
Common grape	1.00	0.68	0.96	1.00	0.83	1.25
Banana	1.00	0.74	0.73	1.00	0.22*	1.64
Plum	1.00	0.47	0.70	1.00	0.88	0.50
Peach	1.00	0.98	1.21	1.00	1.99	1.32
Watermelon	1.00	1.25	0.68	1.00	0.48	0.80
Pear	1.00	0.42	1.60	1.00	1.11	1.31
Fruit cocktail	1.00	0.76	0.85	1.00	1.08	0.64
Citrus fruits	1.00	0.17*	0.20*	1.00	0.45	0.35
Non citrus fruits	1.00	0.92	1.19	1.00	1.23	1.12
Total fruits	1.00	0.43	0.44	1.00	1.88	0.55

(*) Statistically significant (p<0.05).

Logistic regression model adjusted for: age, age at menarche, menopausal status, duration of menses, energy, family history of BC, smoking, total meat, dairy, frequency of exercise and number of live births.

It is an interesting fact that green apples (Granny Smith type, a very popular variety consumed in Uruguay) had a negative and almost significant association (OR=0.55, CI 0.31-1.01), different from red apples (OR=1.31). Considering the taste of each variety, it is likely that the green one could have more vitamin C than the red one. Due to lack of information on this item, we have used values from tables which were assigned to the item "apple" as an only value in their original sources. This point deserves further analysis.

The different analyses show that citrus fruits, usually orange juice above orange and tangerine, were significantly and negatively associated with the risk of BC. This protective effect was stronger among low vegetable consumers, among non smokers and also among normal weight women. Besides, some positive associations concerning moscatel grapes or red apple intakes cannot be precluded as being chance findings. Further studies at a larger scale could be useful to confirm these results.

Studies on fruit consumption and its association with BC have been controversial. Several of the recent reports from prospective studies of diet and cancer have not found the same protective effects of fruits and vegetables that were reported earlier in the epidemiological and case-control studies (reviewed in Riboli and Norat 2003).

Table 5. Odds ratios of breast cancer for each fruit according to BMI level

	Normal weight (<=24.99 kg/m2) Tertiles of fruit intake			Overweight-obesity (>=25.0 kg/m2) Tertiles of fruit intake		
Variable	I	II	III	I	II	III
Orange	1.00	0.68	0.43	1.00	0.50	0.46
Orange juice	1.00	0.23*	0.22*	1.00	0.09*	0.29
Tangerine	1.00	0.70	0.70	1.00	1.70	2.71
Red apple	1.00	1.17	2.15	1.00	0.57	0.45
Green apple	1.00	0.62	0.48	1.00	0.74	0.91
Moscatel grape	1.00	2.70*	0.82	1.00	2.40	1.37
Common grape	1.00	0.79	1.50	1.00	1.22	1.64
Banana	1.00	0.47	1.54	1.00	0.34	0.43
Plum	1.00	0.86	0.40	1.00	0.17*	0.96
Peach	1.00	1.80	1.15	1.00	0.94	1.34
Watermelon	1.00	0.96	0.56	1.00	0.99	1.58
Pear	1.00	0.82	1.18	1.00	0.52	1.85
Fruit cocktail	1.00	1.06	0.76	1.00	0.74	0.96
Citrus fruits	1.00	0.28*	0.19*	1.00	0.25*	0.34
Non citrus fruits	1.00	1.18	1.24	1.00	0.63	0.78
Total fruits	1.00	0.73	0.34*	1.00	0.66	0.42

(*) Statistically significant ($p<0.05$).

Logistic regression model adjusted for: age, age at menarche, menopausal status, duration of menses, energy, family history of BC, smoking, total vegetables, total meat, dairy, frequency of exercise and number of live births.

Methodologic issues concerning mostly the employed instruments (food frequency questionnaires, food diaries, e.g) reveal that inaccurate measurements of fruit and vegetable intake could be a plausible explanation of inconsistencies (Bingham et al, 2003).

The frequently observed lack of association between diet and BC in epidemiological studies requires caution in its interpretation, because diet is assessed with a considerable measurement error in observational studies, and our current diet assessment instruments may not provide sufficiently valid and reliable data to detect small to moderate associations with disease. Similarly, variation in diet within the populations studied may not be sufficiently large to overcome the measurement error that is inherent in self-reported dietary information (Michels K, 2002). Moreover, most participants in epidemiologic studies follow a diet with almost no severe restrictions. Therefore, it is not known whether a more restricted diet might have any major effect on breast cancer incidence. Such dietary regimens are more common in the developed societies and largely prescribe the use of fresh and whole foods, including freshly ground whole grains, plant proteins, and a large variety of organic raw vegetables and fruits (Michels K, 2002). Anyway, based on well-known constituents that are found in vegetables and fruits –like dietary fibre, micronutrients and several phytochemicals- and the interactions among these constituents, it is recognized that they might contribute to the ability of these foods to reduce cancer risk. Obviously, identification of those most effective ones and the mechanisms through they exert they effects represent important challenges in cancer research (Greenwald et al, 2001).

Table 6. Odds ratios of breast cancer for each fruit according to smoking status

	Never smoker			Ever smoker (Current + former)		
	Tertiles of fruit intake			Tertiles of fruit intake		
Variable	I	II	III	I	II	III
Orange	1.00	0.72	0.47*	1.00	1.60	0.65
Orange juice	1.00	0.19*	0.20*	1.00	0.12*	2.63
Tangerine	1.00	1.20	1.74	1.00	0.18	0.22
Red apple	1.00	0.80	1.61	1.00	1.17	0.28
Green apple	1.00	0.57	0.63	1.00	1.78	0.19
Moscatel grape	1.00	2.93*	1.35	1.00	2.50	0.09
Common grape	1.00	0.82	1.47	1.00	1.80	0.83
Banana	1.00	0.42	1.22	1.00	0.34	0.60
Plum	1.00	0.55	0.58	1.00	0.20	0.25
Peach	1.00	1.16	1.11	1.00	7.47	1.14
Watermelon	1.00	0.99	0.79	1.00	1.70	1.11
Pear	1.00	0.73	1.55	1.00	0.12	0.22
Fruit cocktail	1.00	0.80	1.14	1.00	1.68	0.13
Citrus fruits	1.00	0.34*	0.21*	1.00	0.64	0.93
Non citrus fruits	1.00	1.22	1.17	1.00	0.30	0.22
Total fruits	1.00	1.00	0.46	1.00	0.88	0.27

(*) Statistically significant ($p<0.05$).

Logistic regression model adjusted for: age, age at menarche, menopausal status, duration of menses, energy, family history of BC, total vegetables, total meat, dairy, frequency of exercise and number of live births.

As other case-control studies, our work has limitations and strengths. A major limitation is related to the sample size; it would be desirable to analyze a larger one, in order to have enough statistical power for certain results. Another limitation was the lack of validation of the questionnaire, although the instrument was not created de novo. On the other hand, both cases and controls belong to a very homogeneous base subpopulation: they were not only matched by age and residence, but they also proceeded mostly from the same zones within the city of Montevideo (with an urban area ca. 200 sq.km), they belonged to the same healthcare system, and they exhibited similarities concerning most sociodemographic and reproductive variables, all of which means good conditions for the chosen sample, in order to carry out an epidemiologic study.

To be mentioned also among the strengths, we selected as controls community women with normal breasts, not only without cancer –documented through mammograms labeled as Birads 1-; thus, if benign breast diseases had any association with the analyzed dietary items, we avoided the possibility of biasing results due to this. Finally, a high participation was achieved (around 98% of the incident cases below 84 years old during the study period): selection and recall bias appear to be unlikely. Although it is not possible to avoid completely any bias, we think that the results were not chance findings. Anyway, we need caution in the interpretation of results, since generalizability is limited due to the population features: they have high mean ages, high educational level and belong to a mid-to-high socioeconomic class.

The potentiality given by knowledge about fruit intake and the risk of BC within this population that has an extremely high BC incidence at an international level, is promising from the viewpoint of primary prevention of the disease. In previos studies conducted on population admitted at public hospitals in Montevideo, a higher level of protection from fruit consumption than from vegetables consumption was already suggested. Albeith the population groups with lesser income have smaller fruit consumption than the higher strata, every effort in the promotion for its consumption would be extremely useful in attempting to lower the impact of BC as well as with other modern pathologies having cardiovascular and metabolic origin, indeed. When considering recent evidence, it is estimated that around 32% of cancer may be avoidable by changing to a diet rich in fruits and vegetables (Willett 1995). The identification of the active ingredients in such diets for cancer prevention may endorse its use in a wide range of populations. New studies at a larger scale, nevertheless, are required in order to confirm the findings of the present study.

References

Bingham SA, Luben R, Welch A, Wareham N, Khaw KT, Day N: Are imprecise methods obscuring a relation between fat and breast cancer? *Lancet* 2003, 362:212-214.

Breslow NE, Day NE: Statistical methods in cancer research. Volume 1-*The analysis of case-control studies*. IARC scientific publications N°32. IARC, Lyon, 1980.

Comisión Honoraria de Lucha Contra el Cáncer: Conocimientos, creencias, actitudes y prácticas en relación al Cáncer. Cooperación técnica OPP/BID/PNUD. Comisión Honoraria de Lucha Contra el Cáncer, Montevideo, 1993.

De Bruin LS, Josephy PD: Perspectives on the Chemical Etiology of Breast Cancer. *Environ Health Perspect* 2002, 110(suppl 1):119–128.

De Stéfani E, Fierro L, Barrios E, Ronco A: Cancer mortality trends in Uruguay 1953-1991. *Int. J.Cancer* 1994, 56: 634-639.

De Stéfani E, Ronco AL, Mendilaharsu M, Guidobono M, Deneo-Pellegrini H: Meat intake, heterocyclic amines, and risk of breast cancer: a case-control study in Uruguay. *Cancer Epidemiol. Biomarkers Prev.* 1997, 6: 573-581.

De Stéfani E, Correa P, Ronco AL, Mendilaharsu M, Guidobono M, Deneo-Pellegrini H: Dietary fiber and risk of breast cancer. A case-control study in Uruguay. *Nutr.Cancer* 1997, 28(1):14-19.

De Stéfani E, Deneo-Pellegrini H, Mendilaharsu M, Ronco AL: Essential fatty acids and breast cancer: a case-control study in Uruguay. *Int. J. Cancer* 1998, 76:491-494.

Greenwald P, Clifford CK, Milner JA: Diet and cancer prevention. *Eur. J. Cancer* 2001; 37:948-965.

La Vecchia C, Tavani A: Fruit and vegetables, and human cancer. *Eur. J. Cancer Prev.* 1998, 7(1):3-8.

Lichtenstein P, Holm NV, Verkasalo PK, Iliadou A, Kaprio J, Koskenvuo M et al: Environmental and heritable factors in the causation of cancer--analyses of cohorts of twins from Sweden, Denmark, and Finland. *N. Engl. J. Med.* 2000, 343:78-85.

Michels KB: The contribution of the environment (especially diet) to breast cancer risk. *Breast Cancer Res.* 2002, 4:58-61.

Riboli E, Norat T: Epidemiologic evidence of the protective effect of fruit and vegetables on cancer risk. *Am. J. Clin. Nutr.* 2003, 78:559S-569S.

Ronco AL, De Stéfani E, Mendilaharsu M, Deneo-Pellegrini H: Meat, fat and the risk of breast cancer: a case-control study from Uruguay. *Int. J. Cancer* 1996, 65: 328-331.

Ronco AL, De Stéfani E, Boffetta P, Deneo-Pellegrini H, Mendilaharsu M, Leborgne F: Vegetables, fruits, and related nutrients and risk of breast cancer: a case control study in Uruguay. *Nutr. Cancer* 1999, 35(2): 111-119.

Ronco AL, De Stéfani E: Fitoestrógenos y riesgo de cáncer mamario: un estudio caso control. *Rev. Med. Urug.* 1999, 3: 94-102.

Ronco AL, De Stéfani E, Dáttoli R: Dairy foods and risk of breast cancer: a case-control study in Montevideo, Uruguay. *Eur. J. Cancer Prev.* 2002; 11(5):457-463.

Ronco AL, De Stéfani E, Fabra A: White meat intake and the risk of breast cancer: a case-control study in Montevideo, Uruguay. *Nutr. Res.* 2003; 23(2):151-162.

Ronco AL: Use of artificial neural networks in modeling associations of discriminant factors: towards an intelligent selective breast cancer screening. *Artif. Intell. Med.* 1999, 6(3):299-309.

Ronco AL, De Stéfani E: Role of classical and dietary discriminant factors for classification of breast cancer high-risk populations: a study with neural networks. *Cancer Strategy* 1999, 1: 203-209.

Smith-Warner SA, Spiegelman D, Yaun SS, Adami HO, Beeson WL, van den Brandt PA et al: Intake of fruits and vegetables and risk of breast cancer: a pooled analysis of cohort studies. *JAMA* 2001, 285:769–776.

Snyderwine EG: Diet and mammary gland carcinogenesis. *Recent Results Cancer Res.* 1998, 152:3–10.

Stata: Stata User's Guide and Reference Manual. Release 6. Stata Press, College Station, Texas, 1999.

Steinmetz KA, Potter JD: Vegetables, fruit, and cancer prevention: a review. *J. Am. Diet Assoc.* 1996, 96(10):1027-39.

Steinmetz KA, Potter JD: Vegetables, fruit and cancer. I. Epidemiology. *Cancer Causes Control* 1991, 2(5):325-357.

Steinmetz KA, Potter JD: Vegetables, fruit and cancer. II. Mechanisms. *Cancer Causes Control* 1991, 2(6):427-442.

Willett WC, Stampfer MJ: Total energy intake: implications for epidemiologic analyses. *Am. J. Epidemiol.* 1986, 124:17-27.

Willett WC: Diet, nutrition, and avoidable cancer. *Environ. Health Perspect.* 1995; 8:165-70.

World Cancer Research Fund: Food, Nutrition and the prevention of cancer: a global perspective. *World Cancer Research Fund*, Washington DC, 1997, pp.252-287.

In: Frontiers in Breast Cancer Research
Editor: Louis P. Fortugno, pp. 187-195
ISBN: 978-1-60021-671-8

Chapter IX

Role of Mammography in the Diagnosis and Screening of Breast Cancer among an Egyptian Cohort

Sherif Omar[1], Nelly H. Ali-Eldin[2,*] and Hanan Goefel[3]
[1]Surgical Oncology Department, NCI, Cairo University, Egypt
[2]Biostatistics and Epidemiology Department, NCI, Cairo University, Egypt
[3]Cairo-Scan Diagnostic Centre, Cairo Egypt

Abstract

Background: In Egypt, a study on 3747 mastectomies, showed that patients usually had poor presentation in terms of unfavorable histology, high tumor burden, and lymph node metastasis. Because advanced breast cancer has the poorest survival rate and is the most resource intensive to treat, measures to reduce the stage at diagnosis are likely to have the greatest benefit in terms of survival and costs. Mammography is the sole acceptable method for breast cancer screening, but its efficacy is still disputable.

Our objective was to evaluate the potential role of mammography in the diagnosis and screening of breast cancer among a cohort of Egyptian women.

Methods: From July 2002 to December 2003 a total of 7220 mammograms were performed in a private diagnostic centre in Cairo, Egypt and computerized data were retrieved for analysis. Pathology was confirmed in 504 cases.

Results: Screening as baseline, routine or in high risk groups was the basis in 49.4% of mammographic examinations, and diagnosis and follow-up in 50.6%. Median age was 48 (13-88) years and premenopausal represented 51.6%. As a whole, mammography was sensitive in detecting breast cancers in 80.3% of cases. Sensitivity was higher among those above age of 50 year, in postmenopausal women and with diagnostic mammography. Rate of false negatives was 6.6 %. Screening mammography was valuable in early detection of 2 cases with T1 stage tumors.

---

*Correspondance: Nelly H. Ali Eldin. Assist Prof. of Cancer Epidemiology. National Cancer Institute, Cairo University Fom El Khalig, Cairo, Egypt. E mail: nhassan@nci.edu.eg; Telephone: +2 02-5160544 /+2 0101720668; Fax: +2 02-3644720.

Conclusions: Mammography as a diagnostic tool was found to be of fair quality but poor in screening of the breasts among the Egyptian cohort. So, efforts of early detection could begin through public education to increase the awareness of breast cancer health care. Clinical breast examination should be considered as integral component of routine breast care especially in women with limited access to mammography. When needed and if resources permit expand early detection efforts to include mammographic screening.

Keywords: *Breast cancer, mammography, screening, accuracy, and cost effectiveness.*

Introduction

Breast cancer is the most common cause of cancer in women and the second cause of death in the United States [1]. The mortality rate and the possibility of breast conservation are linked to the size of cancer at the time of detection [2] Hospital-based registry at National Cancer Institute, Cairo University, reported 2000 breast cancer cases in the year 2001 with a relative frequency of 36.5% among females [3]. The first regional population-based registry in Egypt [4] illustrated an age-adjusted rate of 49.6 breast cancer case per 100,000 Egyptian women. Although mammographic screening of breast cancer alone or combined with CBE have shown to reduce mortality for about 30% in women over age of 50 years, this reduction is much less evidenced in younger population [5]. Some researchers believe that mammographic screening for breast cancer is controversial as reflected by greatly varying national policies [6]. Others considered the several drawbacks of mammography the major being its tendency for false positive and false negative results [5]. This study aimed at evaluating the potential role of mammographic examination in the diagnosis and screening of breast cancer among a cohort of Egyptian women.

Methods

In a private diagnostic centre in Cairo, Egypt between July 2002 to December 2003, 7220 mammograms have been done for 6585 patients, 30 of them were males (0.5%). It was done using “Senograph” DMR GE conventional mammography ± ultrasound. Ultrasound was used for examining 556 subjects (7.7%) Computerized data included patient name, date of visit and date of birth DOB as identifiers. DOB (age) was unknown in 114 cases. Other data included menopausal status (missed in 26 cases), risk factors for breast cancer, and result of mammography according to BIRAD (*Breast Imaging Reporting and Data*) System (**7**). Results according to BIRAD system were categorized into: 1 = normal breast, 2 = benign lesion, 3 = probably benign, 4 = probably malignant, 5 = malignant lesion.

To calculate accuracy of mammography, cyto-pathologic results after follow-up with the referring physicians and/or phone calls of examined subjects were used to confirm or preclude diagnosis of breast cancer. Pathology was confirmed in 504 cases. To conclude that mammography is sensitive in detecting breast cancer, it had to be either BIRAD category 4 or 5 and to be specific in precluding breast cancer it had to be either 1 or 2. Mammography result with BIRAD category 3 was inconclusive and was not considered in measuring accuracy. Seventy three cases had pathology result (67 malignant and 6 benign or normal) and were BIRAD category 3.

Cost Estimation

A study conducted at NCI, Cairo University showed that direct medical cost of management (diagnosis, treatment and follow-up) of breast cancer increased by an average of 2000 LE for those who end follow-up with recurrence or death compared to those with no evidence of disease NED at end of follow-up [8]. Effectiveness of screening mammography was measured by the net cost of screening minus the treatment savings averted by early detection of cancer cases per year of life saved YLS [9]). Effectiveness was measured also, by the number of target population needed to screen to prevent one death of breast cancer [10]. In this study, cost was estimated as non-profit direct cost of screening mammography, and included number of views, number of time it was done, cost of reading by radiologists, collection, automation and management of data.

Statistical Methods

Chi-square test was used for comparing independent proportions. Confidence interval for proportions was estimated using the following formula p – z * SE to p + z * SE where p = proportion, z = reliability coefficient (1.96 for 95% interval) and SE (standard error) = √ pq / n where q = 1 – p and n = number of group. [11]

Results

Mammographic examination were done for the reason of screening (n = 3569, 49.4%), diagnosis of breast lesion (n = 3151, 43.6%) or follow-up of the breast (n = 500, 6.9%). Screening included first-time or base screening (n = 970, 27.2%), routine screening (n= 1559, 43.7%) and screening of the breast after mastectomy, high risk mastectomy HRM (n=573, 16.1%) and after chemotherapy, high risk chemotherapy HRC (n=467, 13.1%). For those coming for diagnosis of a suspicious breast, clinically they presented with a mass (n = 1737, 55.1%), pain (n = 968, 30.7%), skin changes (n = 322, 10.2%) and others as axillary swelling (n = 89, 2.8%) or asymmetry of the breast (n = 35, 1.1%). The third group came for follow up of breast cyst (n = 246, 49.2%), fibroadenoma (n = 59, 11.8%), breast density (n = 54, 10.8%), calcification (n = 31, 6.2%) and others (n = 110, 22%).

Cohort characteristics and risk factors: males represented small number (n = 30). Median age of the whole cohort was 48 (13-88) years. Median age according to type or reason of mammography was 51 (25-88) among those coming for screeing, 43 (13-87) in patients coming for diagnosis and for follow up median age was 47 (18-78) years. Risk factors in the whole group and categorized by type of mammography are shown in table 1.

Table 1. Risk factors of breast cancer according to type of mammography

Risk factor	Whole group N = 7220 N (%)	Screening N = 3569 N (%)	Diagnostic N = 3151 N (%)	Follow up N = 500 N (%)
Family history				
Fisrt degree	551 (7.6)	334 (9.4)	179 (5.7)	38 (7.6)
Second degree	494 (6.8)	254 (7.1)	196 (6.2)	44 (8.8)
Nulliparity	658 (9.2)	251 (7.0)	358 (11.5)	49 (9.8)
HRT	555 (7.7)	445 (12.5)	71 (2.3)	39 (7.8)
Hysterectomy	596 (8.3)	404 (11.3)	153 (4.9)	39 (7.8)
Antiestrogen	580 (8.0)	554 (15.5)	17 (0.5)	9 (1.8)
Previous cancer	114 (1.6)	91 (2.5)	18 (0.6)	5 (1.0)

HRT = hormonal replacement therapy.

Table 2. Accuracy of mammography

	True positive sensitivity	False negative	True negative Specificity	False positive
Whole group	237/295 (80.3)	58/295 (19.7)	127/136 (93.4)	9/136 (6.6)
By type				
Screening	35/66 (53.0)	31/66 (47.0)	78/83 (94)	5/83 (6)
Diagnostic	186/208 (89.4)	22/208 (10.6)	35/38 (92.1)	3/38 (7.9)
Follow up (FU)	16/21 (76.2)	5/21 (23.8)	14/15 (93.3)	1/15 (6.7)
By age				
< 40 years	25/38 (65.8)	13/38 (34.2)	17/18 (94.4)	1/18 (5.6)
40-<50	72/90 (80.0)	18/90 (20.0)	38/41 (92.7)	3/41 (7.3)
>= 50 years	137/163 (84.0)	26/163 (16.0)	71/76 (93.4)	5/76 (6.6)
Menopause				
Pre-	85/113 (75.2)	28/113 (24.8)	43/47 (91.5)	4/47 (8.5)
Post-	152/182 (83.5)	30/182 (16.5)	84/89 (94.4)	5/89 (5.6)

For the whole group nulliparity (9.2%) was the commonest underlying reason for mammography followed by hysterectomy (8.3%) and antiestrogen treatment (8.0%). Antiestrogent treatment (15.5%), hormonal replacement therapy (12.5%) and hysterectomy (11.3%) were the leading causes of screening normal breast. Associated risk factors for diagnosing suspicious breast lesion was nulliparity (11.5%) followed by fisrt and second degree family history (5.7% and 6.2% respectively)

Accuracy of Mammography

Pathology was confirmed in 504 subjects. True positive rate, false negative, true negative and false positive rate were calculated, and shown in table 2. Seventy three cases were excluded being BIRAD category 3. Number of malignant cases was 295 and normal or benign lesions were 136.

Accuracy as a whole shows false negative rate of 19.7% and false positive rate of 6.6%. When comparing accuracy according to rationale of mammography, results showed that diagnostic mammography had a significantly higher sensitivity than screening mammography (89.4%, 95%CI = 85.2% - 93.6% versus 53%, 95% CI = 41% - 65%) and p value < 0.001. Sensitivity of mammography was higher in those above 50 years (84% and 95% CI = 78.4 - 89.6) than younger age group <40 years (65.8% and 95%CI = 50.8 - 80.8), p = 0.01. Though did not reach significance level, sensitivity of mammography among post-menopausal women was higher (83.5% 95% CI = 78.2 -88.9) than pre-menopausal women (75.2%, 95% CI = 67.3 - 83.1), p = 0.08.

Early Detection and Effectiveness

With the aid of mammography early detection was possible in 11 patients. Pathologic data of these cases showed that:

(a) A case with DCIS came for diagnostic mammography
(b) 2 cases were T1a stage (4 and 5 mm in diameter) and proved to be lymph node LN negative. These 2 cases came for diagnosis of suspicious breast mass.
(c) 2 cases were T1b stage (>0.5 - ≤ 1cm). One of them presented with a mass and was LN positive (< 3 nodes) and the other with pain and was LN negative.
(d) 6 cases were T1c stage (>1cm - < 2cm). Four of them came for diagnosis; of a mass (2/4), painful breast (1/4), and the last with skin changes. The other 2 cases came for routine screening. The first was 54 year (<3 positive LN) and the second was 65 years and LN negative.

Based upon direct cost estimation, the total cost of screening mammography (n = 3569) was calculated to be 214,140 LE. Because screened women were not invited for screening (volunteers) and long term follow-up of screened cohort was not feasible, so it was assumed that the 2 cases (<2 cm masses) of breast cancer detected with routine screening mammography will have >90% chance of surviving the first 5 years [12] and 80% chance of 10 years survival [13]. The net cost of screening mammography would be 210,140 LE cost per year of life saved 21,140 LE. We could summarize effectiveness as the number needed to screen to prevent one death of breast cancer as 3569/2 = 1985.

Risk of Mammography

The frequency of mammography examination in our cohort was recorded in 3907 cases. In 3619 cases it was 1st, 2nd or 3rd mammographic examination. In 239 it was the 4th – 6th visit. Twenty five cases had had 7-9 mammograms and 24 cases had at least 10 (10-14) mammograms. In our study predisposed women to radiation risk (receiving HRT) represented 7.7% (n = 555). Only 13 (2.3%) were initially examined by ultrasound. Out of 1703 cases <40 years, 18.4% have been initially examined by ultrasound. Out of those who had at least 10 mammograms up to the end of this study, one case was treated with hormonal replacement therapy.

Discussion

Among women around the globe breast cancer is both the most common cancer and the leading cause of cancer-related deaths [14]. In Egypt, the NCI hospital-based registry [3] and El-Gharbia regional population-based registry [4] showed that breast cancer ranked the ist among all types of cancer (19.1%) and the first among females with a frequency of 36.5%. In developing countries and those with limited resources, at least half of the women have advanced or metastatic breast cancer at time of diagnosis [14]. A recent study conducted at NCI, Cairo University on 3747 mastectomies showed that 70.6% of patients presented with lymph node metastasis. In the same study median tumor size at diagnosis was 3 (0.5 -20.0) cm. Carcinomas in situ were 1.1% and 8.5% were T1 stage with only 2.4% T1 with negative lymph nodes [15]. Because advanced breast cancer has the poorest survival rate and is the most resource intensive to treat, measures to reduce the stage at diagnosis are likely to have the greatest overall benefit in terms of both survival and costs [14].

It is known that mammography screening represents the only means by which the mortality rate from breast cancer could be modified [9]. The present study represented a starting effort to evaluate the value of mammography as a diagnostic and screening tool of breast cancer among a sector of Egyptian women. In the present study the diagnostic centre is a private one and women who presented to it are preliminary upper and middle income Egyptian; hence they are not representative of the overall Cairo population but nevertheless are an important segment.

The result of our study showed that mammography was equally used as screening (49.4%) and diagnostic/FU (50.6%) tool. This reflects the state of breast health care awareness among examined population. False negative rate of mammography was found to be 19.7%. This result revealed the fact that; these cases would be missed unless the surgeons or primary health care-givers had the suspicion of malignancy. Documented false negative rates are widely variable depending on mammography tool but generally it seems to give rates near to our results. In an Indian study false negative rate ranged from 3% to 20% [16]. In another study which aimed at reviewing accuracy of mammography by reviewing published data it found that mammograms miss approximately 12% to 37% of cancers [17] Results of the present study showed that sensitivity was much affected by the rationale of mammography use. Sensitivity in screening mammography was 53% (41.0 – 65.0) compared to 89.4% (85.2 – 93.6) in diagnostic mammography, $p < 0.001$. This might be explained by extra number of X-ray views performed in the diagnosis of suspicious breast rather than apparently normal one. Most of the cases who came for diagnosis of suspicious breast lesion were clinically examined by a physician before mammography. Screening interval cancer, might explain this low rate [18]. Age was an important factor that associated to accuracy of mammography. Sensitivity of mammography was significantly higher among women above 50 years (84% and 95% CI = 78.4 - 89.6) than younger age group <40 years (65.8% and 95%CI = 50.8 - 80.8), $p = 0.01$. Those who were between 40-50 years did not differ significantly from younger nor older age groups. Influence of age is well established and is well known in controversy around starting age of screening mammography and the screening interval [19]. Several literature reviews of published studies suggest that screening of women less than 50 years of age does not statistically significantly reduce mortality from breast cancer and these results are not explained by screening intervals or patient compliance to screening [20]. The same authors concluded that screening is effective in decreasing mortality from breast cancer for women older than 50 years. For women less than 50, mammography screening programs displace resources that could have a greater benefit in women's health status if used for other purposes [20].

It is generally assumed that radiation risk from mass screening of breast cancer may be neglected. This is questionable in view of the high biological effectiveness of low energy X-rays used in radiography of the breasts. The hormonal replacement therapy HRT should be considered for the unexpected high rates of radiation-induced breast cancer cases. [21] The same author stated that HRT itself makes mammography screening less effective by adversely affecting both the sensitivity and specificity of screening mammography. One study have showed a reduction in sensitivity of screening mammography of between 7% to 21% in the current HRT users [22]. In our study HRT users accounted for 7.7% of examined women with one of them had been screened for more than 10 times in her life.

The cost of screening mammography of the breasts among the Egyptian cohort was found to be high compared to other more privileged countries. In a nationwide Finnish study, the cost of breast carcinoma mammographic screening per YLS was $18,955 ($15,502 to $40,308) [23]. The cost per YLS among the Egyptian cohort was found to be 21,140 LE. Studies of fair qualities or better [10] found the number needed to screen to prevent one death from breast cancer after approximately 14 years of observation to be 1224 (665 to 2564). In this study it was estimated to be 1985. It may not be fair to compare cost effectiveness with more developed countries because in this study it was based upon estimation and probability of surviving rather than long term follow up. On other hand, as a developing country health care resources are limited and economic evaluation plays a critical role in resource allocation, health care policy and clinical decision.

Conclusion and Recommendations

Mammography as a diagnostic tool was found to be of fair quality but poor in screening of the breasts among the Egyptian cohort. Up-till now, the evidence is insufficient to recommend for or against routine CBE alone to screen for breast cancer [24]. So, efforts of early detection in Egypt could begin through public education to increase the awareness of breast cancer health care. Clinical breast examination should be considered as integral component of routine breast care especially in women with limited access to mammography. When resources permit expand early detection efforts to include mammographic screening.

References

[1] Contesso G and Omar Sh. Breast Cancer. *National Cancer Institute*, Cairo University.2001:1-8, 4th ed.

[2] Laundis SH, Murray T, Bolden S : Cancer statistics. CA Cancer 1998. *J. Clin.* 48 (1): 6 – 29.

[3] Cancer Registry at National Cancer Institute, Cairo University. *Oral presentation at National Joint Cancer Conference of the Egyptian Cancer Society (NCI) and Ministry of Health Cancer Centres*. 22-24 March 2002 Luxor – Egypt.

[4] Cancer Profile in Gharbia – Egypt, *Methods and Results,* 1999, December 2002 in collaboration with Middle East Cancer Consorium MECC and Ministry of Health and Population.

[5] Primic-Zakely M,: Screening mammography for early detection of breast cancer. *Ann. Oncol*. 1999; 10 Suppl 6:121-127.

[6] Olzen O, Gotzsche P. Cochrane review on screening for breast cancer with mammography. *The Lancet* 2001;358:1340-42.

[7] American College of Radiology. *Breast Imaging Reporting and Data System* (BI-RADS). 3rd ed. Reston (VA): American College of Radiology; 1998. [Last accessed: 02/06/2003].

[8] Manar M. Moneer: Medical cost estimation study regarding management of the most common malignancies among Egyptian females (aged 18 years and above) attending the National Cancer Institute, Cairo University. *Thesis in Public Health*. Faculty of Medicine, Cairo University, 2000. MD.

[9] Szeto KL, Devlin NJ: The cost-effectiveness of mammography screening evidence from a microsimulation model for New Zealand. *Health Policy*. 1996; Nov;38(2):101-15.

[10] Humphrey LL, Helfand M, Chan BKS, Woolf SH. Breast cancer screening: a summary of the evidence for the U.S. Preventive Services Task Force. *Ann Intern Med.* 2002 Sep 3;137(5 Part 1):347-60.

[11] Kirkwood BR and Sterne JAC: Essential Medical Statistics. 2003 2nd edition by Blackwell *Science Ltd*, USA.

[12] Carter CL, Allen C, Henson DE. Relation of tumor size, lymph node status and survival in 24,740 breast cancer cases. *Cancer* 1989;63:181–187.

[13] Ravdin PM, Siminoff LA, Davis GJ, Mercer MB, Hewlett J, Gerson N, Parker HL.: Computer program to assist in making decisions about adjuvant therapy for women with early breast cancer. *J. Clin. Oncol*. 2001 Feb 15;19(4):980-91.

[14] Anderson BO, Braun S, Carlson RW, Gralow JR, Lagios MD, Lethman C, Schwartmann G, Vargas HI: Overview of breast health care guidelines for countries with limited resources. *Breast J.* 2003 May-Jun; 9 Suppl 2:S42-50.

[15] Nouh MA, Ismail H, Ali El-Din NH, El Bolkainy MN: Lymph node metastasis in breast carcinoma: clinicopathological correlations in 3747 patients. *J. Egypt Natl. Canc Inst.* 2004 Mar;16(1):50-6.

[16] Chabhra S: Breast Cancer screening – an update. Indian *J. Matern. Child Health.* 1995Jul-Sep;6(3):66-70.

[17] Woolf SH: The accuracy and effectiveness of routine population screening with mammography, prostate-specific antigen, and prenatal ultrasound: a review of published scientific evidence. *Int. J. Technol. Assess. Health Care.* 2001 Summer;17(3):375-304.

[18] Stephen WD, Catherine H and Jacques E: *Quantitaive methods for the evaluation of cancer screeing*. Arnolds, Hodder Headline Group, London 2001.1st edition.

[19] Law MR, Morris JK, Wald NJ: The importance of age in screeing for cancer. *J. Med. Screen.* 1999;6(1):16-20.

[20] Navarro AM, Kaplan RM: Mammography screening: prospects and opportunity costs. *Womens Health.* 1996 Winter;2(4):209-33.

[21] Kuni H, Schmitz-Feuerhake I, Dieckmann H.: Mammography screening-neglected aspects of radiation risks. *An Abstract* (Article in German) *Gesundheitswesen*: 2003 Jul; 65(7):443-6.

[22] Evans A: Hormone replacement therapy and mammography screening. *Clin. Radiol.* 2002 Jul; 57(7):563-4.

[23] Leivo T, Sintonen H, Tuominen R, Hakama M, Pukkala E, Heinonen OP. The cost-effectiveness of a nationwide breast carcinoma screening in Finland, 1987-1992. *Cancer.* 1999 Aug 15;86(4):638-46.

[24] U.S. Preventive Services Task Forces (USPSTF). Screening for Breast Cancer: Recommendations and Rationale Updates the 1996 recommendations contained in the *Guide to Clinical Preventive Services*, Second Edition.

In: Frontiers in Breast Cancer Research
Editor: Louis P. Fortugno, pp. 197-223
ISBN: 978-1-60021-671-8

Chapter X

How Fanconi Anemia and Breast Cancer are Connected

***Alex Lyakhovich and Jordi Surrallés*[*]**
Group of Mutagenesis, Department of Genetics and Microbiology, Universitat Autònoma de Barcelona, Bellaterra, Barcelona, Spain;
Centre for Biomedical Research on Rare Diseases (CIBERER), Bellaterra, Spain.

Abstract

Fanconi anaemia (FA) is one of the inherited anemias that characterized by congenital abnormalities, progressive bone marrow failure and cancer susceptibility. It is a recessive disorder: if both parents carry a mutation in the same FA gene, each of their children has a 25 per cent chance of inheriting the defective gene from both parents. Consequently, the child will have FA. Until recently all cloned FA genes considered being orphans, having nothing in common with any other known genes. However, recent discovery that the breast cancer susceptibility gene *BRCA2* is identical to the Fanconi anemia (FA) gene *FANCD1* made possible to reconsider this orphan status. In turn, FANCD2 Fanconi protein recruitment to chromatin is dependent on activation of another breast cancer susceptibility gene BRCA1 which seems to play a role of a switcher of the FA/BRCA pathway regulating chromosomal stability. Although cancer cells with non-functional *BRCA1* or *BRCA2* genes show chromosome damage similar to that in Fanconi anemia cells, it was not clear whether genetic mutations that cause Fanconi can also cause breast cancer. Then what is the connection between Fanconi anemia and breast cancer? Since the discovery of the new FA genes, it is becoming evident that there is a strong, yet unresolved, link between FA and BRCA pathway. For instance, children who inherited two copies of non-functional BRCA2-interecting protein, PALB2 (FANCN) developed a Fanconi anemia phenotype. At the same time, women inheriting one damaged copy of PALB2 have double risk of developing breast cancer. Mutations in another Fanconi gene FANCJ (*BRIP1*) is a risk factor for the breast cancer comprising a class with two breast cancer susceptibility genes, *CHEK2* and *ATM*, which upon exposure to other

* Correspondence concerning this article should be addressed to: Jordi Surrallés, Department of Genetics and Microbiology, Universitat Autonoma de Barcelona, Campus de Bellaterra, Bellaterra, Barcelona 08193, Spain. Tel.: + 34 93 581 18 30; Fax: + 34 93 581 23 87; E-mail: jordi.surralles@uab.es.

environmental risk factors may predispose a woman to cancer. Although all newly discovered FA genes are relatively small contributors to the overall incidence of breast cancers, their cumulative response may be amplified for maintaining the stability of the entire human genome. Accordingly, understanding the connection between the Fanconi genes and BRCA1/2 seems to hold potential for future cancer research.

Introduction

Fanconi Anemia (FA) is an autosomal recessive syndrome characterized by congenital abnormalities, progressive bone marrow failure (BMF), and susceptibility to cancer [1]. The disease is named for the Swiss pediatrician Guido Fanconi (1892-1979) who first described it [2]. In 1927 Fanconi reported a family with 3 brothers having slight stature, skin pigmentation and hypogonadism who had died in childhood from anemia. FA is inherited in an autosomal recessive manner undermining that one copy of an abnormal gene is passed on by each parent. FA occurs in all racial and ethnic groups at an extremely rare incident rates (about 1-5 per 1 000,000 live births) however, some ethnic groups (Ashkenazi Jews, Spanish gypsies) have almost 10 fold higher frequency [3-5].

Table. Fanconi Anemia complementation groups

Gene	DESCRIPTION OF GENES				
	Subtype	Location	Function	Accession Number	Prevalence (%) worldwide
FANCA (FAA , FA1)	A	16q24.3	Forms FA core complex	Z83067	66.0
FANCB	B	Xp22.31	Forms FA core complex	AK091383	0.8
FANCC	C	9q22.3	Forms FA core complex	BC006303	9.6
BRCA2 (FANCD1, FACD, FANCD)	D1	13q12-q13	Forms chromatin complex	U43746	3.3
FANCD2 (FACD, FANCD)	D2	3p25.3	Forms chromatin complex	AF340183	3.3
FANCE (FACE)	E	6p22-p21	Forms FA core complex	AF265210	2.5
FANCF (FAF)	F	11p15	Forms FA core complex	NM_022725	2.1
FANCG (XRCC9)	G	9p13	Forms FA core and chromatin complexes	AJ007669	8.8
FANCI	I		Not cloned	reserved	1.6
FANCJ (BRIP1, BACH1)	J	17q22.2	DEAH/box helicase	AF360549	1.6
FANCL (PHF9)	L	2p16.1	Ubiquitin ligase	AK001197	0.4
FANCM (KIAA1596, Hef)	M	14q21.3	Helicase, translocase	AK001672	0.4
FANCN (PALB2)	N	16p12.1	DNA helicase	NM_024675	>0.1

Comment: *FANCI* gene has not yet been cloned, but is implicated by functional complementation studies. *FANCH* is omitted due to withdrawal of complementation group H (see *Am. J. Hum. Genet. 67*:759-762, 2000). Since *FANCK* sounds like FANCA and may be mistakenly interpreted, the letter K has been missed out; complementation group D was divided into *FANCD1* and *FANCD2*. As described in the text, prevalence of FA for some populations (e.g. Spanish gypsies, Ashkenazi Jews) is different from the total worldwide prevalence.

Patients may be suspected of having the disease if they have particular birth defects, develop decreased blood counts or have a café-au-lait spots on the skin [6-8]. The hypersensitivity of FA cells to chromosomal breakage by cross-linking agents is used for diagnostic purposes to confirm the clinical diagnosis [9,10]. In general, FA is diagnosed between 2 and 15 years of age, but as a rule by age of eight majority of children with FA develops progressive bone marrow failure (aplastic anaemia) and are further predisposed to acute myeloid leukaemia and solid tumors. Moreover, more than half of those who survive BMF tend to develop cancers in areas of the body where cells normally reproduce rapidly, such as the mouth, esophagus, the intestinal and urinary tracts, and the reproductive organs [11].

FA is caused by mutations in at least 13 genes and accordingly is subtyped by 13 complementation groups abbreviated from A to N [12]. Mutations in the A and C genes account for about 75% of patients in the United States with Fanconi anemia, while the rest distribution is disproportional (see Table). For instance, in all Spanish population, over 80% of FA patients are subtyped with FANCA group, while Ashkenazi Jews always reveal FANCC group [13,14]. Overall, FA genes serve to prevent cells from fixing damaged DNA or generating toxic, oxygen free radicals that damage cells. Additional effects include but not limited to abnormal metabolism of xenobiotic compounds and defects in signal transduction pathways.

Until recently most of FA genes considered to be orphan ones as they did not reveal any common functions or conserved structures with each other or with any other known gene in any other organism [15]. Attempts to match gene sequences to any known disease-sensitive genes revealed pure homology and did not suggest a model organism to facilitate this area of research. However, recent discovery that the breast cancer susceptibility gene *BRCA2* is identical to the FA gene *FANCD1* made possible to reconsider this orphan status [16]. Another data showing that recruitment of FANCD2 is dependent on breast cancer susceptibility gene product BRCA1 suggested involvement of FANCD2 into triggering mechanism of the BRCA pathway thus regulating chromosomal stability [17]. Although heterozygous mutations in both *BRCA1* and *BRCA2* genes are characterized by predisposition to breast, ovarian and other cancers, the risk of developing cancer that is associated with *BRCA1* and *BRCA2* cancer-predisposing mutations is not known and appears to be variable even within families of similar ethnic background with the same mutation [18]. It was well studied that cancer cells with non-functional *BRCA1* or *BRCA2* genes show chromosome damage similar to that in Fanconi anemia cells. However, for a long time it was not clear whether genetic mutations that cause Fanconi can also cause breast cancer [7]. Since the discovery of the new FA genes, it is becoming evident that there is a strong, yet unresolved, link between FA and BRCA pathway. For instance, children who inherited two copies of non-functional BRCA2-interacting gene product FANCN (PALB2) develop a Fanconi anemia phenotype [19]. At the same time, women inheriting one damaged copy of *FANCN* have double risk of developing breast cancer. Mutations in another Fanconi gene *FANCJ* (*BRIP1*or *BATCH1*) is a risk factor for the breast cancer comprising a class with two breast cancer susceptibility genes, *CHEK2* and *ATM*, which upon exposure to other environmental risk factors may predispose a woman to cancer [20]. Although all newly discovered FA genes are relatively small contributors to the overall incidence of breast cancers, their cumulative response may be amplified for maintaining the stability of the entire human genome. Accordingly, understanding the connection between the Fanconi and BRCA1/2 genes and gene products seems to hold potential for future cancer research making FA an important genetic model for the study of breast cancer susceptibility and cancer suppression mechanisms.

Communication of FA Gene Products

In accordance with current model, the Fanconi anemia proteins are comprised into several major groups with regard to their known functions. The group which is conventionally called FA-core complex consists of at least eight gene products incorporating FANCA, FANCB, FANCC, FANCE, FANCF, FANCG, FANCL and FANCM proteins and couple recently identified players including FAAP1000 and FAAP24 [21,22]. This complex is mobile and can be regulated by phosphorylation of one of its components [24]. In normal conditions core proteins seem to be functioning in some other parts of cell compartments however, upon exposure to DNA damaging agents (DNA cross-linkers, oxidative damage, UV or ionizing radiation) this complex is assembled by joining FANCA:FANCG and FANCC:FANCE subcomplexes with the help of FANCF [25] following by recruitment of FANCL, an ubiquitin ligase that mediates ubiquitinylation of another FA protein called FANCD2 (see Figure 1A). This ubiquitinylation, preceding phosphorylation in at least two sites, activates FANCD2 and targets it to chromatin, preferentially to the sites of DNA damages [26]. At chromatin FANCD2 forms another FA complex (chromatin complex) interacting with FANCD1 (BRCA2), FANCE and γH2AX [27,28]. Conventionally, when describing multiprotein pathways, scientists agreed to divide all proteins into up- and downstream ones depending on whose action precedes in time. Consecutively, components of a FA core complex should be called upstream of the FANCD2 ubiquitinylation pathway and components of chromatin FA complex incorporating ubiquitinylated FANCD2 - downstream acting proteins. This scheme suffers from some limitations and is only useful when describing cascade of events where each partner's role is precisely defined. Moreover, this should be applied only to one specific pathway as, for example some proteins being called downstream ones, may be upstream in respect to some others from different pathway. For our purposes, however, we are going to use this abbreviation. Monoubiquitinylated FANCD2 is accumulated in chromatin complex at stall replication fork that encounters a DNA cross-link , apparently leading to repair of the cross-link possibly through homologous recombination (HR) and translesion synthesis (TLS) [1]. The cell cycle checkpoint kinase ATR is required for the efficient monoubiquitination of FANCD2, while another checkpoint kinase, ATM, directly phosphorylates FANCD2 at least by two residues and controls the ionizing radiation (IR)-inducible intra-S-phase checkpoint [26]. The turnover of this pathway is terminated by FANCD2 deubiquitination mediated by USP1 [29]. After that step the FA pathway is inactivated. Depending on situation, arrangement of FA core complex could be different. It seems that at least two types of complexes are formed. The first one, as described above, involves presumably FA proteins. The second one, however, may involve interaction of a core FA complex with Topoisomerase III, BLM and FANCM proteins. According to this model, unidentified ubiquitin-conjugating enzyme (E1) transfers ubiquitin molecule to an E2 (yet unknown). In turn, the FANCD2 substrate mediated by ATR-dependent phosphorylations on the FANCD2 protein may bind to FANCL. The BRCA2/FANCD1 protein is connected to the FA pathway by interactions with the FANCG and FANCD2 proteins, both of which co-localise with the RAD51 recombinase, which is regulated by BRCA2. FANCG was found to interact with XRCC3 and is proposed to play a role in building multiprotein complexes that facilitate HR repair [30]. A recently identified component of FA network - γH2AX seems to play a crucial role in FA pathway (see Figure 1B).

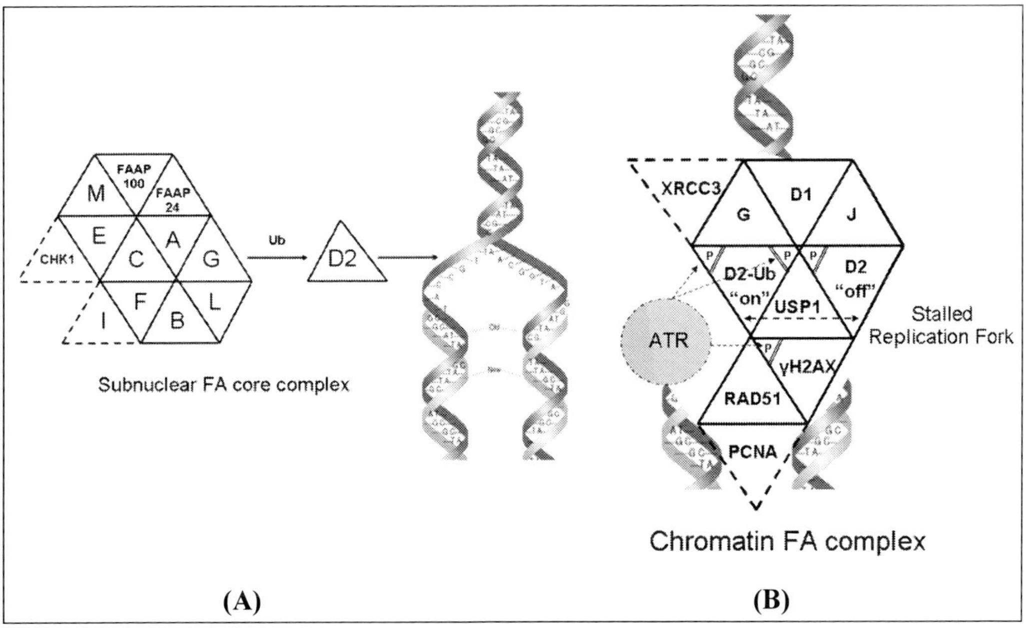

Figure 1. Schematic interaction of the FA pathway. (A) Subnuclear protein core complex contains the FA proteins A, B, C, E, F, G, L, M and possibly I and CHK1 mediate complex formation but do not participate in its formation and therefore are depicted with dotted lines. During S phase, when a replication fork encounters a DNA cross-link, the FA subnuclear complex is sequentially assembled. Formation of this complex is required for ubiquitinylation of FANCD2 followed by its relocation to stalled replication fork. (B) Chromatin FA complex is formed by phosphorylation of γH2AX and FANCD2 by ATR (not included in this complex) followed by ubiquitinylation of FANCD2. It contains BRCA2 and possibly FANCJ. This activation leads to the monoubiquitinaiton of FANCD2, which is then targeted to chromatin containing the cross-link in BRCA1-dependent manner. FANCD2-Ub then loads onto chromatin where it mediates repair of the cross-link possibly through HR and TLS. FANCD2 is then deubiquitinated by USP1, thereby inactivating the pathway.

Although in the cells deficient in H2AX or having non-phosphorylated (mutant) form of γH2AX FANCD2 is normally activated, these cells reveal FA-like phenotype with all similar hallmarks of FA patients including sensitivity to cross-linking agents and impairment to target FANCD2 into the sites of DNA damage [29]. After this long introduction describing FA complex formation, we may now link these events to the subject of our chapter – connection to breast cancer susceptible genes. Since FA complex is associated with chromatin it was suggested that it may function as a sensor of DNA damaging cascades [24]. Recently, two more FA genes have been identified. PALB2 (FANCN) and BRIP1 (FANCJ) function likewise BRCA2/FANCD1 of the FANCD2 activation step. Checkpoint kinase 2 (CHEK2, Chk2) emerges another important signal transducer of cellular responses to DNA damage and functions in a ATM-BRCA2-CHEK2 pathway [31,32]. We know that many components of these cascades involve other breast cancer (BRCA) susceptible genes or genes indirectly regulating BRCA functions. Therefore, finding connection in/between these groups of genes and FA genes would serve additional understanding of how these genes may work together and whether defects in one or several FA genes may amplify misbalance in normal functioning of BRCA.

BRCA Pathway

One of the first evidences for a gene linked to hereditary breast cancer was released by geneticist Mary-Claire King who by studying families that had breast and ovarian cancer history across several generations had positioned a gene on chromosome 17 that might be responsible for breast cancers [33]. In 1994 the gene was finally isolated by the scientists at Myriad Genetics which they called *Breast Cancer 1*, or later *BRCA1*. An altered *BRCA1* has been linked to the development of breast and ovarian cancer [34]. A year later a second gene located on chromosome 13 and called *Breast Cancer 2*, early onset gene (*BRCA2*), was isolated by Richard Wooster´s and Michael Stratton´s groups [35,36]. The big surprise came after discovery that only 5% of breast cancer cases are linked to the *BRCA* genes. In other words, if a woman does not have the altered *BRCA1*, this does not necessarily mean she will be free of breast cancer during her lifetime [37]. To resolve this puzzle it was suggested that the rest 95% of breast cancer patients who are not *BRCA* carriers should have some other mutated genes linked to BRCA. However, attempts to screen women with breast cancers for some unidentified genes that could have mutated before or during cancer's development failed. Since then, researchers have learned that both BRCA1 and 2 gene products interact with other proteins comprising a family collectively known as the BRCA pathway (see Figure 2). BRCA network overlaps with the BASC (BRCA1-associated genome surveillance complex). This complex includes tumor suppressors and DNA damage repair proteins MSH2, MSH6, MLH1, ATM, BLM, and the RAD50-MRE11-NBS1 protein complex. Although the *BRCA* genes themselves appear only slightly connected to common, nonhereditary cancers, emerging evidence suggests that defects in other parts of the BRCA pathway might be critical in driving breast cancers. Let us briefly outline several relevant members of the BRCA network.

BRCA1

The BRCA1 gene is located on chromosome 17 spanning more than 80 kb of genomic DNA and encoding a 7.8-kb transcript composed of 22 coding exons [38]. The normal gene product gives a protein of 1863 amino acids (220 kDa) that contains phosphorylated residues and is located in the nucleus [39]. The transcription of *BRCA1* is induced late in the G1 phase of the cell cycle and remains elevated during the S phase, indicating some role during DNA synthesis [40,41]. A variety of evidence now points to BRCA1 as being directly involved in the DNA repair process. The BRCA1 gene product interacts with the RAD51 protein, a key component in homologous recombination and double-strand break repair [42]. BRCA1 and BRCA2 are associated with each other at sites of DNA synthesis after the induction of DNA damage [43]. In order to study the function of *BRCA1*, homozygous knockout mice were developed. In most cases, the complete loss of function of *BRCA1* results in embryonic lethality characterized by a lack of cell proliferation [44,45]. Finally, *BRCA1* knockout mice can be partially rescued by crossing with a *p53* knockout strain suggesting that these genes crosstalk with the p53 -mediated DNA damage checkpoint [46]. To summarize, *BRCA1* serves as a "caretaker," like p53, maintaining genomic stability [47]. When this function is lost, it probably allows for the accumulation of other genetic defects that are themselves directly responsible for cancer formation.

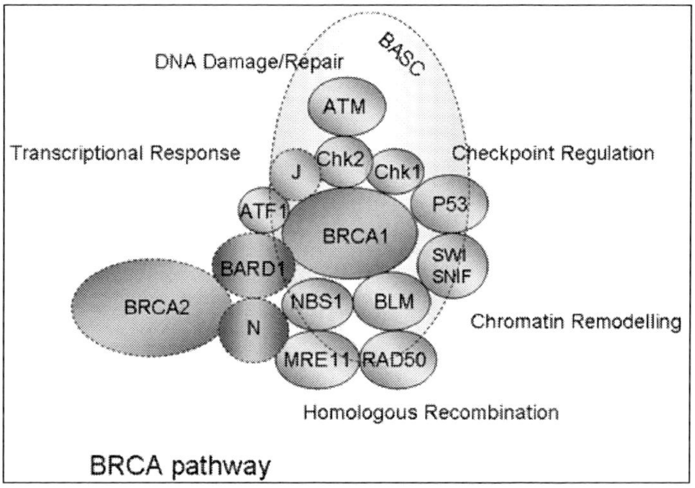

Figure 2. Schematic structure of the BRCA pathway. BRCA and BRCA-related pathways safeguard genetic content, and are interconnected with major intracellular events including checkpoint control, chromatin remodelling, DNA damage recognition, double-strand break repair, checkpoint control, transcription regulation and many others. BASC (BRCA1-associated genome surveillance complex) overlaps with BRCA pathway and includes tumor suppressors and DNA damage repair proteins MSH2, MSH6, MLH1, ATM, BLM, and the RAD50-MRE11-NBS1 protein complex. Functions of FANCN, FANCJ and BRCA2 in BRCA pathway are not well understood and therefore these proteins are depicted with dotted circles.

BRCA2

The *BRCA2* gene belongs to a class of genes known as tumor suppressor genes. It codes for a 380-kd protein and has no recognizable motifs and no apparent relation to the BRCA1. However, both BRCA1 and BRCA2 appear to share a number of functional similarities explaining why mutations in these genes lead to a specific hereditary predisposition to breast and ovarian cancer [48]. BRCA2 is normally located in the nucleus and contains phosphorylated residues [49]. Like *BRCA1*, *BRCA2* is expressed in most tissues and cell types analyzed, indicating that gene expression does not account for the tissue-restricted phenotype of breast and ovarian cancer. BRCA2 is directly involved in the repair of damaged

DNA. Along with several other proteins, including RAD51, it mends DNA lesions caused by radiation or during cell division. It also regulates the activity of other genes and participates in embryonic development. Overall, *BRCA2* appears to be a cancer-causing gene when altered triggering BRCA pathway. Interestingly, hematopoietic phenotype of mice with a hypomorphic mutation in the *Brca2/Fancd1* (*Brca2*$^{\Delta 27/\Delta 27}$) revealed low numbers of hematopoietic colony-forming cells as well as a high incidence of spontaneous chromosomal instability thus making this model the most resembling one to FA disease [50].

P53

One of the tumor-suppressor genes is P53 gene that has structural and functional similarities to the Myc family of protooncogenes [51]. The job of P53 is to prevent (suppress) cells from growing. Alteration or inactivation of p53 by mutation or interaction of p53 with oncogene products of DNA tumor viruses can lead to cancer.

More than 50% of all human breast cancer cells contain a P53 mutation. These cancers are more aggressive and more often fatal [52]. Recent data in zebrafish show that after FANCD2 knocked out, a proportion of the cells undergo p53-mediated apoptosis [54]. At the same time FANCD2 knockout mice developing solid tumors only at adult age reveal early onset of cancer when one of the p53 alleles is deleted [55]. Since P53 is so important for normal cell growth in humans, researchers are continuing to look for ways to diagnose, prevent, and treat cancers associated with P53.

ATM

One of those proteins that are in BRCA network is called *ataxia telangiectasia mutated* (ATM). The biallelic altered form of the *ATM* is directly linked to a childhood disorder of the nervous system called Ataxia Telangiectasia (AT). Like FA patients, AT predisposes children to multiple cancers, especially lymphomas; scientists have also long debated whether one mutated *AT* gene increases the chance of breast cancer. In 1999, geneticist Stephen Elledge and his colleagues reported an intriguing connection between *AT* and *BRCA1* [56]. It was already known that like *BRCA1*, the normal *ATM* gene helps correct DNA damage also playing a role in controlling cell division and breast cancer susceptibility [57]. But Elledge's team discovered that upon DNA damage in normal cells the healthy ATM protein function is amplified resulting in modification of BRCA1 protein to enhance its performance. Link in between ATM and FA/BRCA pathway was further validated upon discovery of ATM-dependent phosphorylation of FANCD2 *in vitro* [58]. It was shown that Serine 222 site was also phosphorylated *in vivo* in an ATM-dependent manner following IR and that FANCD2 phosphorylation is required for activation of an S phase checkpoint. Interestingly, other BRCA family members H2AX, NBS1, and p53 are substrates of ATM kinase and are involved in ATM-dependent DNA damage responses [58,125]. Not surprisingly, that alteration in *ATM* is attributed to cancer predisposition and sensitivity to ionizing radiation.

CHK1

CHK1 is required for checkpoint mediated cell cycle arrest in response to DNA damage or the presence of unreplicated DNA and may also negatively regulate cell cycle progression during unperturbed cell cycles [59]. CHEK1 binds to and phosphorylates CDC25A/B/C, thus inhibiting CDC25 activity and blocking cell cycle progression. It binds to RAD51 enhancing its association with chromatin and promoting DNA repair by HR. Functioning in line with fragile site proteins, CHK1 was implicated in constitutional and cancer chromosome rearrangements suggesting its role in chromosome damage caused by replication stress during early tumorigenesis [60]. In response to DNA damage, Chk1 directly phosphorylates the FANCE subunit of the FA core complex on two conserved sites (Threonine 346 and Serine 374). Phosphorylated FANCE assembles in nuclear foci and colocalizes with FANCD2 [61].

CHK2

CHEK2 (previously known as "CHK2") is a kinase involved in ATM-dependent DNA damage checkpoint. The *Saccharomyces cerevisiae* homolog of Chk2, Rad53, plays a role in the checkpoint response to DNA damage and replication block signals as well as normal cell growth [62]. Rad53 kinase activation is required for arrest at all stages of the cell cycle (G_1/S, intra-S and G_2/M checkpoints) depending on where the DNA damage occurs and for a replication checkpoint that monitors the progress of DNA replication [63]. Rad53 is also important for the relocalization, transcriptional up-regulation, and activation of proteins required for repair [64,65]. BRCA1 is a downstream target of CHK2. Its phosphorylation on Serine 988 is dependent on CHK2 expression and provides link to ATM-CHK2 pathway [66]. CHEK2 acts as a low-penetrance tumor-suppressor gene in breast cancer and makes a significant contribution to familial clustering of breast cancer-including families [67].

RAD50

Identified in a genetic screen for mutants that are sensitive to ionizing radiation *RAD50* is a member of the *RAD52* epistasis group involved in the repair of DSBs [68]. Mutants are defective in the repair of DNA damage caused by ionizing radiation and the alkylating agent methyl methanesulfonate (MMS), in the maintenance of telomere length, in mitotic and meiotic recombination, and in mating-type switching because DSB intermediates are involved in these processes [69,70]. Hypomorphic Rad50 mutant mice (RAD50(S/S) mice) exhibit growth defects and cancer predisposition [71].

RAD51

When a cell divides, the healthy BRCA1 protein interacts with another protein called RAD51 [42]. RAD51 is an enzyme that coordinates recombination and plays an important role in error-free DNA repair by recombination. This protein comprises the RAD51-family which is very similar to bacterial RecA and Saccharomyces cerevisiae Rad51. Alteration in Rad51 is linked to bilateral breast cancer [72]. Rad51 can interact with the ssDNA-binding protein RPA, RAD52 and is also found to interact with BRCA1 and BRCA2. Following treatment with DNA cross-linkers FANCD2 colocalizes with RAD51 and PCNA at the same foci, suggesting that FANCD2 may have a role in the cellular response to stalled replication forks or in the repair of replication-associated DSB [73].

H2AX

Histone H2AX is a minor variant of the highly conserved histone H2A that is part of the histone octamer in the core of the nucleosome [74]. Following a genotoxic insult, ATM or

ATR (depending on the type of DNA damage) phosphorylates H2AX at serine 139 (part of the SQE motif) [75] and phosphorylated H2AX (γ-H2AX) seems to localise at sites of stall replication fork [76,77]. More importantly, several proteins involved in DNA repair including BRCA1/2, Rad51, Mre11, FANCD2 and p53 are recruited to sites of γ-H2AX. Therefore, H2AX functions in the parallel pathway of p53 and NBS1, H2AX, and p53 playing synergistic roles in ATM-dependent DNA damage responses and tumor suppression [78]. Phosphorylation of S129 of Saccharomyces cerevisiae H2A (homologous to S139 in human H2AX) is necessary for efficient processing of DNA repair and is proposed to cause alteration of chromatin structure that facilitates repair. [79]. Recently identified role of H2AX in the FA pathway provides additional bridge to connect FA and BRCA network [28].

NBS1

The human genetic disorder, Nijmegen breakage syndrome (NBS), is characterized by radiosensitivity, immunodeficiency and an increased risk for cancer, particularly B-cell non-Hodgkin lymphoma. The NBS1 gene codes for a protein, nibrin, involved in the in cell cycle checkpoints and is one of the key proteins that participates in recognition and repair of DSBs in humans [80]. NBS1 appears to function both as an activator of ATM to mediate ATM activities after DNA DSB damage [81] and as an interacting partner of FANCD2 [82]. Recent reports linked polymorphisms of the NBS1 gene with risk of sporadic breast cancer [83].

Bridging BRCA and FA Pathways: Mutations of BRCA Pathway

Mutations in BRCA genes play important roles in breast cancer, however the degree of current progress does not give clear answer on the most important question: what types of mutations cause breast cancer? We now know enormous allelic variations in BRCA genes. In more than 600 pathologic variants (different mutations) identified in *BRCA1* only a small number has been found repeatedly in unrelated families. Most *BRCA1* mutations lead to frameshifts resulting in missing or nonfunctional protein. For BRCA2 gene, researchers have identified more than 450 mutations, many of those are insertions or deletions resulting in an abnormally small, nonfunctional version of the BRCA2 protein. About a third of mutations identified in *BRCA1* and *BRCA2* sequencing studies are of uncertain clinical significance [84].

The facts that FA crosstalk with BRCA pathway and that the cell lines homozygous for *BRCA1/2* mutations are hypersensitive to mitomycin-C and the cells from homozygous *BRCA2* mutant mice reveal FA-like phenotype suggested that BRCA1/2 mutations may occur in FA patients and *vise versa.* [16,85-88]. Moreover, accumulating data suggest that only synergetic functioning of FA and BRCA pathways reveal truly functional and protective mechanism against cancer. Indeed, disruption of FA/BRCA pathway may serve as a risk factor for cancer predisposition [89]. Data provided below illustrate some mutations of the main BRCA pathway players most of them with known molecular connexions with FA proteins.

BRCA2 (FANCD1) Mutations

The first breakthrough in connecting breast cancer genes with FA was done by Alan D'Andrea's group showing that cell lines derived from FA-B and FA-D1 patients have biallelic mutations in BRCA2 and express truncated BRCA2 proteins [16]. In the course of mutation screening of the BRCA1 and BRCA2 genes in a hospital based series of patients with risk factors for hereditary breast/ovarian cancer, a germline mutation in the BRCA2 gene (3034del4) was identified in a patient with early onset breast cancer and no strong family history of the disease [90]. Later, in the studies by Arleen Auerbach' group, examination of four kindreds afflicted with Fanconi anemia revealed for the presence of germline BRCA2 deletions (6174delT/C3069X, BRCA2*6174delT/886delGT) or mutations (BRCA2*I2490T/ 5301insA, BRCA2*Q3066X/E1308X) providing a link of those individuals with their breast cancer family history [91]. After that, clinical and molecular description of FANCD1 kindreds, initially identified through a young child with a solid tumor revealed deletion (886-887delGT) and mutations (8447T>A, 4876G>T, 7757T>C) in BRCA2 gene [92]. Some FA patients in families with breast cancer history exhibited the co-occurrence of BRCA2 deletion (5164Δl4,11) and mutations (W2626C, 8106G>C, 5910C>G) and were identified with early onset acute leukaemia and brain tumors [93]. Another paper, describing an individual with a severe FA phenotype who developed AML discovered two biallelic mutations in the FANCD1/BRCA2 gene (3827ΔGT). Mutational screening of *BRCA2* in the two affected brothers revealed two truncating mutations in each child (886ΔGT, 5873C→A) having glioblastoma [94]. The most recent study by Alter *et al.* dealing with analysis of the BRCA2 mutations revealed that missense mutations formed a distinct cluster in a highly conserved region of the BRCA2 protein [95].

ATM Mutations

For a long time *ATM* was a good candidate to be screened for mutations with possible link to breast cancer risk. Recent comprehensive sequencing of *ATM* in 434 familial breast cancer patients revealed seven protein-truncating alleles, two splice mutations, and two missense alleles (one of which appeared in two families) experimentally verified to affect ATM function. In contrast, only two *ATM* sequence variants were found in 521 controls [96].

RAD50 Mutations

A protein-truncating allele of *RAD50* (RAD50 687ΔT) identified in northern Finland cohort provided the first evidence in increased breast cancer risk (approximately 4-fold) [80].

RAD51 Mutations

The BRCA1 and FANCD1 (BRCA2) proteins function in DNA repair in conjunction with RAD51. A single nucleotide polymorphism in the 5' untranslated region of Rad51 (135C/G) increases breast cancer risk in BRCA1 and FANCD1 (BRCA2) carriers. Rad51-135C is a clinically significant modifier of BRCA2 penetrance, specifically in raising breast cancer risk at younger ages [72,97].

H2AX Mutations

It is still not known whether mutations in H2AX, functioning in line with FA pathway has any clinical implications in FA patients, however recent study of hereditary breast cancer families revealed absence of constitutional H2AX gene mutations [98]. So far, our and other attempts to find altered H2AX genes in a cohort of FA patients, including those which subtyping did not attribute patients to any known FA group, indicated that H2AX is unlikely to be mutated in FA. This however, may suggest that for such a strong and evolutionary conserved protein mutation of any type would be lethal and hence the chance of finding individuals with biallelic H2AX mutations would be close to zero.

NBS1 Mutations

Recently, two patients who were initially diagnosed with FA were found to have mutations in NBS1 (657Δl5 and 1089C>A). Surprisingly, they both showed sensitivity to DNA cross-linking agents and ionizing radiation [99]. Another case study reported a family that was initially diagnosed with FA on the basis of increased sensitivity to DNA cross-linking agents. The genetic defect was shown to be a novel mutation in the NBS1 gene (1089C > A) [100]. And the last study of Nordic populations discovered NBS1 Leu150Phe missense mutation affecting a conserved residue in the functionally important BRCA1 carboxy-terminal [80]. To sum up, Nijmegen Breakage Syndrome shares overlapping clinical features with FA.

CHEK2 Mutations

CHEK2 (also known as CHK2) is an additional breast cancer susceptibility gene which encodes a cell-cycle checkpoint kinase that is implicated in DNA repair processes involving BRCA1 and p53. It was shown that delition in *CHEK2* 1100ΔC abrogates the kinase activity and has a frequency of 1.1% in healthy individuals. However, this variant is present in 5.1% of individuals with breast cancer from 718 families that do not carry mutations in BRCA1 or BRCA2 [101]. Other *CHEK2* mutations have been subsequently associated with similarly increased risk of breast cancer [102].

p53 Mutations

Since the discovery that two p53 binding sites are present in the gene coding for the FANCC protein (promoter regions -1295/-1266 and gene region +1828/+1848) there were some reasons to admit that p53 may regulate transcription of some of the FA genes and that mutations in p53 may affect FA pathway [103]. However, mutations of the N-ras and p53 genes studied by a combination of single strand conformation polymorphism (SSCP) analysis and direct sequencing of the PCR product in the bone marrow and/or peripheral blood of FA patients revealed that only normal N-ras and p53 sequences were detected in all cases analyzed suggesting that the genetic mechanisms underlying FA-associated leukemogenesis appear to be independent of N-ras and p53 mutations [104]. In another sudy, however, a greater proportion of patients with Fanconi anemia and SCC were homozygous for Arg72, a p53 polymorphism that may be associated with increased cancer risk [105]. Another link to suggest cooperation of p53 with FA was provided in the study comparing FANCC -/- and Trp53 -/-cells with with FANCC -/-cells and showing an increased inability to maintain the DNA damage-induced G2 checkpoint [106].

Mutations of FA Genes in Breast Cancer Families

Proteins involved into FA complex promote a cascade of biochemical events most of which crosstalk with the DNA damage and repair pathways [107]. Mutation of any upstream protein within the FA complex eventually results to the disruption of FANCD2 monoubiquitination thus impairing DNA repair machinery. In the Western blot picture of the cells undergoing DNA damage, FANCD2 is present as a doublet – the upper band, representing ubiquitinylated FANCD2 (FANCD2-L, where L stands for Large) (see Figure 3). In FA cells, where one of the core complex proteins is defective, only single band of FANCD2-S is present and FANCD2-L is not seen even after treatment with DNA damaging agents. In turn, correction of those cells by transfection with fully functional FA recuperates FA activation. In some cases, FANCD2 gene is defective itself (FA-D2 subtype) thus, neither of FANCD2 forms on a Western can be seen. Consecutively, the correction with FANCD2 vector saves the regular FA pathway. Importantly, detection of mono-ubiquitinated FANCD2 protein by Western blotting along with cell-cycle analyses (G2 arrest after DNA damage) serve as additional instrument to diagnose FA.

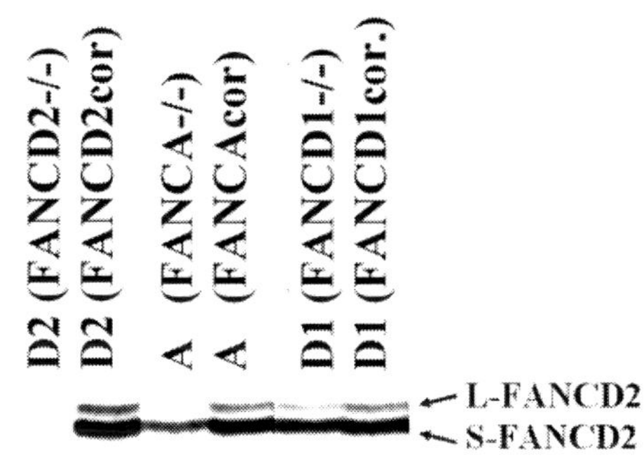

Figure 3. Western blot representing signals from two forms of FANCD2 (L and S) obtained after treatment cells with mytomycin C. Mutations in any upstream FA gene "turn off" FANCD2 monoubiquitinylation (no L-FANCD2 signal is observed). Correction of FANCD2 or FANCA deficient cells with corresponding the full length genes restores FANCD2 capacity to ubiquitinylation. Mutation in any downstream FA genes (e.g. FANCD1) does not affect FANCD2 monoubiquitinylation.

It should be noticed, however, that FANCD2 mutations in the FA-D2 patients are in general hypomorphic and therefore small signals of FANCD2 can be revealed [108]. Only the BRCA2, FANCJ and FANCN proteins act downstream of this mono-ubiquitinated FANCD2 protein, so that FA altered status cannot be detected with Western blotting. Same is true for the genes of the BRCA pathway where two isoforms of FANCD2 are in general unaffected suggesting that FA pathway is either separated from BRCA pathway or that BRCA-dependent transformation of cells into FA phenotype occurs somewhere downstream of the FA complex. Indeed, we know now that FANCD2 protein interacts with BRCA pathway after targeting to chromatin therefore any mutations either in BRCA1 or BRCA2 should not affect FANCD2 activation (though some studies revealed that FANCD2 ubiquitinylation is impaired in BRCA1 deficient cells). Due to rareness of FA disease it is hard to make a large screening for other BRCA family members in FA patients. Probably, some of the BRCA mutations found in specific ethnic groups could involve individuals with FA, however by the time most of the studies were done, it was unnecessary to screen for FA mutations [109-111]. Along with the evidence linking breast cancer and FANCD1 (BRCA2) mutations provided above, we are going to describe some other FA mutations found in patients having breast cancer.

FANCA

FANCA itself is also a potential breast and ovarian cancer susceptibility gene. A novel allele having a tandem duplication of a 13 base pair sequence in the promoter region was identified by screening germline DNA from 352 breast cancer patients and was associated with an increased risk of breast or ovarian cancer. Although this allele with the tandem duplication does not appear to modify breast cancer risk, it may act as a low penetrance protective allele for ovarian cancer [112]. One of the major studies made so far was done to investigate whether heterozygous variants in other FA genes are high penetrance breast cancer susceptibility alleles. Since monoallelic (heterozygous) BRCA2 mutations confer a high risk of breast cancer and are a major cause of familial breast cancer, researchers screened germ-line DNA from 88 BRCAI/2-negative families, each with at least three cases of breast cancer, for mutations in FANCA, FANCC, FANCD2, FANCE, FANCF, and FANCG. Two conservative missense variants (*FANCA* L1143V and FANCE R365K) were identified in family of twin sisters and two additional sisters, all affected with breast cancer before age 55 years. The twins and one sister carried *FANCA* L1143V as did an unaffected brother [113].

FANCN

PALB2 gene product, later identified as FANCN, interacts with BRCA2, and biallelic mutations in PALB2 (2386G →T, 2982insT, 3113G →A, 3113G →A, 3116ΔA, 3116ΔA, 3116ΔA, 3549C →G, 3549C →G, 3549C →G), similar to biallelic BRCA2 mutations, cause Fanconi anemia. Recent study identified monoallelic truncating PALB2 mutations in individuals with familial breast cancer and showed that such mutations confer approximately 2.3-fold higher risk of breast cancer [114]. PALB2 frameshift mutation (c.1592ΔT) is present at significantly elevated frequency in Finnish familial breast cancer cases compared with ancestry-matched population controls [115].

FANCJ

Some more individuals with breast cancer from BRCA1/BRCA2 mutation-negative families turned out to have FANCJ (BRIP1 helicase) mutation. Inactivation of truncating mutations of BRIP1 (141ΔC, 2392C →T, 2008insT, 2255ΔAA, 2108ΔAinsTCC), similar to those in BRCA2, cause Fanconi anemia and confer susceptibility to breast cancer in monoallelic carriers [116]. Later on, FANCJ mutations (658C →T, 718G →A, 725T →C, 1396C →T, 1732T →G, 2392C →T, 1760A →T, 2636G →A, 2896C →T, 2778G →A, 2945T →G, 3552C →T, 3968A →C, 4049C →T) have been found in 21 families with potentially inherited breast/ovarian cancer. It should be noted that all these families were BRCA1/BRCA2 negative, but had at least one case of male breast cancer, two cases of ovarian cancer, or three or more cases of female breast and ovarian cancers again confirming that FANCJ mutations have a moderate risk of breast cancer [117].

FANCD2

Studies of seven SNPs in FANCA, FANCL and FANCD2 in a total of 897 consecutive and non-related sporadic breast cancer cases and 1033 unaffected controls from the Spanish population revealed statistically significant association with sporadic breast cancer located on FANCD2 indicating a relationship between FANCD2 and breast cancer risk. Statistically significant association with sporadic breast cancer has been observed for the variant rs2272125 (L1366L) located on FANCD2 [118]. It was also hypothesised that germline mutations in FANCD2 may account for some of the unexplained multiple-case breast cancer families. Analysis of *FANCD2* in the 33 index cases from 30 breast and ovarian cancer families, and of exons 9 and 19 (containing the ATM phosphorylation site and the FANCD2 monoubiquitination site, respectively) in a further 399 non-*BRCA1/2* index cases, identified 32 germline sequence alterations [118]. And the very last study of breast cancers family members revealed that 19% sporadic breast cancers and 10% BRCA1-related breast cancers were completely FANCD2-negative, indicating that somatic inactivation in FANCD2 may be important in both sporadic and hereditary breast carcinogenesis and that FANCD2 is of independent prognostic value in sporadic breast cancer [119].

Breast Cancer in FA-BRCA Pathway. Connection to Repair and Recombination

Having started from almost unrelated properties and functions, FA genes now turned out to share mutations with the family of breast cancer susceptibility genes. The reason people did not find this link earlier is probably related to the rareness of FA itself as well as to the difficulties in studying FA mutations in large cohorts of FA patients. At the same time, researchers seemed to underestimate importance of FA family paying much of their efforts to decipher mechanistic links among BRCA members rather than finding the bridges to Fanconi and other rare diseases. Luckily, the discovery of FANCD1 as a BRCA2 gene made a breakthrough in this field and the race for finding connection of FA and BRCA began. At that time, scientists suspected only two breast cancer genes *BRCA1* and *BRCA2* responsible for tumorigenesis having in minds that when disturbed, damaged DNA in the cell might go unrepaired eventually leading to unchecked mutations and formation of tumors. Since the discovery of new FA genes, it is becoming evident that there is a strong, yet unresolved, link between FA and BRCA. Finding of BRIP1 as a FANCJ gene made possible to correlate its mutations in some of FA patients with the breast cancer risk factor. Rough estimation now suggests that mutations in *BRIP1* result in a twofold increase in breast cancer. This puts the gene in a class with two other breast cancer susceptibility genes, *CHEK2* and *ATM*, which may predispose a woman to cancer only in the presence of other genetic or environmental risk factors. Women who inherit one damaged copy of a PALB2 (FANCN) gene have double the risk of developing breast cancer. Although PALB2 is a relatively small contributor to the overall incidence of breast cancer in the general population, it is now *the third* FA cancer susceptibility gene to be identified in families where breast cancer is common. Then what is the missing link between FA, BRCA and breast cancer? We now know that in higher eukaryotes there are several mechanisms allowing normal functioning of DNA repair machinery in response to various DNA damaging factors. Some of the BRCA gene products are highly susceptible to ionizing irradiation and most of them to DNA cross-linking agents. At the same time, most of the FA cell lines are hyposensitive to DNA cross-linkers and much less to ionizing radiation. Therefore, some operation involved into the repair machinery seems to exist in between FA and BRCA. In light of this suggestion, recombination of any type might be a potential driving force bridging BRCA and FA on the way to maintain the stability of the cell genome. Until recently, only FANCD1 mutant cells recognized to have a profound impairment in HR repair. However, additional proof for that has been done in the set of studies demonstrating impairment in homologous recombination in FANCA and FANCG cell lines [120]. Other studies using chicken-derived FANCG and FANCC cells showed a dramatic decrease in repair of DSBs by malfunctioning of HR system [121,122]. The functional connection of BRCA gene products with recombination is less studied, however it is known that BRCA2 facilitates the formation of a single-stranded DNA-Rad51 filamentand stabilizes stalled replication forks [123]. FANCD2 ubiquitinylation promotes BRCA2 loading into a chromatin complex [124]. At the same time, USP1 negatively regulates FANCD2 and PCNA monoubiquitination providing connection to BRCA pathway via DNA damage response [29]. Still, HR defects in FA cells seem to be moderate versus BRCA pathway suggesting that the FA path may be not entirely involved in the HR. However, recent cloning of FANCJ and FANCM DNA helicases lends further support to the model where the FA pathway interacts with HR repair proteins and at least partially regulates a subset of their functions in response to DNA cross-links (see Figure 4). There is no need to convince that any alteration in such a complex machinery as being HR may eventually lead to occurrence of different types of cancers therefore confirming the link of FA/BRCA/HR pathway to breast cancer. Recently identified connection of FA genes with breast cancer predisposition and co-occurrence of mutations of BRCA family members with breast cancer make FA/breast cancer/BRCA link even stronger.

Conclusion

Breast cancer shares the top ten of the death casualties worldwide. According to WHO prognoses, one in nine women will develop breast cancer in her. Hereditary breast cancer accounts for nearly 10% of all breast cancers and many studies within the past decade have sought to identify the cause. Eventually, researchers came up to many susceptibility genes starting with two major ones BRCA1 and BRCA2, further embracing the whole class known as BRCA family. Oppositely, Fanconi anemia is one of the rarest diseases on earth attacking only small percentage of individuals, historically was unrelated to any type of breast cancer. However, recent progress uncovered that germline mutations in *BRCA2* may be causative in Fanconi anemia complementation group D1 and the discovery of new Fanconi genes *FANCN*

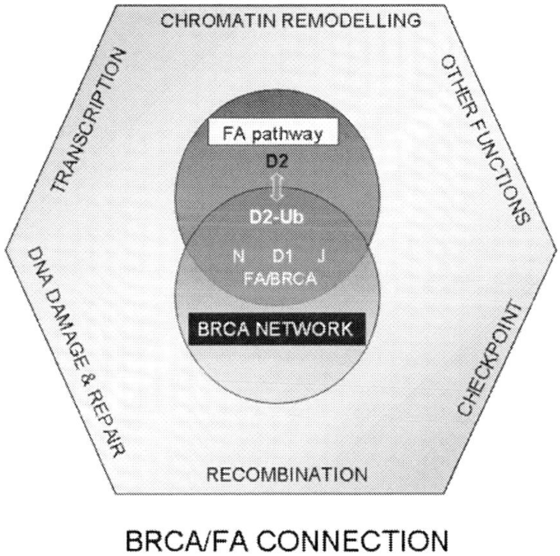

Figure 4. Connection of FA and BRCA pathways. Ubiquitinylation of FANCD2 protein (FA pathway) is crucial both for its loading to chromatin and interaction with the proteins of BRCA pathway. Since the discovery of new FA genes (FANCN, FANCJ, FANCD1/BRCA2) involved into the inheritance of breast cancer risk it is become plausible to suggest that the link connecting FA and BRCA pathway lies somewhere on DNA level and apparently results in controlling other major functions, including homologous recombination (HR), DNA damage/repair, transcription, chromatin remodelling, checkpoint and some other, yet unknown pathways.

and *FANCJ* associated with increased risk of breast cancer totally changed this stereotype. In this chapter we tried to summarize the most recent findings in BRCA/FA field and provide the link to breast cancer predisposition through some of the Fanconi and BRCA genes that now seem to orchestrate one of the main mechanism of genomic integrity - DNA damage/repair and tumor suppression. Evolutionary speaking, genome of any creature has evolved multiple cellular defence mechanisms, including DNA repair and cell cycle checkpoint processes. These defence mechanisms are cell-specific and situation-related as cell must have ways to decide which one to use for a given reason. These requirements imply that signalling networks not only sense the presence of DNA damage, but also receive specific input such as the chemical nature of the damage, the timing of the cell cycle, the type of cell and the location of damage on the DNA. With advances made in mutation screening of newly identified FA genes and clinical characterization of corresponding FA patients it is becoming clear that the clinical differences between different mutations of the same FA gene may be stronger than the symptoms between two different FA genes. This fact probably tells that normal communication of a certain FA gene with any defence-pathway is more important than malfunctioning of any FA genes not leading to disruption of a whole path. We underlined the role of recombination pathway as a platform for functional communication of FA and BRCA genes. Probably, only some of FA and BRCA members are of importance to provide enough stability against cancer predisposition. Mutations in the FA or BRCA pathway may be involved in the development of breast cancers. Importantly, synergistic interaction of some known and unknown FA-BRCA members seems to be the link that defines breast cancer predisposition, therefore studying the cross-talk of the FA- and BRCA-pathways with other proteins involved in DNA repair need to be dissected to identify the nature of such predisposition.

Acknowledgements

Research in JS laboratory is supported the Generalitat de Catalunya (SGR-00197-2002), the La Caixa Fundation Oncology Program (BM05-67-0), Genoma España, the Spanish Ministry of Health and Consumption (projects FIS PI020145, FIS G03/073, FIS PI051205, FIS PI061099 and CIBER-ER CB06/07/0023), the Spanish Ministry of Science and Technology (projects SAF2003-020328, SAF2004-20372-E and SAF2006-3440), the Commission of the European Union (project FI6R-CT-2003-508842) and the European Regional Development Funds.

References

[1] Kennedy, R.D. & D'Andrea, A.D. (2005). The Fanconi anemia/BRCA pathway: new faces in the crowd, *Genes Dev., 19*, 2925–2940.

[2] Fanconi, G. (1927) Familiäre infantile perniziosaartige Anämie (perniziöses Blutbild und Konstitution). *Jahb Kinderheilkd, 117*, 257-280.

[3] Whitney, M.A., Jakobs, P., Kaback, M., Moses, R.E. & Grompe, M. (1994). The Ashkenazi Jewish Fanconi anemia mutation: incidence among patients and carrier frequency in the at-risk population. *Hum Mutat., 3*, 339-334.

[4] Callen, E., Casado, J.A., Tischkowitz, M.D., Bueren, J.A., Creus, A., Marcos, R, Dasi, A., Estella, J.M., Munoz, A., Ortega, J.J., de Winter, J., Joenje, H., Schindler, D., Hanenberg, H., Hodgson, S.V., Mathew, C.G. & Surralles, J. (2005). A common founder mutation in FANCA underlies the world's highest prevalence of Fanconi anemia in Gypsy families from Spain. *Blood, 105*, 1946-1949.

[5] Kutler, D.I. & Auerbach, A.D. (2004). Fanconi anemia in Ashkenazi Jew. Fanconi anemia in Ashkenazi Jews. *Fam Cancer., 3*, 241-248.

[6] Kutler, D.I., Singh, B., Satagopan, J., Batish, S.D., Berwick, M., Giampietro, P.F., Hanenberg, H. & Auerbach, A.D. (2003). A 20-year perspective on the International Fanconi Anemia Registry (IFAR). *Blood, 101*, 1249-1256

[7] Tischkowitz, M.D. & Hodgson, S.V. (2003). Fanconi anaemia. *J Med Genet., 40*, 1-10

[8] Tekin, M., Bodurtha, J.N. & Riccardi, V.M. (2001). Cafe au lait spots: the pediatrician's perspective. *Pediatr Rev., 22*, 82-90.

[9] Auerbach, A.D., Warburton, D., Bloom, A.D. & Chaganti, R.S. (1979). Preliminary communication: prenatal detection of the Fanconi Anemia gene by cytogenetic methods. *Am J Hum Genet., 31*, 77-81

[10] Bagby, G.C., & Alter, B.P. (2006). Fanconi anemia. *Semin Hematol. 43*, 147-145.

[11] D'Andrea, A.D. (2003). The Fanconi road to cancer. *Genes Dev., 17,* 1933-1936

[12] Mathew, C.G. (2006). Fanconi anaemia genes and susceptibility to cancer. *Oncogene*, 25, 5875-5884.

[13] Casado, J.A., Callen, E., Jacome, A., Rio, P., Castella, M., Lobitz, S., Ferro, T., Munoz, A., Sevilla, J., Cantalejo, A., Cela, E., Cervera, J., Sanchez-Calero, J., Badell, I., Estella, J., Dasi, A., Olive, T., Ortega, J.J., Rodriguez-Villa, A., Tapia, M., Molines, A., Madero, L., Segovia, J.C., Nevelling, K., Kalb, R., Schindler, D., Hanenberg, H., Surralles, J. & Bueren, J.A. (2006). A comprehensive strategy for the subtyping of Fanconi Anemia patients: conclusions from the Spanish Fanconi Anemia research network. *J Med Genet.*

[14] Whitney, M.A., Saito, H., Jakobs, P.M., Gibson, R.A., Moses, R.E. & Grompe, M. (1993). A common mutation in the FACC gene causes Fanconi anaemia in Ashkenazi *Jews. Nat Genet., 4*, 202-205.

[15] Blom, E., van de Vrugt, H.J., de Winter, J.P. & Arwert, F. (2002). Evolutionary clues to the molecular function of fanconi anemia genes. *Acta Haematol., 108*, 231-236.

[16] Howlett, N.G., Taniguchi, T., Olson, S., Cox, B., Waisfisz, Q., De Die-Smulders, C., Persky, N., Grompe, M., Joenje, H., Pals, G., Ikeda, H., Fox, E.A. & D'Andrea, A.D. (2002). Biallelic inactivation of BRCA2 in Fanconi anemia. *Science, 297*, 606-609.

[17] Taniguchi, T., Garcia-Higuera, I., Andreassen, P.R., Gregory, R.C., Grompe, M. & D'Andrea, A.D. (2002). S-phase-specific interaction of the Fanconi anemia protein FANCD2 with BRCA1 and RAD51. *Blood, 100*, 2414-2420.

[18] Goldberg, J.I. & Borgen, P.I. (2006). Breast cancer susceptibility testing: past, present and future. *Expert Rev Anticancer Ther., 8*, 1205-1214.

[19] Rahman, N., Seal, S., Thompson, D., Kelly, P., Renwick, A., Elliott, A., Reid, S., Spanova, K., Barfoot, R., Chagtai, T., Jayatilake, H., McGuffog, L., Hanks, S., Evans, D.G., Eccles, D., Easton, D.F. & Stratton, M.R. (2007). PALB2, which encodes a BRCA2-interacting protein, is a breast cancer susceptibility gene. *Nat Genet., 39*, 165-167.

[20] Litman, R., Peng, M., Jin, Z., Zhang, F., Zhang, J., Powell, S., Andreassen, P.R. & Cantor, S.B. (2005). BACH1 is critical for homologous recombination and appears to be the Fanconi anemia gene product FANCJ. *Cancer Cell., 3*, 255-265.

[21] Ciccia, A., Ling, C., Coulthard, R., Yan, Z., Xue, Y., Meetei, A.R., Laghmani, el H., Joenje, H., McDonald, N., de Winter, J.P., Wang, W. & West, S.C. (2007). Identification of FAAP24, a Fanconi anemia core complex protein that interacts with FANCM. *Mol Cell, 25*, 331-343

[22] Niedernhofer, L.J. (2007). The fanconi anemia signalosome anchor. *Mol Cell., 25*, 487-490.

[23] Gurtan, A.M. & D'Andrea, A.D. (2006). Dedicated to the core: understanding the Fanconi anemia complex. *DNA Repair, 5*, 1119-1125.

[24] Kowal, P., Gurtan, A.M., Stuckert, P., D'Andrea, A.D. & Ellenberger, T. (2007). Structural determinants of human FANCF protein that function in the assembly of a DNA damage signalling complex. *J Biol Chem., 282*, 2047-2055

[25] Ho, G.P., Margossian, S., Taniguchi, T. & D'Andrea, A.D. (2006). Phosphorylation of FANCD2 on two novel sites is required for mitomycin C resistance. *Mol Cell Biol., 18*, 7005-7015.

[26] Medhurst, A.L., Laghmani, el H., Steltenpool, J., Ferrer, M., Fontaine, C., de Groot, J., Rooimans, M.A., Scheper, R.J., Meetei, A.R., Wang, W., Joenje, H. & de Winter, J.P. (2006). Evidence for subcomplexes in the Fanconi anemia pathway. *Blood*, *108*, 2072-2080.

[27] Bogliolo, M., Lyakhovich, A., Callen, E., Castella, M., Cappelli, E., Ramirez, M.J., Creus, A., Marcos, R., Kalb, R., Neveling, K., Schindler, D. & Surralles, J. (2007). Histone H2AX and Fanconi anemia FANCD2 function in the same pathway to maintain chromosome stability. *EMBO J.*

[28] Nijman, S.M., Huang, T.T., Dirac, A.M., Brummelkamp, T.R., Kerkhoven, R.M., D'Andrea, A.D. & Bernards, R. (2005). The deubiquitinating enzyme USP1 regulates the Fanconi anemia pathway. *Mol Cell*, *17*, 331-339.

[29] Hussain, S., Wilson, J.B., Blom, E., Thompson, L.H., Sung, P., Gordon, S.M., Kupfer, G.M., Joenje, H., Mathew, C.G. & Jones, N.J. (2006). Tetratricopeptide-motif-mediated interaction of FANCG with recombination proteins XRCC3 and BRCA2. *DNA Repair*, *5*, 629-640.

[30] Nevanlinna, H. & Bartek, J. (2006). The CHEK2 gene and inherited breast cancer susceptibility. *Oncogene*, *25*, 5912-5919.

[31] Rudd, M.F., Sellick, G.S., Webb, E.L., Catovsky, D. & Houlston, R.S. (2006). Variants in the ATM-BRCA2-CHEK2 axis predispose to chronic lymphocytic leukemia. *Blood*, *108*, 638-644.

[32] Hall JM, Friedman L, Guenther C, Lee MK, Weber JL, Black DM, King MC. Closing in on a breast cancer gene on chromosome 17q. *Am J Hum Genet*. 1992 50:1235-1242.

[33] Kuska B. BRCA1 discovery aftermath: no rush for genetic testing. *J Natl Cancer Inst*. 1995 87:1578-1579.

[34] Wooster, R., Neuhausen, S.L., Mangion, J., Quirk, Y., Ford, D., Collins, N., Nguyen, K., Seal, S., Tran, T., Averill, D., et al. (1994). Localization of a breast cancer susceptibility gene, BRCA2, to chromosome 13q12-13. *Science, 265*, 2088-2090.

[35] Cleton-Jansen, A.M., Collins, N., Lakhani, S.R., Weissenbach, J., Devilee, P., Cornelisse, C.J. & Stratton, M.R. (1995). Loss of heterozygosity in sporadic breast tumours at the BRCA2 locus on chromosome 13q12-q13. *Br J Cancer*, *72*, 1241-1244.

[36] Ganguly, A., Leahy, K., Marshall, A.M., Dhulipala, R., Godmilow, L. & Ganguly, T. (1997). Genetic testing for breast cancer susceptibility: frequency of BRCA1 and BRCA2 mutations. *Genet Test.*, *1*, 85-90.

[37] Yoshida, K. & Miki, Y. (2004). Role of BRCA1 and BRCA2 as regulators of DNA repair, transcription, and cell cycle in response to DNA damage. *Cancer Sci.*, *95*, 866-871.

[38] Chen, Y., Farmer, A.A., Chen, C.F., Jones, D.C., Chen, P.L. & Lee, W.H. (1996). BRCA1 is a 220-kDa nuclear phosphoprotein that is expressed and phosphorylated in a cell cycle-dependent manner. *Cancer Res.*, *56*, 3168-3172.

[39] Gudas, J.M., Li, T., Nguyen, H., Jensen. D. & Rauscher, F.J. 3rd, Cowan, K.H. (1996). Cell cycle regulation of BRCA1 messenger RNA in human breast epithelial cells. *Cell Growth Differ.*, *7*, 717-723.

[40] Rajan, J.V., Wang, M., Marquis, S.T. & Chodosh, L.A. (1996). Brca2 is coordinately regulated with Brca1 during proliferation and differentiation in mammary epithelial cells. *Proc Natl Acad Sci.U S A, 93*, 13078-13083.

[41] Scully, R., Chen, J., Plug, A., Xiao, Y., Weaver, D., Feunteun, J., Ashley, T. & Livingston, D.M. (1997). Association of BRCA1 with Rad51 in mitotic and meiotic cells. *Cell, 88*, 265-275.

[42] Chen, J., Silver, D.P., Walpita, D., Cantor, S.B., Gazdar, A.F., Tomlinson, G., Couch, F.J., Weber, B.L., Ashley, T., Livingston, D.M. & Scully, R. (1998). Stable interaction between the products of the BRCA1 and BRCA2 tumor suppressor genes in mitotic and meiotic cells. *Mol Cell, 3*, 317-328.

[43] Hakem, R., de la Pompa, J.L., Sirard, C., Mo, R., Woo, M., Hakem, A., Wakeham, A., Potter, J., Reitmair, A., Billia, F., Firpo, E., Hui, C.C., Roberts, J., Rossant, J. & Mak, T.W. (1996). The tumor suppressor gene Brca1 is required for embryonic cellular proliferation in the mouse. *Cell, 85*, 1009-1023.

[44] Ludwig, T., Chapman, D.L., Papaioannou, V.E. & Efstratiadis, A. (1997). Targeted mutations of breast cancer susceptibility gene homologs in mice: lethal phenotypes of Brca1, Brca2, Brca1/Brca2, Brca1/p53, and Brca2/p53 nullizygous embryos *Genes Dev., 11*, 1226-1241.

[45] Brugarolas, J. & Jacks, T. (1997). Double indemnity: p53, BRCA and cancer. p53 mutation partially rescues developmental arrest in Brca1 and Brca2 null mice, suggesting a role for familial breast cancer genes in DNA damage repair. *Nat Med., 3*, 721-722.

[46] Zhang, H., Tombline, G. & Weber, B.L. (1998). BRCA1, BRCA2, and DNA damage response: collision or collusion? *Cell, 92*, 433-436.

[47] Venkitaraman, A.R. (2001). Functions of BRCA1 and BRCA2 in the biological response to DNA damage. *J Cell Sci.114*, 3591-3598.

[48] Bertwistle, D. & Ashworth, A. (1998). Functions of the BRCA1 and BRCA2 genes. *Curr Opin Genet Dev., 8*, 14-20.

[49] Navarro, S., Meza, N.W., Quintana-Bustamante, O., Casado, J.A., Jacome, A., McAllister, K., Puerto, S., Surralles, J., Segovia, J.C. & Bueren, J.A. (2006). Hematopoietic dysfunction in a mouse model for Fanconi Anemia group D1. *Mol Ther. 14*, 525-535.

[50] Sidransky, D. & Hollstein, M. (1996). Clinical implications of the p53 gene. *Annu Rev Med., 47*, 285-230.

[51] Steeg, P.S. (1992). Suppressor genes in breast cancer: an overview. *Cancer Treat Res., 61*, 45-57.

[52] Liu, T.X., Howlett, N.G., Deng, M., Langenau, D.M., Hsu, K., Rhodes, J., Kanki, J.P., D'Andrea, A.D., & Look, A.T. (2003). Knockdown of zebrafish Fancd2 causes developmental abnormalities via p53-dependent apoptosis. *Dev. Cell, 5*, 903-914.

[53] Houghtaling, S., Granville, L., Akkari, Y., Torimaru, Y., Olson, S., Finegold, M., & Grompe, M. (2005). Heterozygosity for p53 (Trp53+/-) accelerates epithelial tumor formation in Fanconi anemia complementation group D2 (Fancd2) knockout mice. *Cancer Res., 65*, 85-91.

[54] Cortez, D., Wang, Y., Qin, J. & Elledge, S.J. (1999). Requirement of ATM-dependent phosphorylation of BRCA1 in the DNA damage response to double-strand breaks. *Science*, *286*, 1162-1166.

[55] Heikkinen, K., Mansikka, V., Karppinen, S.M., Rapakko, K. & Winqvist, R. (2005). Mutation analysis of the ATR gene in breast and ovarian cancer families. *Breast Cancer Res*. *7*, 495-501.

[56] Taniguchi, T., Garcia-Higuera, I., Xu, B., Andreassen, P.R., Gregory, R.C., Kim, S.T., Lane, W.S., Kastan, M.B. & D'Andrea AD. (2002). Convergence of the fanconi anemia and ataxia telangiectasia signaling pathways. *Cell*, *109*, 459-472.

[57] McCabe, N., Turner, N.C., Lord, C.J., Kluzek, K., Bialkowska, A., Swift, S., Giavara, S., O'connor, M.J., Tutt, A.N., Zdzienicka, M.Z., Smith, G.C. & Ashworth, A.(2006). Deficiency in the Repair of DNA Damage by Homologous Recombination and Sensitivity to Poly(ADP-Ribose) Polymerase Inhibition. *Cancer Res*., *66*, 8109-8115.

[58] Arlt, M.F., Durkin, S.G., Ragland, R.L. & Glover, T.W. (2006).Common fragile sites as targets for chromosome rearrangements. *DNA Repair, 5,* 1126-1135.

[59] Wang, X., Kennedy, R., Ray, K., Stuckert, P., Ellenberger, T. & D'Andrea, A.D. (2007). Chk1-mediated Phosphorylation of FANCE is Required for the Fanconi Anemia/BRCA Pathway. *Mol Cell Biol*.

[60] Foiani, M., Pellicioli, A., Lopes, M., Lucca, C., Ferrari, M., Liberi, G., Muzi Falconi, M., & Plevani, P. (2000). DNA damage checkpoints and DNA replication controls in Saccharomyces cerevisiae. *Mutat. Res. 451*, 187–196.

[61] Weinert, T. A., Kiser, G. L. & Hartwell, L. H. (1994). *Genes Dev., 8*, 652–665.

[62] Huang, M., Zhou, Z. & Elledge, S. J. (1998). *Cell, 94*, 595–605.

[63] Martin, S.G., Laroche, T., Suka, N., Grunstein, M. & Gasser, S. M. (1999). *Cell, 97*, 621–633.

[64] Gibson, S.L., Bindra, R.S. & Glazer PM. (2006). CHK2-dependent phosphorylation of BRCA1 in hypoxia. *Radiat Res*., *166*, 646-651.

[65] Vahteristo, P., Bartkova, J., Eerola, H., Syrjakoski, K., Ojala, S., Kilpivaara, O., Tamminen, A., Kononen, J., Aittomaki, K., Heikkila, P., Holli, K., Blomqvist, C., Bartek, J., Kallioniemi, O.P. & Nevanlinna, H. (2002). A CHEK2 genetic variant contributing to a substantial fraction of familial breast cancer. *Am J Hum Genet*., *71*, 432-438.

[66] Game, J.C. & Mortimer, R.K. (1974). A genetic study of x-ray sensitive mutants in yeast. *Mutat Res., 24*, 281-292.

[67] Symington, L.S. (2002). Role of RAD52 epistasis group genes in homologous recombination and double-strand break repair. *Microbiol Mol Biol Rev., 66*, 630-670.

[68] Krogh, B.O. & Symington, L.S. (2004). Recombination proteins in yeast. *Annu Rev Genet., 38,* 233-271.

[69] Bender, C.F., Sikes, M.L., Sullivan, R., Huye, L.E., Le Beau, M.M., Roth, D.B., Mirzoeva, O.K., Oltz, E.M. & Petrini, J.H. (2002). Cancer predisposition and hematopoietic failure in Rad50(S/S) mice. *Genes Dev*., *16*, 2237-2251.

[70] Kato, M., Yano, K., Matsuo, F., Saito, H., Katagiri, T., Kurumizaka, H., Yoshimoto, M., Kasumi, F., Akiyama, F., Sakamoto, G., Nagawa, H., Nakamura, Y. & Miki, Y.

(2000). Identification of Rad51 alteration in patients with bilateral breast cancer. *J Hum Genet., 45*, 133-137.

[71] Hussain, S., Wilson, J.B., Medhurst, A.L., Hejna, J., Witt, E. & Ananth, S. (2004). Davies A, Masson JY, Moses R, West SC, de Winter JP, Ashworth A, Jones NJ, Mathew CG. Direct interaction of FANCD2 with BRCA2 in DNA damage response pathways. *Hum Mol Genet.,13*,1241-1248.

[72] Redon, C., Pilch, D., Rogakou, E., Sedelnikova, O., Newrock, K. & Bonner, W. (2002). Histone H2A variants H2AX and H2AZ. *Curr Opin Genet Dev., 12*, 162-169.

[73] Burma, S., Chen, B.P., Murphy, M., Kurimasa, A. & Chen, D.J. (2001). ATM phosphorylates histone H2AX in response to DNA double-strand breaks. *J Biol Chem., 276*, 42462–42467.

[74] Rogakou, E.P., Boon, C., Redon, C. & Bonner, W.M. (1999). Megabase chromatin domains involved in DNA double-strand breaks in vivo. *J Cell Biol., 146,* 905–916.

[75] Paull, T.T., Rogakou, E.P., Yamazaki, V., Kirchgessner, C.U., Gellert, M., Bonner, W.M. (2000). A critical role for histone H2AX in recruitment of repair factors to nuclear foci after DNA damage. *Curr Biol., 10*, 886–895.

[76] Kang, J., Ferguson, D., Song, H., Bassing, C., Eckersdorff, M., Alt, F.W. & Xu, Y.(2005). Functional Interaction of H2AX, NBS1, and p53 in ATM-Dependent DNA Damage Responses and Tumor Suppression. *Mol. Cell Biol., 25*, 661-670.

[77] Downs, J.A., Lowndes, N.F. & Jackson, S.P. (2000). A role for Saccharomyces cerevisiae histone H2A in DNA repair. *Nature, 408*, 1001–1004.

[78] Heikkinen, K., Rapakko, K., Karppinen, S.M., Erkko, H., Knuutila, S., Lundan, T., Mannermaa, A., Borresen-Dale, A.L., Borg, A., Barkardottir, R.B., Petrini, J. & Winqvist, R. (2006). RAD50 and NBS1 are breast cancer susceptibility genes associated with genomic instability. *Carcinogenesis, 27*, 1593-1599.

[79] Iijima, K., Komatsu, K., Matsuura, S., Tauchi, H. (2004). The Nijmegen breakage syndrome gene and its role in genome stability. *Chromosoma, 113*, 53-61.

[80] Nakanishi, K., Taniguchi, T., Ranganathan, V., New, H.V., Moreau, L.A., Stotsky, M., Mathew, C.G., Kastan, M.B., Weaver, D.T. & D'Andrea, A.D. (2002). Interaction of FANCD2 and NBS1 in the DNA damage response *Nat Cell Biol., 4*, 913-920.

[81] Lu, J., Wei, Q., Bondy, M.L., Li, D., Brewster, A., Shete, S., Yu, T.K., Sahin, A., Meric-Bernstam, F., Hunt, K.K., Singletary, S.E., Ross, M.I. & Wang, L.E. (2006). Polymorphisms and haplotypes of the NBS1 gene are associated with risk of sporadic breast cancer in non-Hispanic white women <or=55 years. *Carcinogenesis, 27*, 2209-2216.

[82] Shattuck-Eidens, D., Oliphant, A., McClure, M., McBride, C., Gupte, J., Rubano, T., Pruss, D., Tavtigian, S.V., Teng, D.H., Adey, N., Staebell, M., Gumpper, K., Lundstrom, R., Hulick, M., Kelly, M., Holmen, J., Lingenfelter, B., Manley, S., Fujimura, F., Luce, M., Ward, B., Cannon-Albright, L., Steele, L., Offit, K., Thomas, A., et al. (1997). BRCA1 sequence analysis in women at high risk for susceptibility mutations. Risk factor analysis and implications for genetic testing. *JAMA, 278*, 1242-1250.

[83] D'Andrea, A.D. & Grompe, M. (2003). The Fanconi Anaemia/BRCA pathway. *Nat. Rev. Cancer, 3*, 23-34.

[84] Moynahan, M. E., Cui, T. Y. & Jain, M. (2001). Homology-directed DNA repair, mitomycin-c resistance, and chromosome stability is restored with correction of a Brca1 mutation. *Cancer Res.*, *61*, 4842-4850.

[85] Patel, K. J., Yu, V. P., Lee, H., Corcoran, A., Thistletwaite, F. C., Evans, M. J., Colledge, W. H., Friedman, L. S., Ponder, B. A. & Venkitaraman, A. R. (1998). Involvement of Brca2 in DNA repair. *Mol. Cell*, *1*, 347-357.

[86] Connor, F., Bertwistle, D., Mee, P. J., Ross, G.M., Swift, S., Grigorieva, E., Tybulewicz, V. L. & Ashworth, A. (1997). Tumorigenesis and a DNA repair defect in mice with a truncating Brca2 mutation. *Nat. Genet.*, *17*, 423-430.

[87] Lyakhovich, A. & Surralles, J. (2006). Disruption of the Fanconi anemia/BRCA pathway in sporadic cancer. *Cancer Lett.*, *232*, 99-106.

[88] van der Luijt, R. B., van Zon, P. H. A., Jansen, R. P. M., van der Sijs-Bos, C. J. M., Warlam-Rodenhuis, C. C. & Ausems, M. G. E. M. (2001). De novo recurrent germline mutation of the BRCA2 gene in a patient with early onset breast cancer. *J. Med. Genet.* *38*, 102-105.

[89] Offit, K., Levran, O., Mullaney, B., Mah, K., Nafa, K., Batish, S.D., Diotti, R., Schneider, H., Deffenbaugh, A., Scholl, T., Proud, V.K., Robson, M., Norton, L., Ellis, N., Hanenberg, H. & Auerbach, A.D. (2003). Shared genetic susceptibility to breast cancer, brain tumors, and Fanconi anemia. *J Natl Cancer Inst.*, *95*, 1548-1551.

[90] Hirsch, B., Shimamura, A., Moreau, L., Baldinger, S., Hag-alshiekh, M., Bostrom, B., Sencer, S. & D'Andrea, A.D. (2004). Association of biallelic BRCA2/FANCD1 mutations with spontaneous chromosomal instability and solid tumors of childhood. *Blood*, *103*, 2554-2559.

[91] Wagner, J.E., Tolar, J., Levran, O., Scholl, T., Deffenbaugh, A., Satagopan, J., Ben-Porat, L., Mah, K., Batish, S.D., Kutler, D.I., MacMillan, M.L., Hanenberg, H. & Auerbach, A.D. (2004). Germline mutations in BRCA2: shared genetic susceptibility to breast cancer, early onset leukemia, and Fanconi anemia. *Blood*, *103*, 3226-3229.

[92] Reid, S., Renwick, A., Seal, S., Baskcomb, L., Barfoot, R., Jayatilake, H., Pritchard-Jones, K., Stratton, M.R., Ridolfi-Luthy, A. & Rahman, N. (2005). Familial Wilms Tumour Collaboration. Biallelic BRCA2 mutations are associated with multiple malignancies in childhood including familial Wilms tumour. *J Med Genet.*, *42*, 147-145.

[93] Alter, B.P., Rosenberg, P.S. & Brody, LC. (2007). Clinical and molecular features associated with biallelic mutations in FANCD1/BRCA2. *J Med Genet.*, *44*, 1-9.

[94] Renwick, A., Thompson, D., Seal, A., Kelly, P., Chagtai, T., Ahmed, M., North, B., Jayatilake, H., Barfoot R. and Spanova K. *et al.*, (2006). *Nat. Genet.*, *38*, 873–875.

[95] Levy-Lahad, E., Lahad, A., Eisenberg, S., Dagan, E., Paperna, T., Kasinetz, L., Catane, R., Kaufman, B., Beller, U., Renbaum, P. & Gershoni-Baruch, R. (2001). A single nucleotide polymorphism in the RAD51 gene modifies cancer risk in BRCA2 but not BRCA1 carriers. *Proc Natl Acad Sci U S A, 98*, 3232-3236.

[96] Monteiro, A.N., Zhang, S., Phelan, C.M. & Narod, S.A. (2003). Absence of constitutional H2AX gene mutations in 101 hereditary breast cancer families. *J Med Genet., 40*, e51.

[97] Gennery, A.R., Slatter, M.A., Bhattacharya, A., Barge, D., Haigh, S., O'Driscoll, M., Coleman, R., Abinun, M., Flood, T.J., Cant, A.J. & Jeggo, P.A. (2004). The clinical and biological overlap between Nijmegen Breakage Syndrome and Fanconi anemia. *Clin Immunol., 113*, 214-219.

[98] New, H.V., Cale, C.M., Tischkowitz, M., Jones, A., Telfer, P., Veys, P., D'Andrea, A., Mathew, C.G. & Hann, I. (2005). Nijmegen breakage syndrome diagnosed as Fanconi anaemia. *Pediatr Blood Cancer., 44*, 494-499.

[99] Meijers-Heijboer, H., van den Ouweland, A., Klijn, J., Wasielewski, M., de Snoo, A. & Oldenburg, R. (2002). Low-penetrance susceptibility to breast cancer due to CHEK21100delC in noncarriers of BRCA1 or BRCA2 mutations. *Nat. Genet., 31*, 55-59.

[100] Walsh, T., Casadei, S., Coats, K.H., Swisher, E., Stray, S.M., Higgins, J., Roach, K.C., Mandell, J., Lee, M.K. & Ciernikova S. (2006). *JAMA, 295*, 1379–1388.

[101] Liebetrau, W., Budde, A., Savoia, A., Grummt, F. & Hoehn, H. (1997). p53 activates Fanconi anemia group C gene expression. *Hum Mol Genet. 6*, 277-283.

[102] Venkatraj, V.S., Gaidano, G. & Auerbach, A.D. (1994). Clonality studies and N-ras and p53 mutation analysis of hematopoietic cells in Fanconi anemia. *Leukemia, 8*, 1354135-1354138.

[103] Kutler, D.I, Wreesmann, V.B., Goberdhan, A., Ben-Porat, L., Satagopan, J., Ngai, I., Huvos, A.G., Giampietro, P., Levran, O., Pujara, K., Diotti, R., Carlson, D., Huryn, L.A., Auerbach, A.D. & Singh, B. (2003). Human papillomavirus DNA and p53 polymorphisms in squamous cell carcinomas from Fanconi anemia patients. *J Natl Cancer Inst. 95*, 1718-1721.

[104] Freie, B.W., Ciccone, S.L., Li, X., Plett, P.A., Orschell, C.M., Srour, E.F., Hanenberg, H., Schindler, D., Lee, S.H. & Clapp, D.W. (2004). A role for the Fanconi anemia C protein in maintaining the DNA damage-induced G2 checkpoint. *J Biol Chem., 279*, 50986-50989.

[105] Mirchandani, K.D. & D'Andrea, A.D. (2006). The Fanconi anemia/BRCA pathway: a coordinator of cross-link repair. *Exp Cell Res. 312*, 2647- 2653.

[106] Kalb, R, K., Neveling, H., Hoehn, K., Goettsche, S.D., Battish, C., Hunt, M., Berwick, Callén, E., Surrallés, J., Casado, J.A., Bueren, J.A., Dasí, A., Zwaan, C.M., Vervenne, R., Pals, G., de Winter, J., Joenje, H., Grompe, M., Auerbach, A.D., Hanenberg, H. & Schindler, D. (2007). Hypomorphic Mutations in the Central Fanconi Anemia Gene FANCD2 Sustain a Significant Group of FA-D2 Patients with Severe Phenotype. In press, *Am J Hum Genet.*

[107] Struewing, J.P., Lerman, C., Kase, R.G., Giambarresi, T.R. & Tucker, M.A. (1995). Anticipated uptake and impact of genetic testing in hereditary breast and ovarian cancer families. *Cancer Epidemiol Biomarkers Prev., 4*, 169-173.

[108] Struewing, J.P., Brody, L.C., Erdos, M.R., Kase, R.G., Giambarresi, T.R., Smith, S.A., Collins, F.S. & Tucker, M.A. (1995). Detection of eight BRCA1 mutations in 10 breast/ovarian cancer families, including 1 family with male breast cancer. *Am J Hum Genet., 57*, 1-7.

[109] Struewing, J.P., Hartge, P., Wacholder, S., Baker, S.M., Berlin, M., McAdams, M., Timmerman, M.M., Brody, L.C. & Tucker, M.A. (1997). The risk of cancer associated

with specific mutations of BRCA1 and BRCA2 among Ashkenazi Jews. *N Engl J Med., 336*, 1401-1408.

[110] Thompson, E., Dragovic, R.L., Stephenson, S.A., Eccles, D.M., Campbell, I.G. & Dobrovic, A. (2005). A novel duplication polymorphism in the FANCA promoter and its association with breast and ovarian cancer. *BMC Cancer, 5*, 43.

[111] Seal, S., Barfoot, R., Jayatilake, H., Smith, P., Renwick, A., Bascombe, L., McGuffog, L., Evans, D.G., Eccles, D., Easton, D.F., Stratton, M.R. & Rahman, N. (2003). Breast Cancer Susceptibility Collaboration. *Cancer Research*, 8596-8599.

[112] Rahman, N., Seal, S., Thompson, D., Kelly, P., Renwick, A., Elliott, A., Reid, S., Spanova, K., Barfoot, R., Chagtai, T., Jayatilake, H., McGuffog, L., Hanks, S., Evans, D.G., Eccles, D., Easton, D.F. & Stratton, M.R. (2007). PALB2, which encodes a BRCA2-interacting protein, is a breast cancer susceptibility gene. *Nat Genet., 39*, 165-167.

[113] Erkko, H., Xia, B., Nikkila, J., Schleutker, J., Syrjakoski, K., Mannermaa, A., Kallioniemi, A., Pylkas, K., Karppinen, S.M., Rapakko, K., Miron, A., Sheng, Q., Li, G., Mattila, H., Bell, D.W., Haber, D.A., Grip, M., Reiman, M., Jukkola-Vuorinen, A., Mustonen, A., Kere, J., Aaltonen, L.A., Kosma, V.M., Kataja, V., Soini, Y., Drapkin, R.I., Livingston, D.M. & Winqvist, R. (2007). A recurrent mutation in PALB2 in Finnish cancer families. *Nature,* doi:10.1038/nature05609.

[114] Easton, D.F., Stratton, M.R. & Rahman, N. (2006). Truncating mutations in the Fanconi anemia J gene BRIP1 are low-penetrance breast cancer susceptibility alleles. *Nat Genet., 38*, 1239-1241.

[115] Rutter, J.L., Smith, A.M., Davila, M.R., Sigurdson, A.J., Giusti, R.M., Pineda, M.A., Doody, M.M., Tucker, M.A., Greene, M.H., Zhang, J. & Struewing, J.P. (2003). Mutational analysis of the BRCA1-interacting genes ZNF350/ZBRK1 and BRIP1/BACH1 among BRCA1 and BRCA2-negative probands from breast-ovarian cancer families and among early-onset breast cancer cases and reference individuals *Hum Mutat., 22*, 121-128.

[116] Barroso. E., Milne, R.L., Fernandez, P., Zamora, P., Arias, J.I., Benitez, J. & Ribas, G. (2006). FANCD2 associated with sporadic breast cancer risk. *Carcinogenesis, 27*, 1930-1937.

[117] Lewis, A.G., Flanagan, J., Marsh, A., Pupo, G.M., Mann, G., Spurdle, A.B., Lindeman, G.J., Visvader, J.E., Brown, M.A. & Chenevix-Trench, G. (2005). Kathleen Cuningham Foundation Consortium for Research into Familial Breast Cancer.Mutation analysis of FANCD2, BRIP1/BACH1, LMO4 and SFN in familial breast cancer. *Breast Cancer Res., 7*, 1005-1016.

[118] van der Groep, P., Hoelzel, M., Buerger, H., Joenje, H., de Winter, J.P. & van Diest, P.J. (2007). Loss of expression of FANCD2 protein in sporadic and hereditary breast cancer. *Breast Cancer Res Treat.*

[119] Nakanishi, K., Yang, Y.G., Pierce, A.J., Taniguchi, T., Digweed, M., D'Andrea, A.D., Wang, Z.Q. & Jasin, M. (2005). Human Fanconi anemia monoubiquitination pathway promotes homologous DNA repair, *Proc. Natl. Acad. Sci. U. S. A., 102*, 1110–1115.

[120] Yamamoto, K., Ishiai, M., Matsushita, N., Arakawa, H., Lamerdin, J.E., Buerstedde, J.M., Tanimoto, M., Harada, M., Thompson, L.H. & Takata, H. (2003). Fanconi anemia

FANCG protein in mitigating radiation- and enzyme-induced DNA double-strand breaks by homologous recombination in vertebrate cells, *Mol. Cell. Biol., 23*, 5421–5430.

[121] Niedzwiedz, W., Mosedale, G., Johnson, M., Ong, C.Y., Pace P. & Patel, K.J. (2004). The Fanconi anaemia gene FANCC promotes homologous recombination and error-prone DNA repair, *Mol. Cell, 15*, 607–620.

[122] Davies, A.A., Masson, J.Y., McIlwraith, M.J., Stasiak, A.Z., Stasiak, A., Venkitaraman, A.R. & West, S.C. (2001). Role of BRCA2 in control of the RAD51 recombination and DNA repair protein, *Mol. Cell, 7*, 273–282.

[123] Wang, X., Andreassen, P.R. & D'Andrea, A.D. (2004). Functional interaction of monoubiquitinated FANCD2 and BRCA2/FANCD1 in chromatin. *Mol Cell Biol., 24*, 5850-5862.

[124] Pichierri, P. & Rosselli, F. (2004). The DNA crosslink-induced S-phase checkpoint depends on ATR-CHK1 and ATR-NBS1-FANCD2 pathways. *EMBO J., 23*, 1178-1187.

Index

A

B

C

D

E

F

G

H

I

K

L

M

N

O

P

Q

R

S

T

U